NUTRITION
SCIENCE

NUTRITION SCIENCE
(Third Edition)

B. Srilakshmi
M.Sc., M.Ed., M.Phil.

Programme In-charge
M.Sc. (Dietetics and Food Service Management)
Indira Gandhi National Open University
Chennai 600 010

PUBLISHING FOR ONE WORLD

NEW AGE INTERNATIONAL (P) LIMITED, PUBLISHERS
New Delhi • Bangalore • Chennai • Guwahati • Hyderabad
Jalandhar • Kolkata • Lucknow • Mumbai • Ranchi
Visit us at **www.newagepublishers.com**

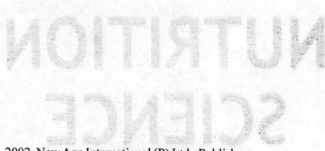

Copyright © 2008, 2006, 2002, New Age International (P) Ltd., Publishers
Published by New Age International (P) Ltd., Publishers
First Edition: 2002
Second Edition: 2006
Third Edition: 2008
Reprint: 2008

Branches:

- 36, Malikarjuna Temple Street, Opp. ICWA, Basavanagudi, **Bangalore**. ✆ (080) 26677815
- 26, Damodaran Street, T. Nagar, **Chennai**. ✆ (044) 24353401
- Hemsen Complex, Mohd. Shah Road, Paltan Bazar, Near Starline Hotel, **Guwahati**. ✆ (0361) 2543669
- No. 105, 1st Floor, Madhiray Kaveri Tower, 3-2-19, Azam Jahi Road, Nimboliadda, **Hyderabad**. ✆ (040) 24652456
- RDB Chambers (Formerly Lotus Cinema) 106A, Ist Floor, S.N. Banerjee Road, **Kolkata**. ✆ (033) 22275247
- 18, Madan Mohan Malviya Marg, **Lucknow**. ✆ (0522) 2209578
- 142C, Victor House, Ground Floor, N.M. Joshi Marg, Lower Parel, **Mumbai**. ✆ (022) 24927869
- 22, Golden House, Daryaganj, **New Delhi**. ✆ (011) 23262370, 23262368

ISBN (10): 81-224-2147-4

ISBN (13): 978-81-224-2147-7

Rs. 225.00

C-08-08-3035

Printed in India at Print 'O' Pack, Delhi.
Typeset at in-house

PUBLISHING FOR ONE WORLD
NEW AGE INTERNATIONAL (P) LIMITED, PUBLISHERS
4835/24, Ansari Road, Daryaganj, New Delhi-110002
Visit us at **www.newagepublishers.com**

To

my father

Dr. K.S. MURTHY, M.Sc., (Hons.) Ph.D.,

who practised

simple living and high thinking

FOREWORD

Nutrition Science, an ever expanding subject with multi-disciplinary roots, is vitally important for the physical, mental and social well-being of all people. Consequently it has a bearing on work efficiency and productivity. Our changing lifestyles and the promotion of a variety of ready-to-eat and fast foods which are commonly available in the market, call for an adequate knowledge of the nutritive value of foods and of appropriate choices to be made to maintain health.

The author has presented this vast subject matter in a systematic and comprehensive manner so as to be relevant to any beginner and to promote a way of life where nutrition has a central place. The learner would do well to have a grip on basics of Physiology and Biochemistry for an understanding of the role of nutrients in the growth and maintenance of the physical structure and of the metabolism of the body as discussed in many chapters. The learners in both the formal and non-formal systems of education would benefit from this presentation.

The context is Indian with reference to the nutritive value of foods, nutritional disorders and assessment of nutritional status of community groups. Research studies by the National Institute of Nutrition and other Indian organisations of repute form the backdrop to the subject matter, wherever relevant. However, the global perspective has not been missed specially with reference to the programmes for preventing nutritional disorders and curing the effects of malnutrition among the vulnerable groups. This book will serve as a valuable source material for anyone interested and involved in healthcare services and community education.

Prof. Philomena R. Reddy
Formerly Vice-Chancellor,
Sri Padmavathi Mahila Visvavidyalayam,
Tirupati (A.P) India.

PREFACE TO THE THIRD EDITION

Nutrition is the science that interprets the relationship of food to the functioning of the living organism. Chemistry and physiology are the basis of Nutrition Science.

A number of current topics of interest in Nutrition have been added in this edition. A new chapter on 'antioxidants' is added as the important of food being realised not only on the nutritive value but also on the health value of food.

Some changes have been made in the order of chapters and chapter titles. This reorganisation is done to make the book more logical and facilitate understanding of the subject.

Information collected through personal visits to places like United States Department of Agriculture, Beltsville, Mary Land, USA and National Institute of Nutrition, Hyderabad, has been incorporated in this edition.

Information is updated by also visiting websites. Websites are given at the end of each chapter to facilitate additional learning. Nutrition related websites are given in chapter "Computer Applications in Nutritive Practice".

New tables like standard heights and weights of Indian children and soluble, insoluble and total dietary fibre content of foods are included. Almost in every chapter new updated tables are given. RDA table for vitamins and minerals given by National Research Council, USA is also included in this edition.

The main deficiency diseases prevalent in India such as protein energy malnutrition, anaemia, vitamin A deficiency and iodine deficiency disorders are continued to be given importance in this edition with additional pictures. This edition also carries pictures of Indian nutritionists.

Picture presentation at the end of this book may create a good 'visual memory' in the minds of students.

This book is designed for undergraduate "Nutrition and Dietetics" students. This book is valuable as reference book for those specialising in medicine, nursing and other paramedical courses.

I would appreciate any feedback or critical comments at e-mail address: s_bayya@yahoo.com.

B. SRILAKSHMI

ACKNOWLEDGEMENTS

In compiling this book, I have extensively referred to a vast number of standard books, journals, proceedings of seminars, conferences and work-shop manuals.

Though many books were referred, special mention must be made of Guthrie's Human Nutrition and Davidson's Human Nutrition and Dietetics. The different publications of the National Institute of Nutrition, Hyderabad, were used liberally in various chapters. I express my deep sense of indebtedness to these scientists and publishers.

I am extremely grateful to Dr. Philomena Reddy, former Vice Chancellor of Sri Padmavathi Mahila Visvavidyalayam, Tirupathi for improving the presentation with her valuable suggestions.

I am grateful to Ms. Krishna Kumari Menon, Senior Research Officer of the National Institute of Nutrition for clarifying the doubts and extending relevant material. The encouragement of Dr. Raghunatha Rao, Assistant Director and Dr. Vijayaraghavan, Deputy Director, National Institute of Nutrition, Hyderabad, is worth mentioning.

The book could not have taken this shape without the critical comments of Prof. (Mrs.) Shivakumar of Women's Christian College, Chennai. I am extremely grateful to her for her willingness to help me.

I am also grateful to WB Saunders Company, Philadelphia, Pennsylvania, USA, for permitting me to use colour pictures of deficiency diseases.

I am indebted to Dr. Susheela Srivastava, Head of the Department of Home Science, J.B.A.S. College for Women, Chennai, for all the encouragement given in achieving my goals.

I am thankful to my students who were more than willing to help me in many ways throughout the development of this book.

I take this opportunity to thank my daughters Mrs. Kranthi and Dr. Swathi and my sons-in-law Mr. Venu and Mr. Naren from USA for their encouragement. I thank my husband Mr. B.V. Rao for his unhesitant support throughout this project. I am grateful of my brothers from USA whose encouraging comments raised my confidence while working on this second edition.

Special acknowledgement to M/s New Age International (P) Limited, Chennai for consenting to bring out this book.

CONTENTS

CHAPTER 1

INTRODUCTION TO NUTRITION SCIENCE

Life can be sustained only with adequate nourishment. Man needs food for growth, development and to lead an active, productive and healthy life.

DEFINITIONS

Nutrition is the science of foods, the nutrients and other substances therein, their action, interaction and balance in relationship to health and disease; the processes by which the organism ingests, digests, absorbs, transports and utilises nutrients and disposes of their end products. In addition, nutrition is concerned with social, economic, cultural and psychological implications of food and eating. In short, nutrition science is the area of knowledge regarding the role of food in the maintenance of health.

Health is defined by the World Health Organisation as the "State of complete physical, mental and social well being and not merely the absence of disease and infirmity".

The essential requisites (or dimensions) of "health" include the following:

- Achievement of optimal growth and development, reflecting the full expression of one's genetic potential.
- Maintenance of the structural integrity and functional efficiency of body tissues necessary for an active and productive life.
- Ability to withstand the inevitable process of ageing with minimal disability and functional impairment, and
- Ability to combat disease, such as
    - *a* resisting infections (immunocompetence)
    - *b* preventing the onset (and retarding the progress) of degenerative diseases and cancer and
    - *c* resisting the effect of environmental toxins and pollutants.
- Mental health
- Social well being is the ability to live in harmony with others.

Nutrients are the constituents in food that must be supplied to the body in suitable amounts. These include carbohydrates, fats, proteins, minerals, vitamins and water. Chemical substances obtained from food and used in the body to provide energy, structural materials and regulating agents to support growth, maintenance and repair of the body's tissues. Nutrients may also reduce the risks of some degenerative diseases.

Nutritional status is the condition of health of the individual as influenced by the utilisation of the nutrients. It can be determined only by the correlation of information obtained through a careful medical and dietary history, a thorough physical examination and appropriate laboratory investigation.

Bionutrition is the new food science that amalgamates and harmoniously blends the basis of the optimal nutrition and diet therapy with the locally available organic resources to cater to "holistic health". It is a far more comprehensive coverage that provides for the diverse essential needs like

- growth needs of the body
- maintenance requirements
- total well being or physical fitness
- preventive treatment by boosting body resistance through improved immune system.
- curative treatment in the case of some chronic maladies like cancers, diabetes and vitamin deficiency.

Bionutrition aims at broad basing the role of nutrition to cover all the health contingencies and then build up organically the inner reserves to combat disease leading to 'assured good health'.

Nutrition security is an access to all the nutrients in optimum quantity for all people at all times to sustain a healthy and active life.

Food bank is a facility that collects and distributes food donations to authorised organisations that feed the hungry.

Malnutrition has been defined as a pathological state resulting from a relative or absolute deficiency or excess of one or more essential nutrients. It comprises four forms:

1. **Undernutrition** is the condition which results when insufficient food is eaten over an extended period of time.

2. **Overnutrition** is the pathological state resulting from the consumption of excessive quantity of food over an extended period of time.

3. **Imbalance** is the pathological state resulting from a disproportion among essential nutrients with or without the absolute deficiency of any nutrient.

4. **Specific deficiency** is the pathological state resulting from a relative or absolute lack of an individual nutrient.

HISTORY

The facts of nutrition are gained by applying the scientific method; that is, setting upon hypothesis, testing the hypothesis, testing hypothesis under carefully controlled conditions, observing the results and interpreting them. The research may take place within the borders of a community or within the walls of a laboratory. Such experiments have contributed to the development of the science of nutrition.

The science of nutrition had its beginnings in the late 18th century with the discovery of the respiratory gases and especially the studies on the nature and the quantification of energy metabolism by Lavoisier, a Frenchman, often referred to as the Father of the Science of Nutrition.

Respiration and Energy Output

Lavoisier (1770–1794) made the great discovery regarding the nature of respiration. He believed that organic substances were oxidised in the body with the production of CO_2 and heat. The studies of Leibig in 1842, showed that it was not carbon and hydrogen which were burnt in the body but carbohydrates, fats and proteins.

Regnault (1849) first determined the respiratory quotient, that is, ratio of volume of CO_2 expired to O_2 consumed in animals. Carl Voit (1862) determined the energy requirements of human adults. Atwater (1873–1900) studied the energy output of human subjects using the human respiration calorimeter and related the energy output to oxygen consumption.

Protein Nutrition

Carl Voit and co-workers (1870–1890) carried out pioneering studies on protein metabolism and protein requirements. They showed that protein consumed in excess, was not stored but oxidised to urea and excreted in urine. Voit and Chittenden (1901) carried out extensive studies on the protein requirements. Folin (1905–1912) conducted studies on protein metabolism. He distinguished two types of protein metabolism (*i*) endogenous, that is, metabolism of tissue proteins and (*ii*) exogenous, that is, metabolism of dietary proteins. The pioneering studies of Hopkins (1906) in England and Osborne and Mendel (1912) in USA showed that rats did not grow on a purified diet containing zein (a protein from maize) as the sole source of protein. Chemical analysis revealed that zein did not contain tryptophan and lysine. They showed that when these two aminoacids were added to zein, rats grew well.

Discovery of Vitamins

Lunin (1881) fed mice on a diet containing casein, milk fat, cane sugar and different inorganic salts. The animals survived for some months and finally lost body weight and died. Eijkman (1897) in Batavia reported that chicken fed on polished rice, developed polyneuritis and addition of rice polishings extract cured the disease. Pekelharing (1905) in Holland, found that mice did not survive on diet based on bread, rice flour, egg albumin, casein, lard and a mixture of salts. Addition of small amounts of milk to the above diet helped to promote growth and maintain the animals in good health. In 1907, Holst and Frolich produced scurvy in guinea pigs by feeding them on a diet based mainly on oats.

Hopkins (1906) found that rats fed on purified mixture of casein, starch, cane sugar, lard and inorganic salts, did not grow and died after some months. Addition of milk in small quantities promoted growth. He postulated the presence of some unknown growth factors in milk which are essential for the growth of rats and called them "accessory factors of the diet" which are now known as 'vitamins'. Funk (1912) coined the name "Vitamine" for the accessory food factors and propounded the famous "Vitamine" theory that natural foods contained distinct anti beri-beri, anti-scurvy, anti-rickets and anti-pellagra "vitamins".

McCollum and Davis (1913) and Osborne and Mendel (1913) independently showed that albino rats fed on a diet containing bread, casein, lard or olive oil, starch and inorganic salts did not grow, but when butter fat or egg yolk fat or cod liver oil was added, good growth occurred. McCollum and Davis designated the factor as "Fat soluble A" and it is now known as Vitamin A. McCollum and co-workers (1916) using purified diets showed that whey of milk contained a factor necessary for the growth of rats. They called it "Water soluble B".

Treatment of Nutritional Disorders with Foods

The relationship between food consumed and the nutritional status of an individual was realised long time back. Importance of milk on growth of dogs is illustrated in Figure 1a.

Baumann (1895) discovered the presence of iodine in thyroid gland. Iodides were used in the treatment of goitre by Coindet in 1820. The use of cod liver oil in the treatment of rickets has been reported in 1824 by Schutter.

Takaki (1887) reported the results of a remarkable investigation in which he showed that addition of meat, vegetables, condensed milk and barley to a ration based mainly on raw milled rice, helped to prevent the occurrence of beri beri among sailors in the Japanese Navy.

James Lind (1753) clearly established that scurvy can be prevented or cured by the provision of fresh fruits or vegetables among sailors in the British Navy. From 1795 onwards the British Navy introduced lime juice as part of sailor's ration.

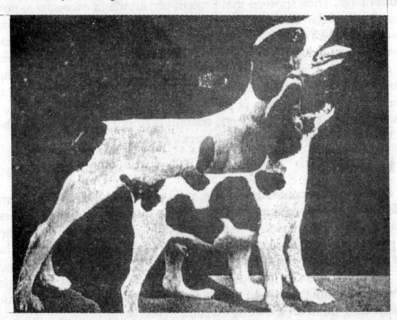

Figure 1a. Milk made the difference. These puppies from the same litter were of the same size at weaning time. After weaning, both were fed as much bread and cooked cereal as they would eat with some meat added. The big dog also received milk every day, but the small dog received none.

Source: Proudfit TF, Corinne H Robinson 1957, Nutrition and diet therapy. The Macmillan Company, New York.

Goldberger (1915) in USA found that addition of milk and eggs to a poor maize diet prevented the occurrence of pellagra among inmates in an institution. He also produced pellagra among human volunteers by feeding them on a poor diet consisting of maize, wheat flour, potato, salt pork and syrup for a period of 6 months and found that addition of 200 g meat or 30 g brewer's yeast or 2 pints of milk can cure the disease. Cicely Williams demonstrated in 1935 that kwashiorkor in children is caused by protein deficiency and can be cured by feeding milk.

Table 1.1: Scientists and Their Contribution to Nutrition Science

Year	Scientist	Contribution
1713	Lernery	Recognised iron as constituent of body.
1747	Lind	Proved oranges and lemons cure scurvy.
1770–1794	Lavoisier	Studied energy metabolism and nature of respiration. Father of science of nutrition.
1800	Lecanu	Identified iron in haemoglobin
1820	Coindet	Used iodine in the treatment of goitre
1824	Shutter	Use of cod liver oil in the treatment of rickets
1838	Mulder	Introduced the term protein means to take first place
1842	Liebig	Showed that no carbon and hydrogen were burnt in body but carbohydrate, protein and fat.
1849	Regnault	Determined Respiratory Quotient
1862	Carl Voit	Studied energy requirement of human adults
1870–1890	Carl Voit and co-workers	Studied protein metabolism and protein requirement
1887	Takaki	Prevention of beri beri.
1883	Rubner	Demonstrated relationship between the surface area and heat production.
1895	Baumann	Presence of iodine in thyroid gland
1897	Eijkman	Chicken when fed polished rice developed polyneuritis
1899	Sherman	Interested in protein and calcium requirements.
1873–1900	Atwater	Energy output studied using human respiration calorimeter
1901	Voit and Chittenden	Studied protein requirements.
1901	Hopkins and Cole	Isolated tryptophan
1905	Pakelharing	Diet based on bread, rice flour, egg albumin, casein, lard and a mixture of fats, mice did not survive. A small amount of milk fed to the above helped to promote growth.
1906	Hopkins	Found out vitamins as "accessory factors of the diet".
1909	McCollum and Davis	Discovered fat soluble substance is necessary for growth.
1909	Osborne and Mendel	Nutritive value of isolated proteins
1905–1912	Folin	Studied protein metabolism
1912	Funk	Coined the name "Vitamine".
1913	Mendel and Osborne	Rats did not grow on a purified diet containing Zein as sole source of protein.
1915	Mendel	Divided proteins into 2 classes; failed to allow growth, allowed growth.
1915	Dubois	Estimated surface area of body.
1915	Goldberger	Found protein of milk and egg to a poor maize diet can prevent pellagra.
1916	McCollum and co-workers	'Fat soluble A' is necessary for growth of rat.
1918	Mellanby	Proved fat soluble substance with antirachetic property (cod liver oil)

Contd....

Year	Scientist	Contribution
1919	Osborne, Mendel and Ferry	Developed Protein Efficiency Ratio method.
1921	Tanner	Tryptophan can cure pellagra.
1922	Evans and Bishops	Vitamin E essential is for reproduction of rats.
1925	Mitchell	Developed Biological value method.
1926	Minet and Murphy	Pernicious anaemia can be cured by feeding at least 0.3 kg/day of raw liver.
1929	Burr and Burr	Showed that rats on fat free diet developed dermatitis.
1929	Hopkins and Eijkman	Won Nobel prize for accessory food factors
1931	Lucy Wills	Found megaloblastic anaemia in pregnant women
1934	Dam	Discovered vitamin K.
1935	Cicely Williams	Kwashiorkor is caused by protein deficiency and cured by feeding milk.
1935	William C. Rose	Contributed to amino acid nutrition
1937	Elvejhem	Isolated nicotimamide from liver
1937	Royal Lee	Conceived endocardiograph, a tool for graphing heart sounds and a means for measuring nutritional status.
1954	Paul Gyorgy	Discovered Bifidus factor.
1955	Miller and Bender	Developed Net Protein Utilization method
1957	Bender and Doell	Developed Net Protein Ratio method
1963	Hansen	Found importance of linoleic acid.
1971	Lappe	Found complementary value of vegetable proteins.
1985	Burkett	Low intake of cereal fibre could increase hardness of stool
1991	Lappe	Complementary proteins need not be in the same meal to improve quality of protein.

NUTRITION RESEARCH IN INDIA

Nutrition Research began in India as the "Beri Beri Enquiry" unit in 1918 under Sir Robert McCarrison at Coonor Pasteur Institute. Then later it was called a "Deficiency Disease Enquiry" unit and expanded to full fledged Nutrition Research Laboratories. Under the leadership of Aykroyd studies were conducted on the nutritive value of various Indian food stuffs. Field studies on the diet and nutritional status of people in different parts of the country were also done.

Patwardhan "the first Indian Director" of Nutrition Research Laboratories expanded the scope of nutrition research programme to clinical, biochemical and public health aspects. Later Gopalan established food toxicology, endocrinology and genetics departments. Field studies gained more importance. S.G. Srikantia did community based studies, particularly research on the problems related to the vulnerable groups. New lines of research such as functional consequences of growth retardation, nutritional assessment, drug-nutrient interaction were started. Later research focus was on iron fortified salt, double fortified salt and iodised salt. In 1970, in recognition of the work being done, the institute was renamed as National Institute of Nutrition.

Rajammal Devdas was the Vice Chancellor of the Avinashilingam Deemed University. She was the force behind the supplementary feeding programme. She was pioneer for nutrition eduction in India. She believed that this was one of the most promising and effective strategies to overcome malnutrition among children.

M.S. Swaminathan is the " Father of green revolution". He was awarded World Food Prize in 1987, the Tyler-Honda prize in 1991, United Nations Environment Programme, UNEP, Sasakawa award in 1994. He was Director General of the Indian Council of Agriculture Research during 1972-78 and headed the International Rice Research Institute from 1982 to 1988.

Lately studies have been initiated on the interaction of nutrition with degenerative diseases and cancer both from experimental and epidemiological angles.

Computerisation of data processing by National Nutrition Monitoring Bureau (NNMB) and a modern infrastructure facility for breeding and supply of pathogen free laboratory animals are recent endeavours.

Nutrition research is conducted not only at National Institute of Nutrition, Hyderabad but also at Central Food Technological Research Institute, Mysore, units of Indian Council of Medical Research and Indian Council of Agricultural Research.

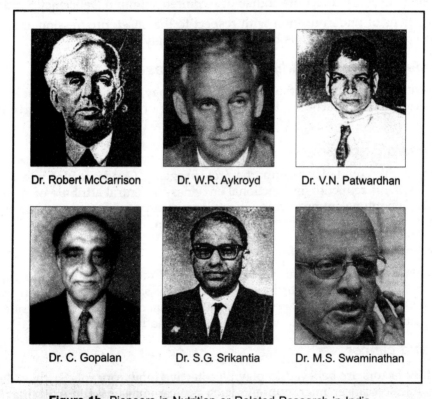

Dr. Robert McCarrison   Dr. W.R. Aykroyd   Dr. V.N. Patwardhan

Dr. C. Gopalan   Dr. S.G. Srikantia   Dr. M.S. Swaminathan

Figure 1b. Pioneers in Nutrition or Related Research in India.

The Nutrition department of various Home Science and Medical Colleges also contribute to nutrition research.

RECENT FINDINGS

The frontiers of Nutrition Science would now seem to extend far beyond the earlier confines of "growth, development, maintenance and repair" to include such other aspects of health as immunocompetence, ageing, mental well being and prevention and retardation of degenerative diseases and cancer.

Nutrition and Immunity

There is now evidence that undernutrition can affect both the nonspecific as well as the "antigen specific" components of the immune system and with respect to the latter it could impair both humoral immunity and cellular immunity. T-cell, B-cell and macrophage lineage subsets of the immune system can all be affected. Several nutrients such as proteins, lipids and micronutrients such as zinc, iron, copper, vitamin A and vitamin B_6 have been shown to affect immune responses through their action on different components of the immune system. Morbidity in undernutrition is attributable to the fact that undernutrition facilitates the onset of infections, aggravates their course and deleteriously affects their outcome. Response to immunization could be sub-optimal in undernourished communities.

High neonatal mortality in low birth weight infants is a direct result of their impaired immunological status attributable to maternal malnutrition during pregnancy. Nutrition deficiency may adversely affect the course of Acquired Immuno Deficiency Syndrome.

The implications of undernutrition with respect to the onset, progression and outcome of several infectious diseases are thus becoming increasingly clear.

Foetal Undernutrition and Adult Chronic Disease

Another recent contribution from the field of epidemiology, pointing to a possible aetiological role of undernutrition in early life is the development of chronic degenerative diseases in adulthood.

Nutrition and old age

Nutrition apparently could play an important role in ageing. Good nutrition retards the ageing process and prevents reduction in functional enzymes—a central attribute of ageing. It helps in overcoming suboptimal immuno competence largely responsible for increased vulnerability to infection in old age and in improving mental function.

Nutrition and atherosclerosis

The convergence of evidence from epidemiological, clinicopathological and experimental studies points to a major role of nutritional factors in the pathogenesis of atherosclerosis and coronary heart disease. Apart from weight and abdominal obesity, fat and essential fatty acid intake and many other nutritional factors are related to atherosclerosis.

Nutrition and cancer

Certain dietary factors are believed to play a protective inhibitory role, such as dietary fibre with respect to colon cancer, micronutrients such as β-carotene, vitamin A, riboflavin, vitamin C, iron, zinc and selenium with respect to cancers of epithelial origin—especially those of alimentary and respiratory tract. Vegetables and fruits (especially of the yellow and green variety) rich in such micronutrients are protective against such cancers of epithelial origin. Micronutrients in the diet, particularly antioxidant vitamins appear to play a pivotal role in reducing damage resulting from environmental exposure and may act synergistically to enhance several protective mechanisms against carcinogenesis.

Several bodies such as the National Research Council in the United States and the World Health Organisation directed their attention to nutrients and foods that have a positive role in maintaining health and in delaying age-related disorders such as cancer, cataract and coronary heart diseases.

Nutraceuticals

The word combines "nutrition" and "pharmaceuticals" to mean that food extracts can be used as preventive drugs or food supplements. Science has added knowledge about the disease preventing phytonutrients present in food stuffs.

The major phytonutrients identified to have nutraceutical properties include terpenes, phytosterol, phenols and theols. Terpenes represent the largest class of phytonutrients. They are found in green foods, soya products and grains.

These nutraceuticals help in preventing many degenerative diseases like diabetes mellitus, atherosclerosis and cancer and play a role in general well being of the individual. People are also recognising the virtue of vegetarianism and role of vegetables and fruits and antioxidants in the prevention of degenerative diseases.

Debate continues, however, as to whether nutrients consumed in amounts above the recommended dietary allowances can provide benefit beyond the traditional functional role of preventing deficiency disorders and associated biochemical and metabolic abnormalities.

Advanced knowledge in Nutrition science has made the people to understand the importance of breast feeding and fibre in the diet.

Knowledge generated in immunology, molecular biology, oncology, geriatrics and phytochemistry during the last three decades has now provided new insights and opened up new vistas in the science of nutrition.

FUTURE RESEARCH

According to C. Gopalan the following is the agenda for the future nutrition research:

- Problems related to poverty and undernutrition.
- Nutrition problems related to chronic diseases, e.g. cancer and degenerative diseases.
- Problems related to new developmental technologies e.g., environmental degradation and food contamination.
- Problems arising from demographic transition e.g., nutrition and ageing.
- Other research areas of possible future importance e.g., nutrition and behaviour, nutrition and work efficiency, nutrition and drugs and nutrition and AIDS.

Further advances in nutrition science may be expected with the wider application of the modern tool of biotechnology and genetic engineering. Nutrition research must now attract geneticists, molecular biologists as much as it must attract clinicians and epidemiologists.

The new frontier of nutrition science is Nutrigenomics.

Nutrigenomics is the understanding of the effects of nutrients in molecular level processes in the body as well as the variable effects of nutrients and non-nutritive dietary phytochemicals have on each individual person (Nancy Fogg-Johnson).

Vast segments of populations of the Third World are today in various stages of developmental transition. Incidence of chronic degenerative diseases has been reported. There are population that are not as yet rid of their problems of undernutrition at one end of the spectrum and problems of chronic degenerative diseases, generally related to affluence at the other end. It would now appear that nutritional factors play an important part with respect to pathogenesis of the prevailing disease profiles at both ends of the age spectrum. This greatly increases the ambit of nutrition science and its practical significance.

National nutrition week is celebrated around 5th September.

National Science day is celebrated on 28th February.

QUESTIONS

1. Define the following:
   i. Nutritional status
   ii. Malnutrition
   iii. Health
2. Explain the contribution of the following scientists for the science of nutrition:
   i. Lavoisier
   ii. Carl Voit
   iii. Atwater
   iv. Osborne and Mendel
3. How were foods used as part of treatment?
4. Name two scientists of 19th century who observed respiration.
5. What are nutraceuticals? Explain their importance.
6. How did the discovery of vitamins take place?
7. Explain "Nutrition Research in India".
8. Discuss the recent advances in nutrition research.
9. Bring out the relationship between nutrition and health.

SUGGESTED READINGS

- Passomore R, Memories of the Coonoor Laboratories, 1937-1940, 1946, Proceedings of Nutrition Society of India, **41**, 1994
- Food and Nutrition Information Centre : http://www.nalusda.gov/fnic.html
- Nutrition : Concepts and Controversies : www.wadsworth.com/nutrition/prod/allprod.html
- National Institute of Nutrition: www.ninindia.org

CHAPTER 2

RECOMMENDED DIETARY ALLOWANCES

The dietary allowances of nutrients for a country's population are recommended based on the current knowledge of nutritional requirements of different age and sex groups and the country's food and dietary habits. Dietary allowances are also influenced by activity of an individual.

Nutrient requirement can be defined as the minimum amount of the absorbed nutrient that is necessary for maintaining the normal physiological functions of the body.

Recommended Dietary Allowances (RDA) is defined as the average daily dietary intake level that is sufficient to meet the nutrient requirement of nearly all (97-98 per cent) healthy individuals in a particular life stage and gender group.

RDA are periodically revised and updated in the light of new emerging knowledge and newer concepts concerning human nutrient requirements. The RDA was revised by Expert Group of Indian Council of Medical Research, ICMR, in 1988. Table 2.1 gives the RDA for Indians which was revised in 1988.

FACTORS AFFECTING RDA

Variability in Nutrient Requirements

Human nutrient requirements depend on the age and sex of the individual. An adult man requires nutrients for maintenance while infants and children need them for both maintenance and growth. Nutrient requirements during childhood are proportional to the children's growth rate. Among adults nutrient requirements are related to the body weight and size. Among women, during the reproductive age, due to blood loss during menstrual period, requirements of certain nutrients like iron are higher than those for men. Women require additional quantities of nutrients during pregnancy to sustain foetal growth and during lactation for milk secretion. There are inter individual differences in nutrient requirements even between individuals of the same age, sex and body weight. The coefficient of variation in nutrient requirements between individuals is currently assumed to be around 12.5 per cent.

In recommending nutrient intake for a given population, the variability in requirements is considered and a safety factor to cover such variability is included.

Dietary Factors

Bioavailability: The physiological requirements of nutrients are expressed in terms of the absorbed nutrients. The absorption or the bioavailability of nutrients from a diet can vary widely, depending upon the nutrient and the quality of the diet. The factor of bioavailability assumes significance in the case of certain nutrients like protein, iron, calcium, zinc, β-carotene and vitamin B_{12}. Absorption

Table 2.1: ICMR Recommended dietary allowances per day for Indians

Group	Particulars	Body wt. Kg	Net energy kcal	Protein g.	Fat g.	Calcium mg.	Iron mg.	Vit. A Retinol μg.	Vit. A β-carotene μg.	Thiamin mg.	Riboflavin mg.	Nicotinic acid mg.	Pyri-doxin mg.	Ascorbic acid mg.	Folic acid μg.	Vit. B-12 μg.
Man	Sedentary work	60	2425	60	20	400	28	600	2400	1.2	1.4	16	2.0	40	100	1
	Moderate work		2875							1.4	1.6	18				
	Heavy work		3800							1.6	1.9	21				
Woman	Sedentary work	50	1875	50	20	400	30	600	2400	0.9	1.1	12	2.0	40	100	1
	Moderate work		2225							1.1	1.3	14				
	Heavy work		2925							1.2	1.5	16				
	Pregnant woman	50	+300	+15	30	1000	38	600	2400	+0.2	+0.2	+2	2.5	40	400	1
	Lactation 0-6 months	50	+550	+25	45	1000	30	950	3800	+0.3	+0.3	+4	2.5	80	150	1.5
	6-12 months		+400	+18						+0.2	+0.2	+3				
Infants	0-6 months	5.4	108/kg	2.05/kg		500		350	1200	55μg/kg	65μg/kg	710μg/kg	0.1	25	25	0.2
	6-12 months	8.6	98/kg	1.65/kg						50μg/kg	60μg/kg	650μg/kg	0.4			
Children	1-3 years	12.2	1240	22		400	12	400		0.6	0.7	8		40	30	
	4-6 years	19.0	1690	30	25	400	18	400	1600	0.9	1.0	11		40	40	
	7-9 years	26.9	1950	41			26	600	2400	1.0	1.2	13		40	60	0.2-1.0
Boys	10-12 years	35.4	2190	54		600	34	600	2400	1.1	1.3	15		40		
Girls	10-12 years	31.5	1970	57		600	19	600	2400	1.0	1.2	13		40		
Boys	13-15 years	47.8	2450	70	22	600	41	600	2400	1.2	1.5	16	1.6	40	70	0.2-1.0
Girls	13-15 years	46.7	2060	65	22	600	28	600	2400	1.0	1.2	14		40		
Boys	16-18 years	57.1	2640	78	22	600	50	600	2400	1.3	1.6	17	2.0	40	100	0.2-1.0
Girls	16-18 years	49.9	2060	63	22	500	30	600	2400	1.0	1.2	14		40	100	0.2-1.0

of nutrients from diets predominantly based on plant foods is often inferior to that from diets based largely on foods of animal origin. Many inhibitory factors present in plant foods like tannins, phytates and antitrypsin factors interfere with absorption of nutrients.

Interrelationship between nutrients: There are close interrelationships between metabolism of nutrients. Establishment of the requirements for a particular nutrient is complicated by numerous interrelationships with other nutrients in the diet. The body does not work in water tight compartments. There is always multi nutrient relationship. Certain relationships are well established like calcium and vitamin D and certain others not so well understood. Interrelationships can be of several types:

- Precursor interrelationship – Trytophan to niacin
- Chemical combination or reaction – Vitamin C and iron
- Noncompetitive metabolic interrelationship – Folic acid and iron
- Competitive interrelationship – Zinc and copper
- Exchange interrelationship – Vitamin E and selenium

The level of intake of one nutrient can influence the requirement of the other. Some well known interrelationships are given in Table 2.2.

Table 2.2: Dietary Components that Influence Nutrient Requirement

Nutrient	Influence by dietary components
Protein	Requirement related to calories when the latter are deficient.
Essential amino acids	Utilisation curtailed if any essential amino acid is deficient.
Phenylalanine	Requirement inversely related to tyrosine intake.
Methionine	Requirement inversely related to cystine intake.
Valine, leucine, Isoleucine	Requirement of each is increased by excess of other branched chain amino acids.
Vitamin E.	Requirement proportional to intake of polyunsaturated fat.
Thiamin	Requirement proportional to calorie intake.
Niacin	Requirement inversely related to tryptophan intake.
Vitamin B_6	Requirement increases by protein intake.
Folacin	Requirement increases by alcohol intake.
Calcium	Urinary excretion increases by high protein intake.
Calcium	Absorption decreases by fats.
Nonhaeme iron	Absorption improved by vitamin C or sulfur containing amino acids.
Copper	Absorption decreased by calcium, requirement increased by excess dietary zinc.

Energy intake must be adequate for proper utilisation of protein. When energy intake is reduced, protein utilisation is impaired. Since several B-complex vitamins take part in energy and protein metabolism, their requirements depend upon the intake of energy and protein. Thus the requirements of B-vitamin, thiamin, riboflavin and niacin are infact expressed in relation to energy requirements and that of pyridoxine in relation to protein requirement. The absorption and utilisation of iron depends upon an adequate intake of ascorbic acid. There are also metabolic inter conversions of nutrients in the body which are considered while establishing their requirements. The well known examples of such conversions are — conversion of tryptophan into niacin and of β-carotene into retinol. There is exchange interrelationship between vitamin E and selenium.

METHODS USED FOR DERIVING RDA

Number of methods have been employed for determining the human nutrient requirements. Dietary intake, growth studies, nutrient balance and obligatory loss of nutrients, nutrient turnover and depletion and repletion studies are conducted.

Dietary intakes: This approach has been used in arriving at the energy requirements of children. Energy intakes of normally growing healthy children are utilised for this purpose.

Growth: The requirements of any particular nutrient or the breast milk intake, for satisfactory growth has been utilised for defining requirements in early infancy.

Nutrient balance: The minimum intake of nutrient for equilibrium (intake = output) in adults and nutrient retention consistent with satisfactory growth in children have been used widely for arriving at the protein requirements.

Obligatory loss of nutrients: The minimal loss of any nutrient or of its metabolic products (namely nitrogenous end products in the case of proteins) through normal routes of elimination—urine, faeces and sweat — is determined on a diet devoid of or very low in the nutrient. This information is used to determine the amount of nutrient to be consumed daily through the diet to replace the obligatory loss. In infants and children, growth requirements are added to the above maintenance requirements.

Factorial approach: In this approach, the requirements for different functions are assessed separately and added to arrive at the total daily requirement. This is the basis of arriving at energy requirement.

Nutrient turnover: Data from turnover of nutrients in healthy persons, using isotopically labelled nutrients have been employed in arriving at requirements of certain nutrients. Requirements of vitamin A and vitamin C, iron and vitamin B_{12} have been determined on this basis. Stable isotopes are particularly useful in infants, children and in women, during pregnancy and lactation where radioisotopes are contra indicated.

Depletion and repletion studies: This approach has been employed in arriving at the requirement of water soluble vitamins. The levels of vitamin or its coenzyme in serum or tissue (erythrocytes, leucocytes) are used as a biochemical marker of the vitamin status. Requirement of ascorbic acid, thiamin, riboflavin, niacin and pyridoxine have been established employing this approach. The subjects are first fed a diet very low in the nutrient under study till the biochemical parameters reach a low level (depleted) after which response to feeding graded doses of the nutrient is determined. The level at which responses increase (repleted) rapidly is an indication of requirement.

REQUIREMENTS AND RDA

To translate the nutrient requirements into recommended dietary intakes or allowance (RDA), allowances for bioavailability and interindividual variations must be made. The RDA includes a margin of safety to take into account possible losses of nutrients during cooking and storage and to provide a buffer against increased requirement during illness and other stages of nutritional stress. .

In practice a level of intake corresponding to mean +2 standard deviations of the requirement which covers 97.5% of population is chosen to define RDA (Figure 2a). This level is also termed as safe level of intake and the chance of finding this level inadequate for any individual is only 2.5%. On the contrary, 97.5% of a given population will have their actual requirements equal to or below the RDA. The coefficient of variation i.e., standard deviation usually employed to arrive at RDA is 12.5%. Therefore, RDA is 25% higher than the average of the mean requirement. Most individual RDA is higher than their actual minimal requirement.

$$RDA = \frac{\text{Physiological minimum requirement}}{\text{Fraction of the nutrient available from the diet}} \times 1.25$$

While prescribing the RDA for a given nutrient, the intakes of all the other nutrients are considered to be at a safe level. The individuals in a population for RDA which is fixed are considered to be well nourished and healthy. RDA is therefore, not applicable to undernourished/malnourished individuals or for those suffering from diseases or infective morbidity.

Recommended dietary allowance (RDAs)

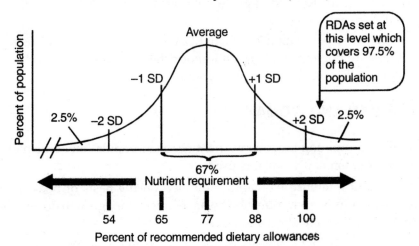

$$RDA = \text{mean} + 2 \times \text{coefficient of variation (15\%) or SD (standard deviation)}$$

$$\text{Average requirement} = RDA \times \frac{100}{130} = 77\% \, RDA$$

Figure 2a. Distribution of actual nutrient requirements with coefficient of variation of 15% around the mean requirement.

Source: Guthrie Helen A. and Mary Frances Piociano, 1999, Human Nutrition, WCB McGraw-Hill Boston.

PRACTICAL APPLICATIONS OF RDA

The nutrient requirements and the recommended dietary intakes of nutrients have several practical applications. Important among them are:

- To assess the adequacy of national food supplies and to plan for food production both in terms of quantity and quality e.g., agriculture planning.
- To provide dietary guidelines for healthy living individuals and groups and to formulate balanced diets.

- RDA can also be used for judging the adequacy of intake of individuals or groups in a preliminary way. In the case of adult individuals RDA has to be adjusted for the actual body weight while assessing the adequacy of intake.

However, RDA cannot be used for estimating the extent of nutrient deficiencies or inadequacies in the population. For this purpose a level of intake at or below M-2SD level can be used to estimate the number of individuals with inadequate nutrient intake. Such dietary assessment should be supplemented with data from anthropometric, biochemical or clinical assessment to establish the extent of undernutrition / malnutrition in the population ascribable solely to dietary inadequacies.

Mean values of heights and weights of Indian boys and girls are given in Tables 2.4 and 2.5.

RDAs are operative under the following conditions :

- While prescribing the RDA for a given nutrient the intakes of all the other nutrients are considered to be at a safe level.
- The individuals in a population for whom RDA is fixed are all well-nourished and healthy. RDA is therefore not applicable to undernourished/malnourished individuals or those suffering from diseases or infective morbidity.

REFERENCE MAN AND WOMAN

For the purpose of computing the total nutrient needs of population at the national level, the concept of reference man and woman is used.

Reference man and reference woman are defined on the basis of body weights of well-nourished healthy adults in each country who have satisfactory growth during their childhood and are currently leading a healthy and active life.

Reference man is between 20-39 years of age, with normal weight. He is free from disease and physically fit for active work. On each working day, he is employed for 8 hours in occupation that usually involves moderate activity. While not at work, he spends 8 hours in bed, 4-6 hours sitting and moving about and 2-4 hours in walking and in active recreation or household duties.

Reference woman is between 20-39 years of age and healthy and active with normal weight. She may be engaged for 8 hours in general household work, in light industry or in any other moderately active work. Apart from 8 hours in bed she spends 4-6 hours sitting or moving around in light activity and 2 hours in walking or active recreation or household chores.

Reference body weights of Indian adult man and woman are 60 kg and 50 kg, respectively for heights of 163 cm and 151 cm, respectively. In case of children, the body weights of well-nourished healthy children with normal growth are used as reference body weights.

INDIAN STANDARDS FOR HEIGHTS AND WEIGHTS

Body weights and heights of childrens reflect their state of health and growth rate while adult weight and height represent what can be attained by an individual with normal growth.

The nutrition goal of any country would be to provide adequate nutrition and health support to its population so that they attain their full genetic potential in growth and development.

Presently available anthropometric data on well-to-do Indian children indicate that their heights and weights correspond to National Centre for Health Statistics (NCHS) standards upto the age of 14 years in the case of boys and 12 years in the case of girls.

The weights and heights of children aged between 0 and 18 years that are used for computing requirements are given in Table 2.3.

Table 2.3: Mean values of heights and weights of well-to-do Indian Children

Age (Years)	Boys		Girls	
	Height (cm)	Weight (kg)	Height (cm)	Weight (kg)
1+	80.07	10.54	78.09	9.98
2+	90.01	12.51	87.93	11.67
3+	98.36	14.78	96.21	13.79
4+	104.70	16.12	104.19	15.85
5+	113.51	19.33	112.24	18.67
6+	118.90	22.14	117.73	21.56
7+	123.32	24.46	122.65	24.45
8+	127.86	26.42	127.22	25.97
9+	133.63	30.00	133.08	29.82
10+	138.45	32.29	138.90	33.58
11+	143.35	35.26	145.00	37.17
12+	148.91	38.78	150.98	42.97
13+	154.94	42.88	153.44	44.54
14+	161.70	48.26	155.04	46.70
15+	165.33	52.15	155.98	48.75
16+	168.40	55.54	156.00	49.75
17+	173.00	57.91		
18+	172.05	58.38		
19+	172.14	58.90		
20+	171.75	59.64		
21+	172.40	59.74		
22+	171.63	60.14		

Data from 1+ to 4+ age groups were collected in Hyderabad and for the remaining age group it was taken from different parts of the country.

Source: A report of the Expert group of the Indian Council of Medical Research, 2000, Nutrient requirements and recommended dietary allowances for Indians, ICMR.

Table 2.4 gives reference body weights of Indians of different age groups.

Table 2.4: Reference Body Weights (kg) of Indians of different age groups

	Age (years)	Male	Female
Infants	0 – ½	5.4	5.4
	½ – 1	8.6	8.6
Children	1 – 3	12.61	11.81
	4 – 6	19.20	18.69
	7 – 9	27.00	26.75
	10 – 12	35.54	37.91
Adolescents	13 – 15	47.88	46.66
	16 – 18	57.28	49.92
Adults	20 – 50	60.00	50.00

Source: A report of the Expert Group of the Indian Council of Medical Research, 2000, Nutrient requirements and recommended dietary allowances for Indians, ICMR.

DETERMINATION OF RDA OF DIFFERENT NUTRIENTS

Energy

Unlike other nutrients, RDA for energy represents only the average daily requirement corresponding to the average daily expenditure of an individual with defined body size, age and level of activity. No safe allowance is provided in case of RDA for energy since both inadequate and excess energy intakes are considered harmful.

Proteins

Protein intake to maintain N equilibrium in adults and positive N balance in children to provide for growth are used as criteria for estimating protein requirements. Based on the International data on N balance studies in different population groups, protein requirements of human beings have been suggested by International Organisations, in terms of high quality protein, namely egg or milk proteins. Lower the quality, higher is the requirement. Protein RDA for Indians is determined on the fact that the diet is based on cereals and legumes and so NPU as 65. Recommended protein intake is that they are valid only when energy intakes are adequate.

Fat

The upper safe limit should not exceed 30 en% (10 en% from invisible fat and 20 en% from visible fat) to avoid health risks like cardiovascular disease and obesity. It is therefore, desirable that the daily intake of added fat by adults should be kept below 50 g/day.

Minerals

Calcium and Phosphorus : Long term calcium balance studies among population groups consuming moderate levels of calcium indicate that calcium balance can be achieved with intakes of 300-500 mg/day. The desirable ratio of Ca:P is 1:1, during infancy where the ratio should be 1:1.5.

Iodine : The minimal requirement of iodine of adults of both sexes is considered to be in the range of 50-75 µg/day. However, safe allowance of iodine for both sexes is set at 150 µg/day.

Iron : Iron requirements are established by determining body iron loss through long term turnover studies in adult men. Dietary iron absorption varies from 3-10 per cent depending upon the quality of diet.

Vitamins

The requirements of vitamins in adults have been determined either by turnover studies or through depletion and repletion studies. The requirements for other age groups are derived by the factorial method by adding the additional requirment for growth in case of children for foetal growth during pregnancy and for milk output during lactation. The requirements of most B vitamins such as thiamin, riboflavin and niacin are related to the dietary energy intake and hence their requirements are expressed per 1000 kcal of energy intake.

Table 2.5: Basis of estimating human nutrient requirements

Nutrient	Criteria of requirement	Method of assessment
Energy	Intake to maintain energy balance	Factorial
Protein	Minimum intake for N equilibrium	N balance
Iron	Minimum absorbed iron to keep iron balance	Turnover
Fat	Minimum intake to prevent EFA deficiency	Biochemical/Clinical study
Calcium	Minimal intake to maintain calcium equilibrium	Long-term Ca balance
Vitamin A	Minimum intake to correct dark adaptation	Depletion and Repletion
Vitamin C	Minimum intake to correct scurvy or biochemical deficiency.	- do -
Thiamin	Minimum to correct biochemical deficiency	- do -
Riboflavin	- do -	- do -
Niacin	- do -	- do -
Folate	Minimum intake for haematological response	- do -
Vitamin B_{12}	- do -	Turnover/clinical Response

Source: Narasinga Rao, B.S., 1998, Nutrient requirements and recommended dietary allowances. (Edited) Bamji S. Mehtab et al.,Textbook of Human Nutrition, Oxford & IBH Publishing Co. Pvt. Ltd., New Delhi.

UNSOLVED QUESTIONS

There are some unsolved questions related to RDA.

- Individual variation in the requirement of nutrients
- Difference in RDA between breast fed and bottle fed infants

- RDA is not available for all nutrients. Estimations of nutrients in food are not standardised.
- Bilingualism in the units of nutrients causes confusion *e.g.,* k cal/MJ; milli moles, m E.q., mg.

Acceptance of RDA means that the diet of every individual would be different from others. This is unreasonable and impractical.

All members of the family tend to consume from the same pot. Dietary guidelines unlike RDA, depend on using food consumption pattern. Limitations of applicability of RDA for different purposes must be understood.

QUESTIONS

1. What is RDA? How is it different from requirements?
2. What are the methods used to determine the RDA of different nutrients.
3. Explain the factors affecting RDA.
4. Discuss how nutritional requirements are affected by interrelationships of nutrients.
5. Give the RDA for the following:
   - Adult man doing sedentary work
   - A girl aged 14
   - Pregnant woman who is in the last trimester of pregnancy.
6. Define reference man and reference woman.
7. Define factorial method.
8. Explain the problems involved in using RDA for planning diets.

SUGGESTED READINGS

- Dietary reference intakes: www.nap.edu

CHAPTER 3

CARBOHYDRATES

Carbohydrates, lipids and proteins are naturally occurring bulk nutrients present in almost all foods in differing quantities.

Carbohydrates are sugars or polymers of sugars such as starch, that can be hydrolysed to simple sugars by the action of digestive enzymes or by heating with dilute acids. Generally, but not always, the hydrogen and oxygen in them are in the proportions to form water; hence the term carbohydrate.

CLASSIFICATION

The dietary carbohydrates are classified as:-

1. Free sugars, to include the monosaccharides and disaccharides and their acid and alcohol derivatives;

2. Carbohydrates, other than free sugars that are soluble in 80% aqueous ethanol under prescribed conditions, for which the term, short chain carbohydrates, is proposed; and

3. Carbohydrates insoluble in 80% ethanol under the prescribed conditions for which the term 'polysaccharides' is retained.

Free sugars

Monosaccharides : These are compounds that cannot be hydrolysed to simpler compounds. Hexoses have dietary importance. Glucose, galactose, fructose and mannose have the same empirical formula, $C_6H_{12}O_6$. Glucose also known as dextrose, grape sugar or corn sugar is found in sweet fruits such as grapes, berries and oranges and in some vegetables such as sweet corn and carrots. It is prepared commercially as corn syrup or in its crystalline form by the hydrolysis of starch with acids. Glucose is the chief end product of the digestion of the disaccharides and polysaccharides. It is the form of carbohydrate circulating in the blood and it is utilized by the cell for energy. Fructose or fruit sugar is a highly soluble sugar that dose not readily crystallise. It is found in honey, ripe fruits and some vegetables. It is also a product of the hydrolysis of sucrose. Galactose is not found free in nature. Its only source is lactose which on hydrolysis yields glucose and galactose. The structure of glucose is given in Figure 3a.

Disaccharides : Sucrose, lactose and maltose are formed when two hexoses are combined with the loss of one molecule of water, the empirical formula being $C_{12}H_{22}O_{11}$. They are split to simple sugars by acid hydrolysis or by digestive enzymes. Sucrose is found in cane or beet sugar, sorghum molasses and maple sugar. Many fruits and some vegetables contain small amounts of sucrose.

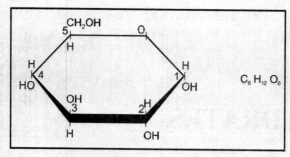

Figure 3a. The structure of glucose

Lactose or milk sugar is a disaccharide of glucose and glatose produced by mammals and is the only carbohydrate of animal origin of significance in the diet.

Maltose is a disaccharide of glucose and does not occur to any appreciable extent in foods. It is an intermediate product in the hydrolysis of starch or malting and fermentation of grain and is present in beer and malted breakfast cereals. It is also used with dextrins as the source of carbohydrate for some infant formulas.

Trehalose is a disaccharide of glucose and is known as the mushroom sugar, since it constitutes up to 15 percent of the dry matter of mushrooms. Trehalose is also present in insects.

Sugar alcohols : Sugar alcohols, also called polyols are found in nature and are prepared commercially. The sugar alcohols are not digested or absorbed in the small intestine but are fermented by the large gut microflora and thus contributes less energy. They are not digested by the bacteria in the mouth therefore are non-cariogenic.

Table 3.1: Classification of Dietary Carbohydrate

Class	Components	Comments
Free sugars	Mono and disaccharides	Associated with high blood glucose and insulin, links with diabetes; coronary heart disease, cancer and the ageing process
Innulin	Sugar alcohols	Sparingly absorbed Partly metabolised
Short-chain carbohydrates **Polysaccharides**	Oligosaccharides Innulin	May be fermented in the large bowel. Innulin and fructooligosaccharides have been shown to stimulate growth of potentially beneficial bifido bacteria
Starch	Rapidly digestible starch RDS, (Includes maltodextrins)	RDS and RAG* associated with high blood glucose and insulin. Links with diabetes, coronary heart disease, cancer and the ageing process
	Slowly digestible starch, SDS.	Only moderate influence on blood glucose and insulin Nutritionally the most desirable form of starch
	Resistant Starch, RS.	Desirability/safety of increase in foods requires further evaluation
Nonstarch Polysaccharides NSP	Cell-wall NSP in unrefined plant foods, dietary fibre.	Encapsulate and thus slow rate of digestion and absorption of sugars and starch.

*RAG (rapidly available glucose) = RDS + free glucose + glucose from sucrose.

Source: Garrow, J.S., et al., 2000, Human nutrition and Dietetics, Churchill Livingstone, Edinburgh.

Sugar acids : The sugar acids rarely occur as free compounds in nature but are abundant as constituents of polysaccharides such as pectin.

Short Chain Carbohydrates (SCC)

Short chain carbohydrates are the dietary carbohydrates other than free sugars (and malto - dextrins) are soluble in 80% ethanol under prescribed conditions. That the naturally occurring oligosaccharides raffinose, stachyose and verbascose, small polysaccharides such as inulin and other fructans are included in this category. Semisynthetic and synthetic carbohydrates like polydextrose and fructo-oligosaccharides are also considered as short chain carbohydrates.

The SCC are not susceptible to hydrolysis by endogenous enzymes but they may be fermented by the microflora in the large intestine. Fructo-oligosaccharides, inulin and some other SCC have been shown to selectively stimulate the growth of bifido bacteria, which is potentially beneficial to health.

Polysaccharides

Starch : Starch is the main storage polysaccharides of plants and is found in considerable amounts in dietary staples such as cereal grains, potatoes and plantains. Starch is the major carbohydrate in the human diet. Starch consists of two types of polysaccharides, amylose and amylopectin and the relative amounts vary in different starches. In waxy corn 2 percent amylose is present whereas high amylose corn starch contains 80 percent starch.

The amylose and amylopectin chains in the granules have a semi-crystalline structure which retards their digestion by pancreatic amylase.

Rapidly Digestible Starch (RDS) is rapidly and completely digested and absorbed in the small intestine. RDS mainly of amorphous and dispersed starch and occurs typically in starchy foods that have been cooked by moist heat, for example, bread and potatoes.

Slowly Digestible Starch, like RDS, is completely digested in the small intestine but more slowly. This category includes starch that is poorly accessible to enzymes, such as a portion of that in partly milled grains and seeds and in foods with a dense structure, for example, pasta, and a high proportion of the granular starch in raw foods.

Table 3.2: Nutritional Classification of Starch

Class	Example of occurrence	Site of digestion and absorption	Glycaemic response
Rapidly Digestible Starch, RDS	Processed foods	Small intestine	Large
Slowly Digestible Starch SDS	Legumes, pasta, muesli	Small intestine	Small
Resistant Starch, RS			
Physically inaccessible, RS_1	Whole grains	Large intestine (fermented)	None
Resistant granules, RS_2	Unripe banana		
Retrograded amylose, RS_3	Processed foods		

Source: Garrow , J.S. et al., 2000, Human Nutrition and Dietetics, Churchill, Livingstone, Edinburgh.

Resistant starch is defined as the starch and starch degradation products that escapes digestion in the small intestine and becomes available for fermentation by the microflora in the large intestine. Physically inaccessible starch which may be found in whole or partly milled grains and seeds and in some very dense types of processed starchy foods, e.g. pasta, is termed RS. Starch that escapes digestion in the small intestine because the granules in, for example, raw potato and banana starch are intrinsically highly resistant to hydrolysis by pancreatic amylase is termed RS_2. The third category RS_3 is mainly retrograded amylose formed during the cooling of gelatinized starch. Most moist heated starchy foods will therefore contain some RS_3 upon cooling.

Rate of digestion is related to the nature of the food itself, and physiological factors which include the extent of chewing, the concentration of amylase in the gut, and transit time through the stomach and small intestine.

The proportions of RDS, SDS and RS vary greatly between foods, depending partly on the source of starch, but largely on the type and extent of processing the food has undergone. The amounts and types of starch in foods are of great importance to health.

Dextrins are degradation products of starch in which the polymers have been broken down to smaller units by partial hydrolysis. They are the main source of carbohydrate in proprietary preparations used as oral supplements for tube feeding. Liquid glucose is a mixture of dextrins, maltose, glucose and water. These products are a means of giving carbohydrates in an easily assimilated form to patients who are seriously ill. Dextrins are larger molecules than sucrose or glucose and have less osmotic effect weight for weight and less likely to cause osmolar diarrhoea.

Non-starch Polysaccharides : Non-starch polysaccharides consist of the polysaccharides other than starch that are insoluble in 80% ethanol. In relation to human nutrition, the principal NSP are those that comprise approximately 90% of plant cell walls.

Plant NSP are often separated into cellulose [β(1–4)glucan] and non-cellulose polysaccharides. The latter are a very heterogeneous group whose main constituents sugars are arabinose , xylose, mannose, galactose , glucose and uronic acids.

Wheat NSP are slowly and incompletely fermented; they are able to bind considerable amounts of water and serve to increase faecal bulk. Compared to wheat products, oats contain a greater proportion of soluble NSP and the main fraction is a β-glucan, measured as soluble NSP glucose. Apples and carrots are typical of fruits and vegetables in general in having high levels of soluble NSP. The main fraction in these foods is pectin, which is measured mostly as soluble NSP uronic acids. In general cereal products contain more xylose than arabinose, while fruits and vegetables contain less xylose than arabinose. From the rmentation of various types of NSP short chain fatty acids are produced.

FUNCTIONS

Source of energy: Carbohydrates are least expensive source of energy to the body. Every gram of carbohydrate, sugar or starch, when oxidized yields on an average 4 kilo calories. Since Indians consume large quantity of cereals, most of the requirement of energy is met by carbohydrates.

Protein sparing action: The body uses carbohydrate as a source of energy, when they are adequately supplied in the diet, sparing protein for tissue building. If diet does not supply adequate calories, the dietary protein is oxidised as a source of energy. There is also breakdown of tissue proteins to a greater extent. This function of carbohydrate of serving as a source of energy and preventing dietary protein from being oxidised is called protein sparing action.

Oxidation of fats: In oxidation of fats the acetyl Co A formed from the oxidation of fatty acids reacts with oxaloacetic acid from carbohydrate and amino acid metabolism to form citric acid which is oxidised through the TCA cycle back to oxaloacetic acid through a series of reactions. Hence, for β-oxidatiom of fats, carbohydrate is essential. If adequate amount of carbohydrate is not consumed, intermediary products of fat oxidation are accumulated. Acetone, acetoacetic acid and β-hydroxy butyric acid accumulate and produce ketosis.

Indispensability for nervous system: The main source of energy for central nervous system is glucose. Prolonged hypoglycaemia can lead to irreversible damage to the brain tissue.

Role in muscle : Carbohydrates are the major source of energy for muscular work. During muscular contraction, glycogen is broken down to lactic acid through glycolysis. During the recovery period, lactic acid is first oxidised to pyruvic acid and then to acetyl CoA which is then oxidized to CO_2 and H_2O, thus producing energy for muscular work.

Role in liver : These include detoxifying action and regulating influence of protein and fat metabolism. Liver is rich in glycogen and is more resistant to certain poisons such as carbon tetrachloride, alcohol, arsenic and toxins of bacteria. The rate of oxidation of amino acids in liver is diminished if abundant supply of carbohydrates are available.

Source of energy for heart muscle : The heart muscle mainly uses glucose as source of energy. In hypoglycemia a definite adverse change in the working of the heart has been observed.

Synthesis of ribose from glucose : The pentose ribose is present in RNA and in many nucleotides. It is formed in the body from glucose by Hexose Mono Phosphate pathway.

Conversion to fat : Excess of calories fed in diet in the form of carbohydrate is stored as fat in the adipose tissue. When the body is in need of energy it can be realised from the adipose tissue.

Promotes growth of desirable bacteria: Lactose has several functions in the gastrointestinal tract. It promotes the growth of desirable bacteria, some of which are useful in the synthesis of B-complex vitamins. Lactose also enhances the absorption of calcium.

Contribution of dietary fibre: Dietary fibre gives no nutrients to the body. It stimulates the peristaltic movement. It helps in preventing many degenerative diseases.

Biosynthesis of amino acids: The carbon skeleton for the synthesis of alanine, aspartic acid and glutamic acid are provided by glucose during its oxidation, from pyruvic acid, oxalo acetic acid and α-ketoglutaric acid respectively.

DIGESTION

Digestion of polysaccharides begins in the mouth by the enzyme, ptyalin or α-amylase. The action of ptyalin may continue for a short period in the stomach till the gastric acidity inactivates the enzyme. Polysaccharides are partially hydrolysed to dextrin and maltose by the pancreatic amalyse. Maltose along with other disaccharides such as lactose and sucrose are hydrolysed by maltase, lactase and sucrase of intestinal juice respectively for the conversion to glucose, galactose and fructose.

Table 3.3: Action of Digestive Enzymes on Carbohydrates

Source	Enzyme	Product
Salivary gland	Salivary α-amylase	Hydrolyses α-(1-4) linkage producing α-limited dextrins, maltotriose and maltose
Pancreas	Pancreatic α-amylase	Hydrolyses α-(1-4) linkages producing α-limited dextrins maltotriose and maltose
Intestinal mucosa	Maltase	Hydrolyses maltose and maltotriose to glucose
	Lactase	Hydrolyses lactose to galactose and glucose
	Sucrase	Hydrolyses sucrose to glucose and fructose
	α-limited dextrinase	Hydrolyses starch to glucose

Source : Guthrie Helen A. and Mary Frances Picciano, 1995, Human Nutrition, WCB McGraw-Hill, Boston.

Starch contained within discrete structures such as whole grains and seeds is physically inaccessible to pancreatic amylase. Crushing, chopping and milling all increase the accessibility of the starch, that is, the rate of digestion influenced by the final particle size. In foods such as pasta, starch hydrolysis is retarded by the density of the product, which decreases enzyme access. Physical inaccessibility may cause the rate of starch hydrolysis to be so slow that some starch enters the large intestine. In extreme cases, starch contained within discrete structures may be excreted in the faeces.

Cooking facilitates the hydrolysis of starch through gelatinisation and dispersion of the starch granules. However, foods eaten raw retain their starch as granules, which show varying degrees of resistance to digestion. Raw starch from cereals is digested slowly within the small intestine, giving a modest glycaemic reponse. Raw starch from banana and potato shows a greater degree of resistance, up to 90% passing undigested through the small intestine.

Retrogradation also retards digestion and retrograded starch, mainly amylose, from processed cereal and potato products has been shown to pass through the intestine.

Raw white wheat flour, which consists mainly of ungelatinised starch granules, is digested relatively slowly. Baking the flour into short bread, which involves cooking in the presence of very little water, results in limited disruption of the granular structure and gives a product that is also digested slowly. On the other hand, baking the flour into bread, a process that requires a long cooking time in the presence of water, leads to extensive gelatinisation of the starch granules and results in a rapidly digestible product.

ABSORPTION

Carbohydrates are absorbed into the blood stream as glucose, galactose and fructose. By way of the capillaries of the villi, the simple sugars enter the portal circulation and are transported to the liver. Here the fructose and galactose are converted to glycogen for storage. The glycogen is reconverted to glucose as needed by body.

The rate of absorption of different monosaccharides taking glucose as 100, galactose is 110; fructose is 43; xylose is 15; and arabinose is 9. It is evident that glucose and galactose are absorbed at a faster rate than fructose and the pentoses are absorbed slowly. It has been found that the high rate of absorption of glucose and galactose is due to the fact that they are actively transported while fructose and pentoses are absorbed by diffusion.

Several methods are used either singly or in combination to transport monosaccharides across the intestinal mucosa into the splanchic capillaries. These transport system include diffusion, facilitated (or carrier-mediated) diffusion and active transport; the third is distinguished by the need for energy input.

The monosaccharides glucose, fructose and galactose are transported across the epithelial cells and enter the portal vein. Free concentrations in the intestine or at the mucosal surface are likely to be high enough for passive or facilitated absorption. But as concentrations fall, active transport against a concentration gradient becomes necessary, which requires energy. Active transport is carrier-mediated and the carrier is a specific transport protein which is an integral part of the membrane to the traversed.

The absorption of glucose is affected by the amount of sodium (Na^+) ions in the intestinal lumen. A high Na^+ concentration facilitates glucose influx into the intestinal mucosal cell, whereas a low Na^+ concentration inhibits influx. This is because glucose and sodium share the same cotransporter carrier protein. Intracellular Na^+ concentration is low relative to the external concentration, thus Na^+ moves into the cell down its concentration gradient . Glucose moves along with the Na^+ and is released inside the cell. The glucose transport mechanism also transports galactose. Fructose is transported via a different carrier and its absorption is independent of Na^+. Some fructose is converted to glucose in the mucosal cells. The rate of absorption is almost equal for glucose and galactose, but fructose is absorbed about half as rapidly. About 97–98 per cent of the carbohydrate is digested and absorbed.

Factors Affecting Absorption

The absorption of digested carbohydrates is influenced by the following:

- The rate at which the carbohydrate enters the small intestine affects its absorption. The rate of entry depends upon the mobility of the stomach and the control of the duodenal sphincter muscle and the pyloric valve.
- The type of the food mixture present influences the degree of competition for absorptive sites and available carrier transport system.
- Absorption is also influenced by the condition of intestinal membrane and the time carbohydrate is held in contact with the membrane. Any abnormal mucosal tissue (enteritis, celiac diseases), or an abnormally rapid movement of the carbohydrate along the intestine (diarrhoea), hinders absorption.
- Normal endocrine activity of the anterior pituitory and the related functioning of the thyroid is necessary for normal absorption. In addition, the adrenal cortex hormones regulate the body sodium exchange, which indirectly influences the operation of the sodium pump.
- The rate of absorption of carbohydrates is decreased in the presence of intact plant cell walls, the dense physical structure of starchy foods and the presence of proteins and fats.
- Small intestinal absorption is slowed by increased meal frequency (nibbling).

METABOLISM

Metabolism involves all those processes by which the nutrients are used for energy.

Direct utilisation: Glucose can be utilised by all the tissues of the body. Glucose should be made accessible to all the cells of the body as the major source of energy. Although fats can also be oxidised to release energy, certain cells, especially the nerve cells and brain tissues cannot function without the availability of glucose from carbohydrate.

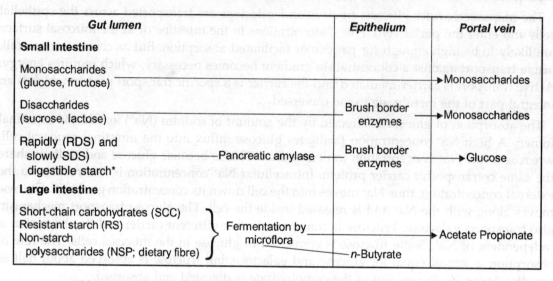

*More marked glycemic response with RDS than with SDS.

Figure 3b. The digestion and utilization of dietary carbohydrates.

Source: Garrow , J.S.,et al., 2000. Human Nutrition and Dietetics, Churchill, Livingstone, Edinburgh.

Glucose undergoes oxidation with the help of the enzymes in the body, to yield carbon-dioxide, water and heat, which is captured in the high energy chemical bonds of specified compounds like Adenosine Tri Phosphate (ATP), which in turn can be enzymatically broken down to release the useful energy, as and when the cells need it.

Glucose is broken down in several steps to two molecules of pyruvate which in turn is converted to acetyl coenzyme A, in the process releasing a small amount of ATP. Next, acetyl Co A enters the TCA Cycle which also involves a series of reactions to release carbon-dioxide, and hydrogen atoms which enter the electron transport system to release ATP.

The complete oxidation of one molecule of glucose produces 36 ATP molecules, 6 molecules of CO_2 and 6 molecules of H_2O.

Conversion into glycogen: Whenever more carbohydrate is supplied in the diet than is needed immediately for energy, both the muscle and liver synthesise glycogen from the extra glucose. The body stores only a limited amount of glycogen. The liver glycogen stores are quickly converted to glucose to be used for energy. Muscle glycogen, however, is used only to supply the muscle with energy via glucose and does not affect blood glucose levels.

About 150 g of glycogen is stored in muscle, this amount can be increased five fold with physical training. The glycogen store in human liver is about 90 g and is involved in the hormonal control of blood sugar.

Conversion into fat: Steady excess intake of the carbohydrate through the diet, is turned into fat and deposited in the adipose tissues of the body.

MAINTENANCE OF BLOOD GLUCOSE LEVELS

Normal blood glucose levels are important for the feeling of well-being, because the brain and other nervous tissues are dependent on blood glucose for energy. Glycogen is not stored in nervous tissue.

The fasting blood glucose level is between 80–100 mg/dl of blood. After eating a meal, containing carbohydrates, blood glucose level normally rises to 130–140 mg/dl at 1 hour, but returns to the fasting level 2 hours after the meal.

If the blood glucose levels fall to low levels (30–50 mg/dl), the body is in hypoglycaemic condition. The brain is deprived of its source of energy and the person experiences symptoms like fatigue, lightheadedness, jitteriness, irritability, sweating, headaches etc. If the levels become even lower, fainting, coma and death ensue. Therefore, it is imperative to maintain normal blood glucose levels.

The liver is the most crucial organ in the metabolism of carbohydrates. It is an energy "traffic cop", routing glucose to where it is needed in the body or changing it to glycogen for storage until needed; which occurs immediately following a meal rich in carbohydrates. As time lapses, body cells remove glucose from blood to use for energy, and blood levels of glucose go down. The body maintains normal blood glucose levels even when there is no carbohydrate in the diet, by converting noncarbohydrate substances to glucose. Gluconeogenesis occurs in the liver and kidneys. During total starvation, gluconeogenesis is the chief mechanism by which blood glucose levels are maintained.

RAPIDLY AVAILABLE GLUCOSE VALUES

Repidly Available Glucose is the sum free glucose, glucose from sucrose and glucose from RAS—Rapidly Available Strach. The values are expressed as grams of glucose per 100g of food as eaten. Meals with a high RAG value will result in elevated levels of blood glucose, i.e., a large glycaemic response and subsequently raised levels of circulating insulin. Unlike glycaemic inded, RAG values give information on the amount of carbohydrate consumed.

Glucose is made available to the circulation by:
- the absorbed sugars from the diet
- glycogenolysis
- gluconeogenesis
- to a lesser extent, the reconversion of pyruvic and lactic acids formed in the glycolytic pathway.

Several hormones control the supply of glucose to the blood.

Six pathways are available for the removal of glucose from the blood:

- the continuous uptake of glucose by every cell in the body and its oxidation for energy
- the conversion of glucose to glycogen by the liver (glycogenesis)
- the synthesis of fats from glucose (lipogenesis)
- the synthesis of numerous carbohydrate derivatives
- glycolysis in the red blood cells and
- elimination of glucose in the urine when the renal threshold is exceeded.

Hormonal Control of Blood Sugar Levels

A number of mechanisms function to maintain blood glucose at a remarkably constant level (70–100 mg/dl) under fasting condition. Many hormones are involved in regulating blood sugar levels.

Insulin: It is produced by the β-cells of the islets of Langerhans in the pancreas. It has been called the "feasting hormone" because its liberation is enhanced by a high glucose level in the blood. The mechanism by which insulin lowers blood glucose involves an increase in the rate of glucose utilisation for oxidation by increasing facilitated diffusion of glucose into muscle and adipose cells. Insulin increases glycogenesis and glucose is stored as glycogen in the liver and muscle cells. Insulin enhances lipogenesis by the uptake of glucose by adipose and liver cells for conversion into fat.

Glucagon: It is produced by the α cells of the islets of Langerhans. It has an effect exactly opposite to that of insulin. It causes a rise in the amount of sugar in blood by increasing glycogenolysis by activating the enzyme phosphorylase. It enhances gluconeogenesis from amino acids and lactate. Insulin and glucagon may thus be considered antagonists and their opposing effects at least in part maintain carbohydrate metabolism in a steady state.

Epinephrine (adrenaline) : It is a hormone secreted by the chromaffin cells of the adrenal medulla. It favours the breakdown of liver and muscle glycogen to yield blood glucose (glycogenolysis) and decreases the release of insulin from the pancreas, thus raising the blood sugar. Secretion of epinephrine is increased during anger or fear, and the subsequent glucose formation provides extra energy for crisis response.

Glucocorticoids : These steroid hormones elaborated by the adrenal cortex also influence blood glucose levels by stimulating gluconeogenesis. These hormones reduce glucose utilisation in the extrahepatic tissue and also increase the rate at which protein is converted into glucose, thus counteracting the action of insulin.

Thyroxine : Severe lowering of blood glucose concentration increases thyroxine secretion. Thyroid hormones enhance the action of epinephrine. Hepatic glycogenolysis and gluconeogenesis are increased, leading to a rise in blood glucose concentration. Thyroxine also increases the rate of hexose absorption from the intestine.

Growth hormone : This is elaborated by the anterior pituitary gland. This raises blood glucose level by increasing amino acid uptake and protein synthesis by all cells by diminishing cellular uptake and increasing the mobilisation of fat for energy.

Table 3.4: Hormonal Maintenance of Blood Glucose

Hormone	Action
• Insulin	• ↑ Glucose oxidation in cells
	• ↑ Glycogenesis
	• ↑ Lipogenesis
	• ↓ Glycogenolysis
• Glucagon	• ↑ Glycogenolysis
	• ↑ Gluconeogenesis
• Epinephrine	• ↑ Glycogenolysis
	• ↓ Release of insulin
• Glucocorticoids	• ↑ Gluconeogenesis
	• ↓ Utilisation of glucose
	• ↑ Protein catabolism
	• ↑ Uptake of amino acids by the liver
• Thyroxine	• ↑ Glycogenolysis
	• ↑ Gluconeogenesis
	• ↑ Hexose absorption
• Growth hormone	• ↑ Protein synthesis
	• ↓ Cellular uptake of glucose
	• ↑ Mobilisation of fat

Insulin reduces the blood sugar whereas all the other hormones are antogonist to insulin.

RECOMMENDED DIETARY ALLOWANCES

Wide variation in allowance of carbohydrate is compatible with health because of the interrelationship with fatty acids and amino acids in meeting the energy needs of the body. The minimum requirement of carbohydrate is 100 g. This is desirable to prevent ketosis. Normal balanced diet contains a much higher amount than this. ICMR has not given any specific recommendations for carbohydrate. However, in a balanced diet sixty per cent of total calories can be from carbohydrates. In a 2000 kcal diet 275–300 g of carbohydrate is recommended. Only 10% should be from sugar and rest should come from complex carbohydrates.

SOURCES

The sources of different carbohydrates are given in Table 3.5.

Table 3.5: Sources of Carbohydrates

Carbohydrate	Sources
FREE SUGARS	
Monosaccharides	
Glucose	Fruits, honey
Fructose	Fruits honey
Galactose	Milk
Xylose	Fruits, vegetables, cereals
Disaccharides	
Sucrose	Cane and beet sugars, molasses
Lactose	Milk and milk products
Maltose	Malt products
Trehalose	Mushrooms
Sugar alcohols	
Sorbitol	Cherries
Xylitol	Fruits and vegetables
Sugar acids	
D-Galacturonic acid	Pectin
SHORT CHAIN CARBOHYDRATES	
Raffinose	Sugar beets, kidney beans, lentils and navy beans
Stachyose	Beans
POLYSACCHARIDES	
Digestible	
Rapidly digestible starch	Processed foods
Slowly digestible starch	Legumes, pasta
Resistant starch	
Physically inaccessible	Whole grains
Resistant granules	Unripe banana
Retrograded amylose	Cooked starches
Indigestible	
Cellulose	Bran, whole wheat flour
Hemicellulose	Stalks and leaves of vegetables, outer covering of seeds

The percentage carbohydrate content of some foods is given in Table 3.6. Pure sugars are almost 100 per cent carbohydrate. Syrups, jellies and jams contain 65 to 80 per cent. Ethanol in beers, wines and hard liquors is product by anaerobic fermentation on carbohydrates.

Table 3.6: Carbohydrate Content of Foods

Name of Food Stuff	Carbohydrate g/100g
Sugar	99
Jaggery	95
Sago	87
Rice	78
Dates dried	76
Wheat flour, whole	69
Red gram dal	58
Skimmed milk powder	51
Whole milk powder	38
Potato	23

DIETARY FIBRE

Dietary fibre is defined as that portion of food derived from plant cells, which is resistant to hydrolysis/digestion by the elementary enzyme system in human beings. It consists of hemicelluloses, cellulose, lignins, oligosaccharides, pectins, gums and waxes.

Some bacteria in the large intestine can degrade some components of fibre releasing products, that can be absorbed into the body and used as energy source.

Two categories of fibre are found in food. Crude fibre is defined as the residue remaining after the treatment with hot sulphuric acid, alkali and alcohol. The major component of crude fibre is a polysaccharide called cellulose. Crude fibre is a component of dietary fibre. Several other carbohydrate and related compounds called pectins, hemicellulose and lignins are the second category found in plant foods and are also resistant to digestion. These together with cellulose are collectively known as dietary fibre.

Insoluble fibres are indigestible and insoluble in water. Soluble fibres are indigestible but soluble in water.

Total Dietary Fibre and Energy content of foods

Current estimates of energy contents of foods assumes that only the "crude fibre" is indigestible. In the present conventional methods of food analysis, the rest of the fibre is included as a part of dietary carbohydrate which is computed by difference. This is by deducting the protein, fat, moisture, crude fibre and ash content per 100 g from 100. By this procedure dietary fibre excluding the crude fibre is assumed to yield 4 kcal/g. Dietary fibre content of food is several fold higher than "crude fibre" hence there could be overestimates. There is a need to reevaluate the energy content of foods after taking into account their total dietary fibre content.

Table 3.7: Sources of Different Fibres

Fibre	Occurrence	Source
Insoluble fibres		
Cellulose	Cell wall constituent	Whole wheat flour, bran, vegetables
Hemi cellulose	Secretions, cell wall material	Bran and whole gram
Lignin	Woody part of plants	Mature vegetables, wheat and fruits like strawberries
Soluble fibres		
Gums	Special cell secretions	Oats, legumes and guar (made from cluster beans), barley
Pectins	Intracellular cementing material	Apples, guavas, citrus fruits, carrots, strawberries

PHYSIOLOGICAL EFFECTS

The effect of fibre on the gastro intestinal tract is influenced by the characteristics of the fibre itself, the particle size, the interaction between fibre and other dietary components and bacterial flora.

Nutrient absorption: Dietary fibre is susceptible to physical disintegration during processing, cooking and mastication into fine particles. Consequent size reduction and dispersal of soluble fibre like β-glucans and pectins in the aqueous phase appears to be causing a delay in the uptake of absorbable nutrients by the epithelial cells that line the mucosa. Delay in absorption can lead to eventual excretion of nutrients.

Barrier to digestion: Inspite of adequate processing, cooking and mastication a part of the structure enveloping the nutrients remains intact and slows down the whole process of digestion and acts as a physical barrier between nutrients and digestive enzymes in the intestine. Legume seeds have relatively thick walls resisting breakdown during processing and cooking and therefore legumes constitute one of the lowest glycaemic response foods, that is, reduced rate of absorption of glucose.

Nutrient binding: Many cell wall polysaccharides and lignins interact with metal ions–iron, calcium and zinc in the aqueous phase of the intestinal contents. This can result in conversion of soluble minerals into unabsorbable forms to be excreted.

Diets with high levels of legumes, oats and whole wheat have undesirable effects on mineral absorption. One of the probable reasons for the above findings could be presence of phytic substances in these sources along with polysaccharide and they do possess strong mineral binding capacity.

Chang et al. (1994) reported that pH had an influence on cation binding by these fibres and invariably more exogenous calcium was found to be bound at higher pH levels.

Adsorption of organic molecules : The organic molecules that can be adsorbed to dietary fibre include bile acids, neutral sterols, carcinogens and toxic compounds.

Some types of soluble dietary fibre have the ability to adsorb bile acids. This adsorption has been suggested to be the mechanism of increased faecal bile acid excretion resulting in decreased levels of serum and tissue cholesterol. Lignin component of the foods is principally responsible for the bile acid binding.

Mobility of intestinal contents: Presence of soluble dietary fibers increase the viscosity of the intestinal contents, decrease the peristalitic movements of the gut, thereby reducing the chances of nutrients to move towards the villi network for efficient absorption. In such a situation the process of physical mixing achieved by peristalitic motion is replaced by simple diffusion, a comparatively slower process. This becomes the rate limiting step in nutrient conveyance across the mucosal surface. Such a condition may not hamper movement of simple and low molecular weight nutrients.

But large molecular complexes from fatty acids, bile salts and cholesterol miscelles cannot easily go through the molecular sieve formed by soluble nonstarch polysaccharides, thus slowing down the process of nutrient absorption. This in turn increases the time required and surface area needed for absorption along the length of the small bowel. The rate at which the nutrients appear in the circulation is reduced under such conditions, while exposure of gut surface to the nutrients is increased, triggering release of regulatory hormones which stimulate growth of mucosal cells.

Faecal output: Dietary fibre increases faecal bulk and frequency of stool. Wheat bran due to its high insoluble fibre content and presence of highly lignified tissues, resist colon fermentation, thus increasing the dry matter content of faeces. Besides that, ability to retain water during transit contributes to soft stools and ease of defaecation. Processing and cooking reduces the bulking effect due to physical disruption of the fibre structure. Coarse bran is effective in increasing bulk and ease of defaecation but fine bran often has little effect.

The faecal weight on western diet is 80–160 g/day. Whereas Indian vegetarian diet gives rise to 225 g/day of faeces. When dietary fibre is supplemented the faecal weight can rise to 470 g/day.

Faecal transit: After ingesting food, it takes about 4–12 hrs for the undigested portion to reach the colon. Complex plant foods not disrupted adequately, take longer time to pass through the stomach and small intestine. Soluble non-absorbing sugars such as lactulose and oligosaccharides pass through very fast. Soluble fibres with the viscosity increasing property slow down passage and delay gastric emptying. A high intake of dietary fibre generally causes reduced transit time in the colon and faster bowl emptying. This is attributed to accelerated colonic mobility by increased intraluminal mass. Higher the faecal bulk, lower will be the transit time in the large intestine.

Reduced transit time could be the result from the stimulation of the mucosa by mechanical effect or perhaps by the byproducts of bacterial fermentation.

If transit time is shortened, there could be less time for exposure of the mucosa to harmful toxicants. Also there could be less time for bacteria to produce harmful substances.

Table 3.8: Influence of dietary fibre on gastrointestinal tract.

Site	Activity
Mouth	Stimulates saliva secretion.
Stomach	Dilutes contents, delays gastric emptying.
Small intestine	Dilutes contents, delays absorption.
Large intestine	Dilutes contents, forms substrate for bacteria, traps water, binds cations.
Stool	Softens, enlarges prevents straining.

Fermentability: There are about 500 species of microbes in the caecum and colon. These microbes mostly are anaerobic in nature and they ferment the fibres, especially the soluble fibre and produce energy for their survival. They generally produce acetate, propionate and butyrate which are transported across the colonic mucosa. Butyrate is the main substrate for growth and metabolism of mucosal cells, while acetate and propionate after absorption are metabolised by liver to generate energy.

Flatus is sometimes wrongly associated with dietary fibre consumption. Incorporation of wheat causes slight increase in the flatus.

ROLE OF FIBRE IN HUMAN NUTRITION

Effect on upper gastro intestinal tract: Coronary Heart Disease CHD, diabetes mellitus and obesity are considered most significant health handicaps that can be alleviated by increased consumption of dietary fibre. Regular intake of dietary fibre at apporprate levels is reported to be effective in counteracting many of the risk factors associated with CHD such as increased apolipoprotein B and consequently increase in Low Density Lipoprotein (LDL) cholesterol, elevated serum cholesterol levels, high levels of blood serum fibrinogen, hypertension, obesity and diabetes mellitus.

Dietary fibre reduces serum fibrinogen levels which inturn lower the risk of blood clot formation and myocardial infarction.

Soluble dietary fibre supplementation reduces serum cholesterol levels significantly. Pectin and gums chelate with bile acids and steroid materials. This chelating effect helps in the reduction of blood cholesterol level. Oat products are found to be very efficient in this respect due to their high β-glucan content. Insoluble fibres do not have this property. Hypocholesteraemic effect was also observed using dietary fibre extracted from dry skins of onions and garlic. One of the postulations was that cholesterol synthesis is inhibited by acetic, propionic and butyric acids, generated by colon bacteria and concurrent clearance of LDL cholesterol. Soluble fibres like hydroxy methyl cellulose which are not known to be fermented in the colon lower cholesterol levels, especially LDL cholesterol in plasma because of their viscous property and increase in excretion of steroids.

The soluble dietary fibre fraction of fenugreek seeds is known for its hypoglycaemic effects in experimental animals as well as humans. Viscous fibres may impair mixing of intestinal contents, thereby impair digestion due to limited access of the food to the enzymes. Hence, the hypoglycaemic effect of dietary fibre could be due to the delaying of starch hydrolysis and glucose absorption and also improvement in glucose utilisation and insulin sensitivity in target tissues.

High intake of fibre by obese individuals cuts down fat in the diet and hence calories. Fibre promotes sensation of satiety.

Effect on large intestine: The colonic bacteria acting on dietary fibre produce short chain fatty acids and their cell mass contributes in the formation of stool. Dietary fibre increases stool weight and decreases intestinal transit time significantly.

Dietary fibre provides relief to the disorders like constipation, diverticulitis, irritable bowel syndrome, gall stones, and colorectal cancer.

Increased dietary fibre intake, especially the insoluble type with high water holding capacity and non-susceptibility to colonic fermentation can reduce the incidence of constipation. While coarse fibre is excellent for increasing the stool bulk, reducing its particle size adversely affects this property. Cereal brans are more effective than fruits and vegetables, for relieving constipation.

Individuals with stool weights of less than 100 g per day can be benefited by a dietary fibre intake of 18 g/day regularly.

Burkitt (1985) postulated that low intake of cereal fibre in regular diet could cause excessive straining and increased hardness of stool. Haemorrhoids and diverticulosis are more prevalent among populations with low fibre intake. Coarse bran was found to be most effective in treating diverticulosis. Figure 3c shows the effect of fibre on the softness of stool.

Burkitt (1985) also observed that varicose vein is predominant in communities known to pass small volume and firm consistency stools. Coarsely ground insoluble fibre consumption is considered as a potential treatment for varicose veins affected patients. Excessive straining during defaecation causing increased intra abdominable pressure can cause varicose veins.

Obesity, diabetes mellitus and hypertriglyceridemia have a bearing on the development of gall stones. It is possible that the beneficial effect of diet supplement like bran, gum, pectin and oats might be due to their ability to control levels of deoxycholic acid probably by hastening its transit in the human system. Since dietary fibre is useful to prevent obesity, diabetes mellitus and hypertriglyceradenia, it may also exert an influence in preventing gall stones.

Dietary fibre can provide protection against colon cancer by increasing the stool weight, by diluting the colonic contents and by reducing the transit time. Dietary fibre also influences the colonic microbial metabolism, influences fermentation in the colon and the production and distribution of short chain fatty acids in the colon. It modifies pH, increases the faecal nitrogen and influence on bile acid and mutagens in the colon. Fibre influences faecal enzymes.

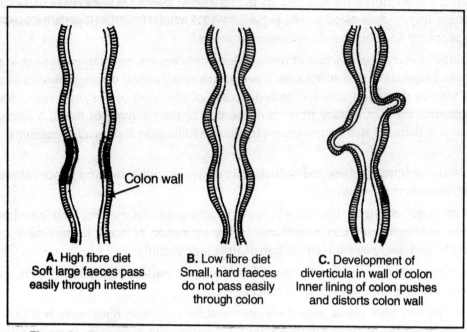

Figure 3c. The effect of fibre and lack of fibre in the diet on stool formation.

Dietary fibre prevents breast cancer in preadolescent girls who consume more fibre can cut their risk of early onset of menstruation by half. Delaying menstruation provides a protection against breast cancer later. Early menarche for girls 12 and under is associated with a 10 to 15 per cent higher risk of breast cancer in life. Vegetarians, who eat high fibre, excrete more oestrogen.

Fibre rich foods are usually low in fat. On high fibre diets one is less likely to over eat. Traditional cooking habits retain fibre.

Table 3.9: Role of fibre in preventing diseases

Disease	Type of Fibre involved	Physiological Mechanism
Constipation Diverticulitis Irritable bowel syndrome Varicose veins Piles (Haemorrhoids)	Insoluble fibre Cellulose Cereal bran	1. Increases the water holding capacity. 2. Increases stool weight. 3. Reduces the transit time. Enhances gastric motility. 4. Volatile fatty acids which are released by the bacteria have a laxative effect. 5. Faster bowel emptying due to increased intra lumenal mass bulk. 6. Decreases intra colonic pressure.
Cancer of the large intestine	Insoluble fibre	1. Changes in the population of microbes in the GI tract. 2. Increases binding of intestinal bile acids. 3. Food residue remains in the colon for less time for carcinogen to be absorbed. 4. Increases stool weight and volume.

Contd...

5. Increases frequency of defaecation.

6. Bulk and water of the faeces may dilute the carcinogens to a non-toxic level.

7. Fibre induced effects on faecal enzymes.

8. Production and distribution of short chain fatty acids in the colon resulting in pH modification.

9. Increases faecal nitrogen.

10. Influence on bile acid and mutagens in the colon.

11. Adsorbing cancer producing hydrocarbons (lignins).

Coronary Heart Disease Gall stones	Soluble fibre, β-glucan content, oats, skin, pectin. Guargum, psyllium, husk, beans, fruits & vegetables.	1. Cholesterol synthesis in inhibited by acetic, propionic and butyric acids produced by bacterial fermentation.
		2. Clearance of LDL cholesterol.
		3. Slows gastric emptying and binds bile acids.
		4. Increases excretion of steroids.
		5. Reduces serum fibrinogen and therefore reduces blood clot formation.
		6. Reduces fatty acid absorption.
		7. Lowers the blood pressure through increased absorption of calcium and magnesium.
		8. Fibre binds faecal bile acids and increases excretion of bile acid derived cholesterol.
Diabetes Mellitus	Soluble fibre, legume seed coverings.	1. Rate of glucose absorption is decreased because of physical barrier for the outer coatings of legumes.
		2. Reduces the requirement of insulin.
		3. Increases peripheral insulin sensitivity.
		4. Alters gut hormones to enhance glucose metabolism in liver.
Obesity	Soluble fibre	1. Gastric emptying is delayed and feeling of satiety is increased.
		2. Diets high in fibre are low in calories.

Table 3.10: Limitations of Excess Consumption of Fibres

Disease	Type of Fibre	Physiological Mechanism
Increased risk of colonic cancer	Soluble fibres such as gum arabic, carrageenan, which are used as stabilisers and emulsifiers in food industry.	1. Reduce the ability of insoluble fibres to absorb and excrete carcinogen.
		2. Soluble fibres are digested by colonic bacteria. The carcinogen formed can be deposited on the mucosal cells.
		3. Soluble fibre may cross the intestinal epithelium and carry with it carcinogens in solution.
Decreased absorption of minerals like calcium, iron, magnesium, zinc	Insoluble fibres, seed coats	Phytate found in seed coat of legumes has the ability to bind metal ions like calcium, copper, iron and zinc and make them insoluble.

Limitations of excess consumption of fibres : Vegetarians who eat high fibre excrete more oestrogen. It may cause abdominal discomfort and diarrhoea due to bacterial action in colon. Other limitations are given in Table 3.10.

RECOMMENDED DIETARY ALLOWANCES

Recommended allowance for fibre is 30 g/day or 12 g/1000 kcal for a normal healthy adult. The proportion of soluble to insoluble fibre should be 1:2 and the intake is preferred through diet made up of various sources. It is advisable to device 50 per cent each of the daily requirement of dietary fibre equally from cereal and fruit and vegetable sources for optimum effect. American diabetic association recommends 25–38 g of dietary fibre per day per person suffering from diabetes. Indian diets provide 50-100g/day when whole grain cereals, pulses and vegetables are consumed daily.

SOURCES

Studies conducted at National Institute of Nutrition showed that dietary fibre content increases as the maturity of green leafy vegetables increase. No effect of cooking on dietary fibre content. Majority of fruits had 30% of dietary fibre as soluble dietary fibre.

Refined and processed foods contain very low amounts of dietary fibre and sugar, oil, milk and meat do not contain any dietary fibre.

Though foods of plant origin in the diet contribute to most of the dietary fibre requirements, individually the extent of intake is influenced by a number of factors like the nature of source, maturity, moisture content, proportion in the diet and the mode of processing and preparation. Total dietary fibre content in these sources may vary from about 1 to 5 per cent.

Some of the natural sources of dietary fibre are listed in Table 3.11. Most fruits and vegetables in fresh state have fibre. Total Dietary Fibre values in the range 1 to 2.2 percent or with an average moisture content of 85 per cent in the fresh condition. TDF content could be between 6 to 17 per cent on dry matter basis.

Fibre rich foods are usually low in fat. On high fibre diets one is less likely to overeat.

Table 3.11: Dietary Fibre Content of Foods g/100 g

Name of the food stuff	Total Dietary Fibre	Insoluble Dietary Fibre	Soluble Dietary Fibre
	g	g	g
Cereals, grains and products			
Bajra	11.3	9.1	2.2
Jowar	9.7	8.0	1.7
Maize, dry	11.9	11.0	0.9
Ragi	11.5	9.9	1.6
Rice	4.1	3.2	0.9
Wheat	12.5	9.6	2.9
Pulses and legumes			
Bengal gram, whole	28.3	25.2	3.1

Contd...

Name of the food stuff	Total Dietary Fibre	Insoluble Dietary Fibre	Soluble Dietary Fibre
	g	g	g
Bengal gram, dhal	15.3	12.7	2.6
Black gram, dhal	11.7	7.6	4.1
Black gram, whole	20.3	15.4	4.9
Green gram, whole	16.7	14.7	2.0
Green gram, dhal	8.2	6.5	1.7
Lentil, whole	15.8	13.5	2.3
Lentil, dhal	10.3	8.3	2.0
Red gram, dhal	9.1	6.8	2.3
Red gram, whole	22.6	19.8	2.8
Leafy vegetables			
Agathi	8.4	6.3	2.1
Amaranth	4.0	3.1	0.9
Ambat chukka	3.2	2.4	0.8
Cabbage	2.8	2.0	0.8
Colocasia, green	6.6	5.1	1.5
Coriander	4.3	3.0	1.3
Curry leaves	16.3	13.4	2.9
Drumstick	9.0	6.8	2.2
Fenugreek	4.7	3.2	1.5
Gogu	3.8	2.6	1.2
Mayalu	2.5	1.6	0.9
Mint	6.3	5.0	1.3
Paruppu keerai	3.9	2.9	1.0
Ponnaganni	7.9	6.9	1.0
Spinach	2.5	1.8	0.7
Tamarind leaves, tender	10.6	9.4	1.2
Roots and tubers			
Beetroot	3.5	2.6	0.9
Carrot	4.4	3.0	1.4
Potato	1.7	1.1	0.6
Radish	2.3	1.8	0.5
Sweet potato	3.9	2.6	1.3
Yam	4.2	3.2	1.0
Colocasia	3.0	2.3	0.7
Other vegetables			
Bananapith	2.2	2.0	0.2
Bitter gourd	4.3	3.2	1.1
Bottlegourd	2.0	1.7	0.3
Brinjal	6.3	4.6	1.7
Broad bean	8.9	6.7	2.1
Cauliflower	3.7	2.6	1.1

Contd...

Name of the food stuff	Total Dietary Fibre g	Insoluble Dietary Fibre g	Soluble Dietary Fibre g
Chochomarrow	1.3	0.9	0.4
Cluster bean	5.7	4.2	1.5
Cucumber	2.6	2.0	0.6
Keera, green	1.1	0.8	0.3
Drumstick	5.8	4.8	1.0
Giant chillies	2.2	2.0	0.2
Kovai	2.5	1.5	1.0
Ladies finger	3.6	2.6	1.0
Mango, raw	3.0	1.4	1.6
Onion stalks	5.1	3.7	1.4
Peas, green	8.6	7.2	1.4
Plantain, green	3.5	2.6	0.9
Ridge gourd	1.9	1.4	0.5
Snake gourd	2.1	1.6	0.5
Tomato	1.7	1.2	0.5
Nuts and oilseeds			
Soya bean	23.0	17.9	5.1
Coconut fresh	13.6	12.7	0.9
Gingelly seeds	16.8	13.6	3.2
Groundnut	11.0	8.5	2.5
Mustard	13.6	10.2	3.4
Fruits			
Papaya	2.6	1.3	1.3
Zizyphus	3.8	2.8	1.0
Amla	7.3	5.8	1.5
Apple	3.2	2.3	0.9
Banana	1.8	1.1	0.7
Cherry	1.5	0.9	0.6
Dates, dry	8.3	6.9	1.4
Dates, fresh	7.7	6.9	0.8
Fig	5.0	2.6	2.4
Grapes, green	1.2	0.8	0.4
Guava	8.5	7.1	1.4
Jackfruit	3.5	2.1	1.4
Jambu	3.5	2.6	0.9
Sweetlime	2.7	1.3	1.4
Mango	2.0	1.0	1.0
Musk melon	0.8	0.5	0.3
Water melon	0.6	0.3	0.3
Orange	1.1	0.6	0.5
Peach	1.6	1.1	0.5

Contd...

Name of the food stuff	Total Dietary Fibre	Insoluble Dietary Fibre	Soluble Dietary Fibre
	g	g	g
Pear	4.3	4.0	0.3
Pineapple	2.8	2.3	0.5
Plum	2.8	1.7	1.1
Pomegranate	2.8	2.3	0.5
Sapota	10.9	9.1	1.8
Custard apple	5.5	4.0	1.5
Strawberry	2.3	1.6	0.7

Source : Gopalan C. et al, 2004, Nutritive Value of Indian Foods, National Institute of Nutrition, Hyderabad.

As food is processed and cooked to varying degrees the dietary fibre component in it is expected to undergo some changes. During milling, polishing, flaking, grinding, puffing and other primary processing operations the dietary fibre in food is not affected to any significant extent chemically but reduction of particle size does influence the behavior in the gastro-intestinal tract. Bringing down the particle size from 800 to 160 micron reduced the water holding capacity of wheat bran by 43 per cent and the glycocholate binding capacity by 19 per cent.

Commercial preparations in concentrated forms, containing very high levels of total dietary fibre obtained from different plant sources are now available in the market.

QUESTIONS

1. Explain the functions of carbohydrate.
2. Discuss the role of different hormones in maintaining normal blood sugar level.
3. What is dietary fibre? How is it different from crude fibre?
4. What are the physiological effects of fibre? Explain the role of fibre in human nutrition.
5. Give the sources, components and requirements of fibres.
6. Describe the clinical effects of fibre in the following conditions:
   a. Diverticular disease
   b. Hyperlipidemia
   c. Diabetes mellitus
   d. Colon cancer.
7. What are non-starch polysaccharides?
8. What are soluble fibres and insoluble fibres?
9. What percentage of kilocalories should come from carbohydrates?
10. What is the normal range of blood glucose levels? How do foods affect the blood sugar level?
11. What is glycaemic index of foods?
12. What are the important differences between the three classes of carbohydrates?
13. Give the nutritional classification of starch.
14. In what form and where is carbohydrate stored in the body?

15. What are the conditions associated with a lack of dietary fibre?
16. Name the specific enzymes involved in the digestion of polysaccharides and disaccharides.
17. How are monoccharides absorbed?
18. What are RAG values ? Why are they better than GI values?
19. What are short chain carbohydrates?

SUGGESTED READING

* Jenkins David J.A., 2002. *High-complex carbohydrate or Lente carbohydrate foods?* The American Journal of Medicine, **113** (9B)

* Ramulu P. and P. Udayasekhara Rao, 2003. Dietary fibre content of fruits and vegetables, Nutrition News, National Institute of Nutrition, **24**, 3

* Information on Fibre and Sugars : ificinfo.health.org.

* Better health : http://www.betterhealth.com

* Englyst H.N. and Cummings J.H, 1985, Digestion of the Polysaccharides of some cereal foods in the human small intestine. Am. J. clin. Nutr **42**

CHAPTER 4

LIPIDS

The term lipid is applied to a group of naturally occurring substances characterised by their insolubility in water and their solubility in such "fat solvents" as ether, chloroform, boiling alcohol and benzene. Chemically, the lipids are either esters of fatty acids or substances capable of forming such esters. The word 'lipid' is used when discussing the metabolism of fats in the body whereas the term 'fats' is used the fatty component of foods and diets.

Fats like carbohydrates are composed of the three elements carbon, hydrogen and oxygen. The lower amount of oxygen in relation to the other two elements results in fat being a more concentrated source of energy than carbohydrates.

Lipids are very wide spread in nature among all vegetable and animal matter. Some compounds of this group, such as phosphatide and sterols are found in all living cells where, with the proteins and carbohydrates they form an essential part of the colloidal complex of protoplasm. Complex lipids are also found in large quantities in brain and nervous tissues.

CLASSIFICATION

Simple Lipids

These are esters of fatty acids with certain alcohols. They are usually further classified according to the nature of the alcohols.

Fats and oils: These are esters of fatty acids and glycerol. They can be triacylglycerols diacyl glycerol or monoacylglycerols.

Waxes: These are esters of fatty acids with long chain aliphatic alcohols or with cyclic alcohols. These may be subdivided into true waxes, cholesterol esters, vitamin A and its carotenoid esters and vitamin D esters.

Compound Lipids

The compound lipids are esters of fatty acids which on hydrolysis yield other substances in addition to fatty acids and an alcohol.

Phospholipids: These are lipids which on hydrolysis yield fatty acids, phosphoric acid, an alcohol and a nitrogenous base e.g., lecithin, cephalin and sphingomyelin.

Glycolipids: Glycolipids can be subclassified into cerebrosides and gangliosides. They are so named because they have a carbohydrate component within their structure like phospholipids, their physiological role is principally structured, contributing little as an energy source. They occur in the medullary sheaths of nerves and in brain tissue, particularly the white matter.

A cerebroside is characterised by the linking of ceramide to a monosaccharide unit such as glucose or galactose.

Gangliosides resemble cerebrosides except that the single monosaccharide unit of the cerebroside is replaced by an oligosaccharide. Gangliosides provide the carbohydrate determinants of the human blood groups A, B and O.

Aminolipids, sulpholipids: The sulpholipids yield sulphuric acid on hydrolysis. Similar to cerebrosides except that sulphuric acid is present as cerebronic acid ester.

Lipoproteins: These compounds found in mammalian plasma are composed of lipid material bound to proteins. The lipid mostly consists of cholesterol esters and phospholipids containing principally stearic, palmitic and oleic acids although palmitoleic, linoleic and arachidonic acids have been identified.

Derived Lipids

These are substances liberated during hydrolysis of simple and compound lipids which still retain the properties of lipids.

CHEMICAL COMPOSITION

Triglycerides

Triglycerides or triacylglycerols are the main form of fats both in foodstuffs and in the storage depots of most animals. They are esters of glycerol and fatty acids.

Figure 4a illustrates a typical example. In this, there is a saturated fatty acid at position 1 on the glycerol molecule and an unsaturated fatty acid in position 2. This is typical of nearly all triglycerides. The fatty acid at position 3 may be either saturated or unsaturated.

Fatty Acids

Over 40 different fatty acids are found in nature. Fatty acids have the basic formula $CH_3(CH_2)n$ COOH where n can be any even number from 2 to 24. Three classes of fatty acids are described according to the number of double bonds between the carbon atoms. In a saturated fatty acid there are none; in an unsaturated fatty acid there may be one (monoenoic acids) or two or more (polyenoic acids) double bonds.

Table 4.1 shows the important natural fatty acids and their occurrence.

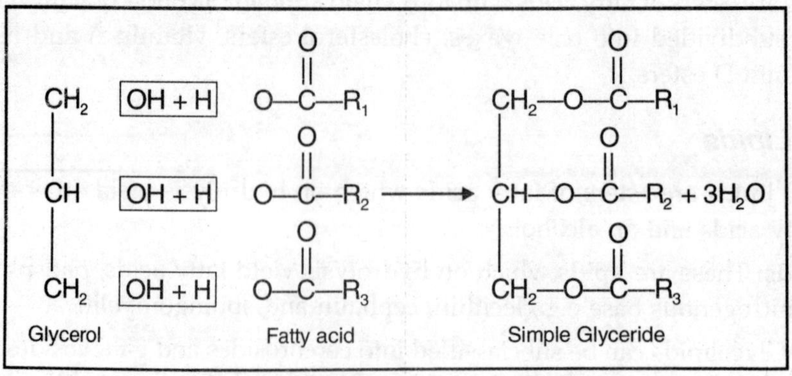

Figure 4a. The structure of triglyceride.

Table 4.1: The important natural fatty acids and their occurrence

Fatty acids	C atoms and double bonds	Occurrence
Saturated acids		
Short chain		
Butyric acid	$C_4 : 0$	Butter
Caproic acid	$C_6 : 0$	Butter, coconut oil
Caprylic acid	$C_8 : 0$	Butter, coconut oil
Medium chain		
Capric acid	$C_{10} : 0$	Butter, coconut oil
Lauric acid	$C_{12} : 0$	Butter, coconut oil
Myristic acid	$C_{14} : 0$	Butter, vegetable foods
Long chain		
Palmitic acid	$C_{16} : 0$	Most vegetable and animal fats
Stearic acid	$C_{18} : 0$	Most vegetable and animal fats
Arachidic acid	$C_{20} : 0$	Butter, lard, peanut oil
Behenic acid	$C_{22} : 0$	Vegetable oils
Unsaturated fatty acids		
Monounsaturated fatty acids		
Palmitoleic acid	$C_{16} : 1$	Olive oil, fish oil, beef fat
Oleic acid	$C_{18} : 1$	Olive oil, Canola oil
Erucic acid	$C_{22} : 1$	Rape seed oil, Canola oil
Polyunsaturated fatty acids		
Linoleic acid	$C_{18} : 2(n-6)$	Vegetable seed oils (Safflower, corn, soyabean, cotton seed)
α-Linolenic acid	$C_{18} : 3(n-3)$	Vegetable seed oils (Soyabean oil)
Arachidonic acid	$C_{20} : 4(n-6)$	Fat and phosphatide fractions of animal tissues particularly liver; lard, meat
Eicosapentaenoic acid	$C_{20} : 5(n-3)$	Fish oils, Shell fish
Docosahexaenoic acid	$C_{22} : 6(n-3)$	Fish oils, shell fish

Double bonds identified relative to the methyl end use the terms 'n' or 'ω' (omega) to indicate distance of the first bond along the carbon chain. ω-6 fatty acids are polyunsaturated fatty acids that have the first double bond on the sixth carbon atom from the methyl ($-CH_3$) end of the carbon chain. ω-3 fatty acids are polyunsaturated fatty acids that have the first double bond on the third carbon atom from the methyl ($-CH_3$) end of the carbon chain.

The four main dietary fatty acids are known as n-3, n-6, n-7 and n-9. The fatty acids with n-7 and n-9 cannot function as essential fatty acids. Biological functions of fatty acids depend on their property of being amphipathic.

The chemical composition of fatty acids alters their physical properties. Chain lengthening and desaturation may give them advantage as structural components of cell membranes. Water solubility depends on chain length. Only caprylic acid and those with shorter chains are soluble in water. The melting point is related to both chain length and unsaturation. Vegetable oils have long chain polyunsaturated fatty acids.

The unsaturated fatty acids found in both plants and animals are in the cis form. Trans forms are not incorporated into structural lipids and cannot function as essential fatty acids, but they are oxidised and serve as fuels for the tissues.

Medium Chain Fatty Acids

These are saturated fatty acids with a chain length between 10 and 14 carbons. They are found in Medium Chain Triglycerides (MCT). They are short enough to be water soluble, require less bile salts for solubilisation, are not re-esterified in the enterocyte and are transported as free fatty acid, bound to albumin, through the portal system. Because the portal blood flow rate is about 250 times faster than lymph flow, MCT are digested quickly and are not likely to be affected by intestinal factors that inhibit fat absorption. Medium chain fatty acids are not stored in adipose tissue but are oxidised to acetic acid. Natural MCT occur in milk fat, coconut oil and palm kernel oil. Clinically, MCT oil is used for patients with fat malabsorption or in catabolic states such as acquired immuno deficiency syndrome and cancer.

FATS IN THE BODY

Phospholipids

As the name implies, lipids belonging to this class contain phosphate as a common component. They also possess one or more fatty acid residues. Phospholipids are categorised into one of two groups called glycerophosphatides and sphingophosphatides, depending on whether their core structure is glycerol or the amino alcohol sphingosine respectively.

Glycerophosphatides : The building block is phosphatidic acid. Phosphatidic acids form a number of derivatives with compounds such as choline, ethanolamine, serine and inositol. Phosphatidylcholine is known by its common name, lecithin.

Glyurophosphatides are very important components of cell membranes. In addition to lending structural support to the membrane, they serve as a source of physiologically active compounds.

Sphingophosphatides: Sphingomyclins are sphingophosphatides occur in plasma membranes of animal cells and are found in particularly large amounts in the myclin sheath of nerve tissues. The sphingomyclins contain a fatty acid residue attached in amide linkage to the amino group of the sphingosine.

Figure 4b shows the structure of a lecithin molecule, a typical phospholipid.

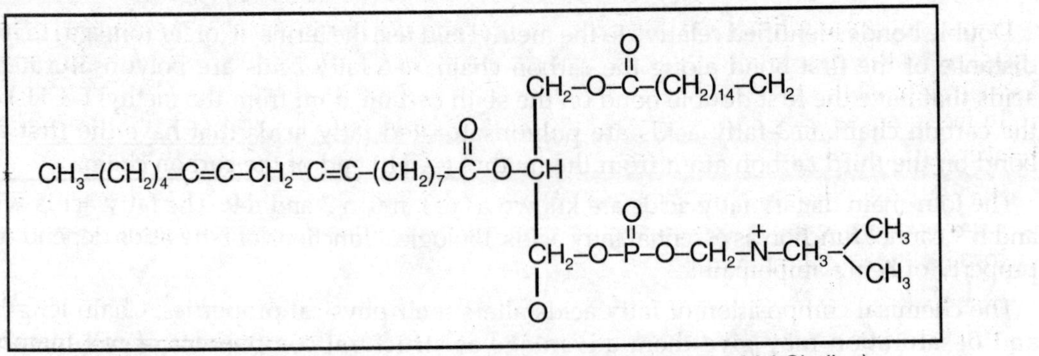

Figure 4b. Structural formula of a typical phospholipid (Phosphatidyl Choline).

Cholesterol

In nature sterols occur in the free state and as esters with fatty acids. Sterols are classified as: (i) Animal sterols e.g., cholesterol, (ii) Plant sterols, e.g., phytosterol and (iii) Mycosterol, e.g., ergosterol.

Cholesterol occurs in all animal and human tissues. The white matter of the brain contains about 14 per cent cholesterol while the grey matter contains 6 per cent on dry basis. Large amounts of cholesterol are also present in sebum secreted by the sebaceous glands.

Cholesterol serves as a precursor for the formation of bile acids. It is present in cell membranes and essential for maintaining the membranes in good condition. It serves as a precursor for the formation of some steroid hormones such as oestrogens, androgens and progesterone. It is also essential for the synthesis of adrenocortical hormones. It is present in large amounts in the nervous tissue and is essential for its function and it serves as a precursor for the formation of dehydrocholesterol (in the skin and some other tissues) which in turn is converted into vitamin D_3 in the body by the action of ultraviolet rays present in the sunlight.

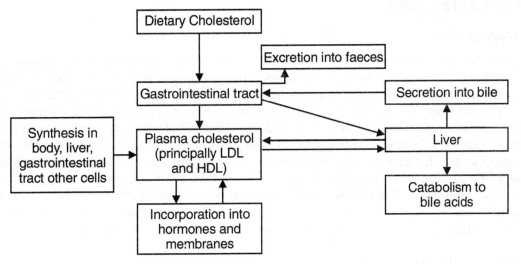

Figure 4c. Metabolism of cholesterol.

Source: Guthrie Helen A. and a Mary Frances Picciano, 1999, Human Nutrition, McGraw Hill, Boston.

Ketone Bodies

In normal human subjects, the degradation of fatty acid to acetyl CoA and the oxidation of acetyl CoA to CO_2 and water take place without appreciable accumulation of the intermediate products. Under some abnormal circumstances e.g., starvation or diabetes mellitus, acetyl CoA accumulates leading to the formation of acetoacetic acid. This, in turn is converted into β-hydroxy butyric acid and acetone. These three products of fat metabolism are known as ketone bodies.

Ketone body formation takes place when large quantities of fats are oxidised to acetyl CoA in subjects who cannot oxidise carbohydrate adequately (diabetics) or who do not get a supply of carbohydrates due to lack of food intake (starvation). The tissues are not able to oxidise the large amounts of acetyl CoA formed through TCA cycle due to lack of oxalo acetate.

Ketosis is a condition in which large amounts of ketone bodies are produced in the liver and circulate in blood when the diet contains less than 100g of carbohydrate. The level of ketone bodies in the blood of a normal person is about 3 mg/100 ml. This value can increase upto 70-80 mg/100 ml in ketosis.

Brown Adipose Tissue

It is involved in metabolism particularly at times when heat generation is necessary. It is active in normal humans but absent from the obese. Brown adipose tissue is characterised by a high content of mitochondria, cytochromes and a well developed blood supply. Metabolic emphasis is placed on oxidation of both glucose and fatty acids. In most new born mammals, brown adipose tissue is responsible for controlling body temperature in a cold weather.

FATS IN THE FOOD

Isoprenoids

These are activated derivatives of isoprene, are an extraordinarily large and diverse groups of lipids built from one or more five-carbon units. Isoprene contains alternating single and double (conjugated) bonds; conjugated bond structures can quench free radicals by accepting or donating electrons. Terpene is a generic term for all compounds synthesised from isoprene precursors. As a group, isoprenoids include essential oils of plants: turpentine from trees and limonene from lemons. Plant pigments that transfer electrons in photosynthesis are also isoprenoids. This group contains lycopene (red pigment in tomatoes) carotenoids (yellow and orange pigments) in pumpkin and carrots and the yellow/green chlorophyll group. Fat soluble vitamins A,D,E and K and the electron transducer, coenzyme Q have isoprenoids structures. Vitamin E, lycopene and β-carotene are effective antioxidants. Non-nutritive phyto-chemicals with antioxidant function usually have an isoprenoid structure.

Visible and Invisible Fats

Visible fats are mainly triacylglycerols. Hidden fats, present in the membranes of plant and animal tissues are mainly phospholipids, glycolipids and cholesterol. Products like butter, ghee, vanaspati and various edible oils such as gingelly oil or groundnut oil are visible fats. Foods like cereals, pulses, oil seeds, nuts, milk, egg and meat contain fat. The fats present in these foods which are not visible are called invisible fat. Part of the requirement of fat is met by invisible fat.

Characteristics of animal and vegetable fats

Vegetable fats contain unsaturated fatty acids and are liquid at room temperature. Animal fats contain more saturated fatty acids and are solid at room temperature. Melting point increases with chain length and lowers considerably on the introduction of double bonds.

Food and body fats contain mixtures of short and long-chain fatty acids and saturated and unsaturated fatty acids.

Only about 5 per cent of fatty acids in food and body fats contain fewer than 14 carbon atoms, coconut oil being an exception.

Animal fats contain 30–60 per cent saturated fatty acids of which palmitic and stearic acids predominate. They contain about 30–50 per cent oleic acid and small amounts of polyunsaturated fatty acids. In general herbivores have harder fats than carnivora and land animals have harder fats than aquatic animals. Lamb and beef fat with their high content of palmitic and stearic acids are much harder than pork and chicken fat which contain some what more of unsaturated fatty acids. Fats from fish have a high proportion of PUFA containing 20 to 24 carbon atoms. The proportion of saturated fatty acids is high in milk fat but this fat is soft because of many short chain fatty acids.

Oleic and linoleic acids predominate in vegetable fats, except for coconut oil. Safflower, corn, cottonseed and soyabean oils are very rich in linoleic acid whereas groundnut and olive oils are rich in oleic acid and correspondingly lower in linoleic acid. Coconut oil contains largely 12-carbon lauric acid, which is liquid at room temperature.

Table 4.2: Distinguishing characteristics of animal and vegetable fats

Characteristic	Animal fat	Vegetable fat
Saturation	Saturated fatty acids. 30 to 60%	Mostly unsaturated fatty acids.
Consistency	Solid at room temperature	Liquid at room temperature
Melting point	High	Low
Carbon atom	>14 (Butter contains short chain) Fish contain 20-24 carbon atoms	<12
Predominating fatty acid	Palmitic and stearic acids	Oleic and linoleic acid (except coconut oil)
Cholesterol	Present	Absent
Examples	Fats in meats, lard, tallow, ruminant adipose tissue, butter, ghee	Vegetable oils. Invisible fat present in plant foods.

FUNCTIONS

The Role of Fat in the Body

Essential constituent of the membrane of every cell: Fat is present not only in the outer membranes of all cells but also in the internal membranes of the nucleus, endoplasmic reticulum and the other membrane bound organelles.

Energy reserve: Fat is the primary form in which energy is stored in the body. One pound (454 g) of stored fat represents 3500 kcal of stored energy. Some fat can be stored within most cells but the body also contains large numbers of specialised fat cells (adipocytes) within fat (adipose) tissue, whose main function is the storage of fat. The number of adipocytes within the body appears to be genetically determined but fat cells can increase in size at any time to accommodate increased stores of fat resulting in obesity.

Within the cells of adipose tissue, fat is stored to the extent of 90 percent largely in the form of globules of triglycerides. These may be the result of the resynthesis of triglyceride from glycerol and fatty acids. When dietary supplies of fat are in excess of bodily requirements or when there is excess carbohydrate or protein resynthesis of triglyceride occurs.

A considerable amount of body fat (about 18 to 24 per cent of body weight in women and 15 to 18 per cent of body weight in men) is normal. People with reserves of fat in excess of these values are considered to be overweight. Excess reserves of fat cannot be excreted and can be reduced by the oxidation of the fat which occurs when there is insufficient intake of calories.

Regulator of body functions: As an essential component of all cell membranes, fats indirectly help to regulate both the flow of materials into and out of the cells and change in cell size and shape such as those involved in growth.

Specific long chain omega-6 and omega-3 unsaturated fatty acids also act as the precursors of a range of hormone like substances, the eicosanoids, involved in the regulation of a wide variety of processes in the body. Eicosanoids include the classes of important physiological regulators known as prostaglandins, prostacyclins, thromboxanes and leukotrienes. Eicosanoids perform many functions, including the regulation of blood pressure, the control of important aspects of the reproductive cycle, the stimulation of pain and fever and the induction of blood clotting.

Prostaglandins, perhaps the best known eicosanoids act within the brain, the wall of blood vessels, certain blood cells and blood platelets. They are involved in promoting conception, inducing labour, effecting spontaneous abortions, regulating the transmission of nervous impulses and regulating blood pressure. Overproduction of some prostaglandins and other eicosanoids from arachidonic acid may cause excessive clotting of the blood and narrowing of the arteries. The risk of these undesirable consequences can be reduced by eicosapentaenoic acid and docosahexaenoic acid which are both omega-3 fatty acids, found in fish oil. These act to decrease the stickiness of the blood platelets involved in clotting, thus reducing the possibility of a clot that could cause a heart attack.

Insulator: Deposits of fat beneath the skin known as the subcutaneous fat, serve as an insulating material for the body and is effective at preventing heat loss. A certain minimal layer of fat is desirable, but too thick, a layer slows down heat loss considerably in hot weather, causing discomfort.

Protector: Deposits of fat surround certain vital organs, such as the kidneys and heart, serving to hold them in position and protect them from physical shock. These protective deposits are the last to be drawn on for energy supplies when energy in the diet is inadequate.

Thus lipids have structural, storage and metabolic functions.

The Role of Fat in the Diet

Source of energy: Fat is the most concentrated source of energy in the diet. Each gram of fat releases 9 kcals of energy, when completely oxidised to carbon dioxide and water.

Satiety value: Fat tends to leave the stomach relatively slowly. It can still be released from the stomach for upto 3.5 hours after a meal with the precise time depending on the size and composition of the meal. This prolonged stay in the stomach helps to delay the onset of hunger pangs and so contributes to a feeling of satiety after a meal. Due to this, moderate fat reducing diets are currently considered more successful in weight control than very low fat diets.

Carrier of fat soluble vitamins: Dietary fat serves as a carrier for vitamins A, D, E and K. Also fat at a level of atleast 10 per cent of total energy intake appears to be required for the absorption of vitamin A precursors from nonfat sources such as carrots. Anything that interferes with absorption or use of fat such as obstruction of bile duct depresses the supply of fat soluble vitamins to the body.

Palatability: The presence of fat in food or its addition to food is responsible for much of the texture and flavour of food. The marbling of fat throughout the lean muscle of a steak contributes greatly to its tenderness and flavour. Frying improves the taste of food. Many of the substances that are responsible for the flavours and aromas of foods are soluble in fat so that fat tends to carry these flavours and aromas and mix them throughout the food as a whole.

DIGESTION AND ABSORPTION

The digestion of fat is initiated by the lingual lipase enzyme. This enzyme mixes with chewed food and hydrolyses fatty acids from triglycerides to form diglycerides as the food travels down the oesophagus to the stomach. Lingual lipase hydrolyses short chain and medium chain triglycerides more readily than it does long chain triglycerides. After entering the stomach, the gastric lipase too hydrolyses short and medium chain triglycerides more quickly than it does long-chain triglycerides.

From the stomach the food mass passes into the small intestine, where the presence of fat stimulates the release of the hormones cholecystokinin and secritin. These hormones in turn stimulate the secretion of pancreatic juice from the pancreas and release of bile, which is synthesised in the liver and stored in and released from the gallbladder. In addition to bile salts and bile pigments, bile contains significant amounts of various phospholipids, including lecithin. As the food mass mixes with bile, the lipid becomes bound within emulsified droplets that are coated in bile salts and bile phospholipids. Pancreatic juice is secreted and it raises the pH value from 5.5 to 6.5 in which pancreatic lipase becomes active.

However, pancreatic lipase cannot act until an enzyme, procolipase (also secreted by the pancreas), becomes activated to colipase by the pancreatic trypsin enzyme. Colipase then combines with pancreatic lipase and the emulsified lipid droplets to permit the lipase to act on the triglycerides within. The pancreatic lipase hydrolyses triglycerides with differing lengths of fatty acid chains to yield free fatty acids and monoglycerides.

Bile micelles (tiny spherical aggregates of lipids and bile salts) then carry the monoglycerides and free fatty acids across what is called the unstirred water layer between the lipid droplets from which they are derived and the membranes of intestinal mucosal cells. This journey is rate limiting step in the entire lipid absorption process.

Once absorbed into the intestinal cell, the longer chain free fatty acids and monoglycerides are combined back in the intestinal lumen. These triglycerides are incorporated into chylomicrons and subsequently released inward to the lymph by the process of exocytosis. Medium and short chain fatty acids (less than 10-12 carbon atoms) are not recombined into triglycerides but are absorbed quickly into the blood capillaries that lead to the portal vein and hence to the liver, a faster means of transport than that taken by the long chain fatty acids.

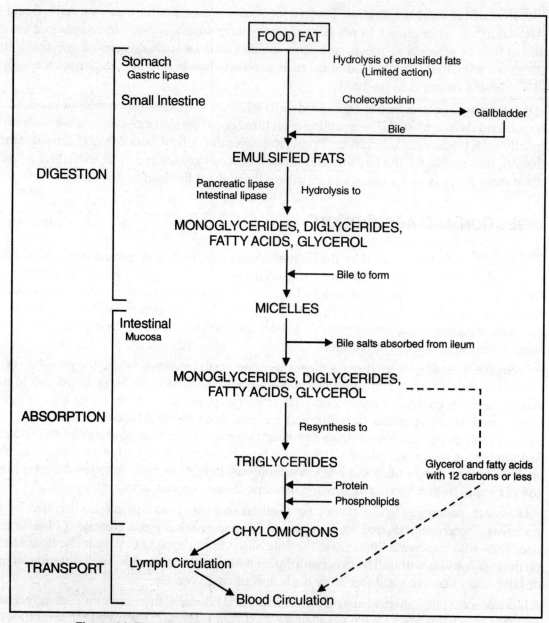

Figure 4d. The digestion, absorption, and transport of fat.

Source: Robinson, C.H., M.R. Lawler, 1982, Normal and therapeutic nutrition, Oxford and IBH Publishing Co., New Delhi.

Long chain fatty acids with higher melting points are absorbed more slowly than those with lower melting points. Transfatty acids are more slowly absorbed than are their cis counterparts though both are well absorbed.

ESSENTIAL FATTY ACIDS

In the course of evolution, human beings lost the ability to make enzymes that catalyse the introduction of double bonds between positions 12–13 and 15–16 as present in linoleic acid and α-linolenic acids which are formed in plants. Yet, these fatty acids are essential to life and must therefore be supplied by the diet. The essential fatty acids are linoleic acid and α-linolenic acid. Arachidonic acid can be formed from linoleic acid. α-linolenic acid can be converted to eicosapentaenoic acid and decosahexaenoic acid.

Linoleic acid → γ-linolenic acid → eicosatrienoic acid → arachidonic acid

Prostaglandine, prostacyclins, thromboxanes and leukotrienes are collectively called eicosanoids because they are derived from 20-carbon precursor fatty acids, the eicosenoic acids. Similar substances are derived from the n-3 family of polyunsaturated fatty acids eicosapentaenoic acid and docosahexaenoic acid.

Table 4.3 Matabolic pathways for the synthesis of various EFAs and their dietary sources and tissue distribution.

Fatty acid	Major members of series	Major dietary sources	Tissue distribution
n-3	Linoleic acid 18 : 3 n-3 ↓	Vegetable oils soy, linseed, leafy vegetables	Minor component of tissues
	Eicosapenta enoic acid 20 : 5 n-3 ↓	Fish and Shell fish	Minor component of tissues
	Docosahexa enoic acid 22 : 6 n-3	Fish and Shell fish	Major component of membrane phospholipids in retinal photoreceptors, cerebral gray matter and sperm.
n-6	Linoleic acid 18 : 2 n-6 ↓	Most vegetable oils	Minor component of tissues.
	Arachidonic acid 20 : 4 n-6 ↓	Meat, liver, Brain	Major component of most membrane phospholipids
	Docosa penta enoic acid 22 : 5 n-6	None	Very low in normal tissues but replaces 22 : 6 n-3 in n-3 fatty acid deficiency
n-6	Oleic acid 18 : 1 n-9 ↓	Animal and vegetable fats	Major component of many tissues including white matter and myelin
	Eicosatri enoic acid	None	Accumulate in epidermis.

Functions

- **Energy stores :** Essential Fatty Acids are found in skin phospholipids and also occur as triglycerides serving as energy stores for sebum precursors. These are oxidised more rapidly than SFA.

- **Bactericidal activity:** The EFAs are involved in the bactericidal activity against common pathogens like staphylococci, streptococci and pneumococci and also are known to be very much involved in the membrane composition of immuno competent cells such as thymus dependent cells (T cells) and B cells. Moreover, the homologous of these fatty acids are known to have bactericidal effect through their ability to disrupt cell wall membranes by their detergent like effect.

- **Growth and development:** The EFAs play a role in foetal growth and early human development.There are significant associations   between dietary intakes of arachidonic acid and docosahexaenoic acid and birth weight, head circumference and placental weight. In EFA deficient animals, conversion of food energy into metabolic energy for growth and maintenance is poor.

Vision and central nervous system: Brain and nervous tissue membrane lipids contain a particularly high proportion of arachidonic acid and DHA. The photo receptor in the retina of the eye also contains a high proportion of the phospholipids containing two DHA moieties.

Health of skin: The major fatty acid of the epidermis is arachidonic acid and it constitutes about nine per cent apart from linoleic and other homologous. Linoleic acid also serves in the epidermis regulating barrier function and it is known to be involved in maintaining the integrity of the skin and fragility of mitochondrial membranes. All the skin functions and maintenance of membrane stability are done mostly by ω-6 fatty acids.

- **Role in cardiovascular disease:** α-linolenic acid is present in fish fat (mackerel and salmon). n-3 fatty acids exert reverse effects on atherogenesis and thrombus formation. Following possible mechanisms are involved.

  — Thromboxane 3, released from platelets has weaker effect on the adhesiveness and vasoconstriction.
  — Prostacyclin and endothelial derived relaxing factors are unimpeded or raised.
  — Fabrinogen levels are lower leading to a decrease in the tendency of clot formation.
  — Increase in fibrinolytic activity.
  — Lowers plasma coagulation factors VII C.
  — Lower the level of homocysteine and triglycerides.
  — Dilates blood vessels and reduces blood pressure.
  — Lowers total Cholesterol and Triglycerides in blood.
  — Lowers the LDL cholesterol but also prevents oxidation.

Thus ω-3 fatty acids have antiinflammatory, antithrombic, antiarrhythmic, hypolipidemic and vasodilatory properties.

Prevent cancer: ω-3 fatty acids have been found to prevent cancer of breast and colon in humans by inhibiting tumour cell growth.

Anti-inflammatory effect: ω-3 rich foods increase the cell membrane content of both EPA and DHA which increases the production of anti-inflammatory group icosanoid. ω-3 fatty acids decrease the production of interleukin-I and tumour necrosis factor (TNF) by down regulating inflammatory response. Fish oil supplementation in patients with inflammatory diseases such as rheumatoid arthritis and inflammatory bowel disorders result in significant improvements. ω-3 fatty acids relax muscles and blood vessels of the uterus and reduce menstrual cramps. They reduce inflammation of mucous memberane of the uterus. Thus they help to reduce abdominal pain before during and after menstrual periods makes delivery easier by virtue of the same action.

Deficiency

This is rare in man. It has been reported, however, in patients fed solely by vein (Total Parenteral Nutrition-TPN) for long periods without fat emulsions. EFA deficiency can occur in fat malabsorption and occasionally in protein calorie malnutrition where there is a deficiency of fat calories.

In 1929, two American nutritionists Burr and Burr showed that young rats when put on a fat-free diet continued to grow normally for upto 8 weeks. But growth then slowed down and stopped altogether by 2 weeks. A squamous dermatitis developed and was most marked over the tail.

The first clear evidence for the nutritional essentiality of linoleic acid was reported by Hansen and colleagues in 1963. Their studies involved infants fed on proprietary milk formulas that were adequate in all other nutrients except linoleic acid. The amounts of linoleic acid varied from 7.3 per cent to 0.1 per cent of total caloric needs. Infants who were fed on the formula with lowest amount of linoleic acid for 3 months developed dry, thick, flaking skin and suffered from retarded growth. The clinical symptoms disappeared when large amount of linoleic acid was provided.

Holman and colleagues reported a case of peripheral neuropathy and blurred vision in a child receiving TPN, devoid of ω-3 fatty acid for 5 months. Recent research in preterm human infants has revealed abnormalities in vision and electro retinogram when the feeding formulas given were low in ω-3 fatty acid.

Deficiency of EFA may cause permanent learning defects and alterations in synaptic functions in the brain.

The normal human skin contains pores which are the openings of microscopic follicles. The secretions of the sebaceous and sweat producing glands enter the follicles and reach the surface through the pores. Hairs emerge from the roots through the same follicles. In follicular hyperkeratosis, the follicles become blocked with plugs of keratin derived from their epithelial lining which has undergone squamous metaplasia. Because of the roughness in appearance the condition has been called, toad skin or phrynoderma. It is characterised by horny papular eruptions on the posterior and lateral aspects of limbs and on the back and buttocks. Phrynoderma can be cured by EFA along with vitamins A and B-complex group.

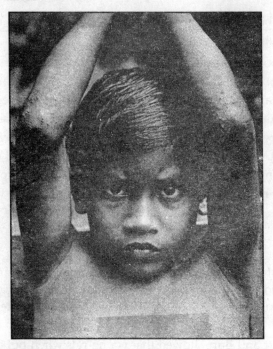
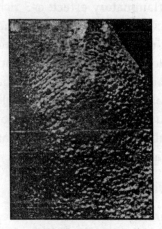

Figure 4e. Phrynoderma: The extensor aspects of the extremities are involved. The horny summits of the keratinised follicles may be seen clearly in the magnified picture.

Source: Passmore R. and M.A. Eastwood, 1990, Davidson and Passmore, Human Nutrition and Dietetics, ELBS, Churchill, Livingstone. Swaminathan, M;1988, Essentials of Food and Nutrition, Volume I, The Bangalore Printing and Publishing Co. Ltd. Bangalore.

Deficiency of EFA can increase the risk of coronary heart disease. Arachidonic acid which is derived from linoleic acid is the precursor of prostaglandins. These are converted to prostacyline which help in vasodilation. In linoleic acid deficiency there are more chances for the thrombus formation and chances of getting coronary heart disease increase.

Essential fatty acid deficiency adversely affects:

- reproduction and lactation
- integrity of the cell membranes and cells
- certain enzyme systems
- transport of cholesterol and
- water balance
- growth
- production of energy by the oxidation of fatty acids

EFA deficiency respond successfully to the application to the skin of lipids containing a high proportion of linoleic acid.

Evaluation of EFA status

The ratio of 20:3 n-9/20:4 n-6 (the triene/tetraene ratio) measured in plasma phospholipids is used as a biochemical index of EFA status. In health the ratio is about 0.1 or less and a ratio of 0.4 indicates EFA deficiency.

Table 4.4: Differing characteristics of ω-3 and ω-6 fatty acid deficiencies

	Fatty acid ω-3	Fatty acid ω-6
Skin	Normal	Skin lesions
Growth	Normal	Retardation
Reproduction	Normal	Failure
Learning	Reduced	Normal
Vision	Electro retino gram abnormal. Impaired vision	Normal

Sources of EFA

Corn, cotton seed, safflower and soyabean oils are good sources of linoleic acid. α-linolenic acid is present not only in fish oils but also found in green leaf vegetable flax seeds, rape seed, soyabean and walnuts. Barley and oats contain appreciable amounts of gamma linolenic acid which lower cholesterol levels. Marine oils are high in n-3 fatty acids and have antiatherogenic properties. The fat in fish and fish oils is predominently the highly unsaturated n-3 fatty acids eicosapenta enoic acid and docosahexaonic acid. Sources of long chain ω-3 fatty acids are primarily marine, cod liver oil, mackerel, salmon as well as crab shrimp and oyster. Egg yolk, especially from chickens fed ω-3 containing feed is also a source of ω-3 fatty acids.

Table 4.5: Essential fatty acid composition of some important edible oils and fats (Values are percentage of total methylester of fatty acid)

Oils and fats	Linoleic acid ω-6	Linolenic acid ω-3
Coconut oil	2.0	–
Corn oil	57.4	–
Cotton seed oil	50.9	–
Groundnut oil	29.9	–
Mustard or Rapeseed oil	18.1	14.5
Olive oil	10.0	–
Palm oil	10.0	–
Palmolein	10.3	0.3
Rice bran oil	34.3	1.4
Safflower oil	73.5	–
Gingelly oil	44.5	–
Soyabean oil	50.7	6.5
Sunflower oil	66.2	–
Butter	2.5	–
Lard	11.0	–
Tallow	4.2	–

Source: Gopalan et al., 2004, Nutritive Value of Indian Foods, National Institute of Nutrition, Hyderabad.

Cereals such as wheat, bajra and maize and pulses such as bengal gram contain only small quantities of oil (2-5%) but this is rich in linoleic acids. It is also found in leafy vegetables, sea weeds and algae. As fish live on algae, fish liver is also rich in linoleic acid. Arachidonic acid is found in milk and butter. From cereals, we get 15 g of invisible fat daily and this meets 50% of EFA requirements. Adequately breast fed infants receive nearly 30g of fat/day of which about 10 per cent is linoleic acid and 1% linolenic acid. Breast milk meets the EFA needs of infant which is about 6 en %. Cow's milk has less quantity of EFA and contains no arachidonic acid, whereas human milk contains arachidonic acid. Cow's milk contains 50 per cent linoleic acid in trans form which is not easily available to infants. In human milk linoleic acid is present in cis form which is readily available. Essential fatty acid content of legumes increase on germination.

RECOMMENDED DIETARY ALLOWANCES

Although a minimum amount of fat is essential to provide EFA, fat intake above a certain level is also undesirable. Studies relating fat intake to cardiovascular diseases, suggest that an intake of fat energy at 30% or more of total calories is undesirable particularly in sedentary individuals. Since in India some 10-15% of this can come from invisible fat, visible fat intake should be kept below 24 en%. This means that daily visible fat intake should be kept below 50 g/day.

WHO suggest that the ratio of n-6 : n-3 should be 5 to 10:1 in the diet.

Table 4.6: Fat RDA of Indians suggested by ICMR

Group desirable	EFA requirement en%	Invisible Fat* en%	Minimum visible fat** en%		Suggested visible fat Intake	
			en%	g/day	g/day	en%
Adults**	3	10	5	12**	20**	9
Older children**	3	10	5	12	22	9
Young children	3	10	5	8	25	15
Pregnant women	4.5	10	12.5	30	30	12.5
Lactating woman	5.7	10	17.5	45	45	17.5

*Contains 20% EFA about 6 per cent would be from cereals and pulses and rest from milk, nutes and spices.

**EFA at least 20 per cent.

***Average of males and females.

SOURCES

Nuts and oil seeds are excellent sources of fat. The visible fats are butter, ghee and oil. Invisible fats are present in cereals, pulses, oilseed, milk and egg. Fruits and vegetables are poor sources of fat; avocado being an exception. Fat content of some foods is given in Table 4.7.

Table 4.7: Fat content of foods

Name of Food stuff	Fat g/100 g
Ghee and oil	100
Butter	81
Coconut dry	62
Cashew nut	40
Groundnut	25
Cheese	23
Avocado	23
Soyabean	19
Egg hen	13

DIETARY FAT AND CORONARY HEART DISEASE

Ancel Keys in 1957 stated emphatically that diet, through its fat content, plays an important role in the incidence of Coronary Heart Disease. This is probably through effect on levels of serum cholesterol and alteration in the tendency for thrombosis and inhibition of fibrinolysis. Sinclair, around the same time, visualised the dual effects of lipids on atherosclerosis and processes of thrombosis and thrombolysis.

Saturated fatty aids C_{12}, C_{14} and C_{16} promote hypercholesterolaemia while C_{14}, C_{16} and C_{18} potentiate thrombogenesis.

Mono Unsaturated Fatty Acids

MUFA are a better replacement for saturated fatty acids than polyunsaturated fatty acids because they are less susceptible to oxidation. Oxidised LDL is taken up by macrophages and deposited in atherosclerotic plagues. Inhibition of LDL oxidation slows the development of atherosclerosis. It was observed that high intake of PUFA resulted in some lowering of HDL-cholesterol along with the levels of total and LDL cholesterol. MUFA is resistant to peroxidation and helps to lower oxidised LDL by preserving HDL level.

Olive oil extensively used in the Mediterrnean region is rich in monounsaturated (18:1) oleic acid 73 (%). Both hyper cholesteolaemia and CHD are less prevalent in Mediterranean countries than in USA, UK, north and central Europe.

More recent studies reveal that high dietary PUFA (ω-6) when SFA intake remains the same, may enhance platelet aggregation while MUFA does not. Further larger proportion of MUFA in diet may be conducive to thrombolysis and may be antiinflammatory as n-3 PUFA. It is now established that substitution of SFA by MUFA lowers both total and LDL cholesterol but not HDL-C. Uncontrolled peroxidation of PUFA in cell membrane may lead to cellular damage while maintenance of a balance with MUFA is conducive to maintain cell function.

In 1979 American Dietetic Association recommended restriction of total fat intake upto 30 en percent equally divided among SFA, MUFA and PUFA (10 en percent each).

—ADA recommended in 1986 raised the proportion of MUFA to 12-14-en percent and consequential reduction of PUFA to 6-8 en percent.

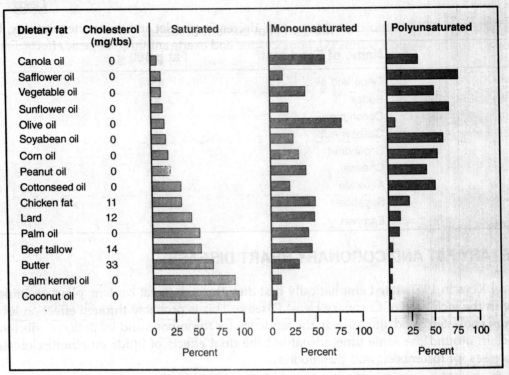

Figure 4f. Fatty acid composition of common food fats.

Source: Sienkiewicz Sizer Frances and Eleanor Noss Whitney, 2000, Nutrition Concepts and Controversies, Wadsworth, Thomson Learning, Belmont.

Poly Unsaturated Fatty Acids

The very low prevalence of CHD among Eskimos inspite of high fat diet has drawn the attention of researchers from the early days of systematic epidemiologic studies. Detailed analysis of plasma lipids of Eskimos by Bang and coworkers highlighted the usefulness of intake of fat of marine fauna. Subsequent observations on inverse relation of death from CHD and fish consumption in Japan and Netherlands called attention for critical analysis of the basis of these observations at molecular levels. These led to the exposition of differential effects of n-3 and n-6 types of dietary PUFA.

Experimental studies revealed that excess intake of n-6 PUFA is associated with increase in insulin resistance in muscles, adipose tissue and liver. Linoleic acid, the principal n-6 PUFA in vegetable oils (corn safflower, sunflower, peanut and sesame)is converted into arachidonic acid which is utilised as a constituent of cell membranes Platelets rich in arachidonic acid release Tx´A$_2$ a potent mediator that enhances platelet adhesiveness, aggregation, increase coagulability, decrease thrombolysis and promote vasoconstriction.

Liponins, products of arachidonic acid, increase glomerular filtration pressure and permeability. Further there may be increase in free radical activity and lipid peroxidation leading to increase in the atherogenic potential of LDL. As a result, any beneficial effect of substitution of n-6 PUFA for SFA is evident only when diet is rich is antioxidants.

Dietary supplementation of n-3 fatty acid, decreases platelet and monocyte reactivity, lowers blood pressure, reduces serum TG, homocystine and exerts antithrombogenic effects. Fatty fish and canola oil preparations substantially lower cardiac events. Intake of 80g salmon once a week or 5.5 g of n-3 fatty acid per month was shown to reduce the risk of primary cardiac arrest by 50 percent.

It is therefore, recommended that proportion of n-6: n-3 PUFA should be kept at 5–10:1 as is the case with breast milk.

Saturated Fatty Acids

Individual saturated fatty acids differ in their ability to change blood LDL-cholesterol levels. Palmitic, myristic and to a lesser degree lauric acids increase the LDL-cholesterol level. In contrast stearic acid and medium to short chain saturated fatty acids do not increase the LDL-cholesterol.

Although milk fat and coconut oil contain short chain fatty acids (9 and 15%) the contents of most althereogenic C_{12}, C_{14}, C_{16}, SFA are high (45 and 73%) particularly in the latter. SFA content of meat fat (46%) is double that of fish oils while it is intermediate in chicken (35%). The only dubious advantage of coconut oil and butter is that these are richer in lauric (C_{12}) and myristic (C_{14}) acids that raise HDL along with LDL cholesterol. Yet both are more atherogenic and thrombogenic than meat fat.

Palm oil contains α tocopherol of alpha tocotrienols and a variety of carotenoides with potent antioxidant properties. Palmitic acid the chief constituent of palm oil, raises serum cholesterol to a much lower extent than myristic acid of coconut oil and dairy fat.

Intake of cholesterol may contribute modestly to plasma cholesterol only when intake of SFA is high.

Further trans fatty acids present in hydrogenated fat have been found to raise Lp (a) levels thus raising the risk of CHD.

Saturated fatty acids contribute to atherogenicity.

Summary of Fat as the Cause of Atherosclerosis

1. High intake of saturated fatty acid can lead to
   (a) ↑ Plasma cholesterol →↑ Atheroma formation.
   (b) ↓ LDL receptors →↑ LDL cholesterol.
   (c) Arrhythmia → Thrombosis.
   (d) ↑ T Lipid oxidation → Injury to coronary arteries.
   (e) ↑ Factor VII level → Thrombosis.
   (f) ↓ Antiaggregatory prostacylin.
   (g) ↓ HDL cholesterol.
   (h) ↑ Plasma triglycerides.
2. High cholesterol intake can lead to.
   (a) ↑ Plasma cholesterol.
   (b) ↑ LDL synthesis.
   (c) ↓ LDL catabolism by cells.

3.   Low ω-3 fatty acid intake can lead to
    (a)   Arrhythmia → Thrombosis.
    (b)   ↑ Fibrinogen → Thrombosis.
                         →↑ Fibrous plaque.
    (c)   ↑ Platelet aggregation → Thrombosis.
    (d)   ↑ Lipoprotein (a) →↑ Fibrous plaque.
    (e)   ↑ Inflammation → injury to coronary arteries.
    (f)   ↑ B.P. → Injury to coronary arteries.

Table 4.8: Summary of fatty acids in atherosclerosis

	SFA	Oleic	n-6	n-3
Blood cholesterol	↓	↓	↓	↓
HDL cholesterol	↓	no change	↓	no change
Triglycerides	↓	no change	no change	↓
Platelet aggregation	g	no change	↓	↓↓↓

Source: Ghafoorunissa, Nutrition aspects of fats in Indian diets, Proceedings of the Nutrition Society of India, 35,1989.

Fat components of diet should be as given in Table 4.9

Table 4.9: Desirable percentage of calories from different fats

Recommended Fat	%of kcal
Total fat	<30
Saturated	8-10
Polyunsaturated	5-8
Monounsaturated	Difference
Ratio ω-6 to ω-3	5–10:1

Table 4.8. shows the effect of saturated and n-6 and n-3 fatty acids in the blood. Table 4.8 gives desirable percentage of calories from different fats.

Recommendation on Fat Components of Diet

National Cholesterol Education programme (USA), Adult Treatment Panel III recommended the following standards (2001) :

Table 4.10: Standards of cholesterol levels

Cholesterol		Comment
LDL Cholesterol	<100	Optimal
	100 – 129	Near optimal
	130 – 159	Borderline high
	160 – 189	High
	≥ 190	Very high

Contd...

Cholesterol	Comment
Total Cholesterol	
< 200	Desirable
200 – 239	Borderline high
≥ 240	High
HDL Cholesterol	
< 40	Low
≥ 60	High

To prevent heart disease one needs to control total energy, total fat and saturated fat and cholesterol content of the diet and proper balance between ω-6/ω-3 fatty acids.

Table 4.11: Recommended combinations of oils for optimal health benefits.

Combinations	Proportions
Groundnut oil + Soyabean oil	2:1
Palmolein oil + Soyabean oil	1:1
Safflower oil + Palmolein oil	1:2
Sunflower oil + Palmolein oil	1:1
Sesame oil + Palmolein oil	1:1
Safflower oil + Groundnut oil Rice Bran oil	2:3
Sunflower oil + Groundnut oil Rice Bran oil	1:3
Sesame oil + Groundnut oil	1:3

Blended oils are the solution to prevent atherosclerosis as no single oil has absolutely desirable composition. Government of India has permitted admixture of any two vegetable oils. Consumption of blended oils could ensure optimum balance of fatty acids in Indian diets.

QUESTIONS

1. Explain the functions of lipids.
2. Discuss the functions and deficiency symptoms of EFA.
3. How are fats digested and absorbed?
4. Give the sources of EFA.
5. Explain the role of fat in the development of atherosclerosis.
6. Write short notes on:
   i. Cholesterol
   ii. Phospholipids
   iii. Ketone bodies
   iv. Isoprenoids

7. Discuss the role of n-3 fatty acids in the prevention of atherosclerosis.
8. What is invisible fat?
9. What is brown adipose tissue?
10. What is the relationship between fat consumption and health problems such as heart disease and cancer?
11. Give examples of food sources of saturated, monounsaturated and polyunsaturated fatty acids.
12. Explain the role of cholesterol in the body.
13. Which foods are to be avoided in low cholesterol diet?
14. Write a note on 'blended' oils.
15. Differentiate the characteristics of ω-6 and ω-3 fatty acids.

SUGGESTED READINGS

- Proceedings of a symposium, 2002, Dietary fat, the Mediterrnean Diet and Health: Reports from scientific Exchanges, 1998 and 2000, The American Journal of Medicine, *113*,

- Simopoulos Artemis P., 1999, Essential fatty acids in health and chronic disease, Am.J. clin. Nutr, **70**,

- Information on Cholesterol : www.healthfinder.gov/searchoptions/topicsaz.htm

- Fats, oils and cholesterol : www.eatright.org/cgi/search.cgi

CHAPTER 5

ENERGY METABOLISM

Energy is the ability to do work. The energy contained within the chemical constituents of food can be either trapped within the chemical constituents of the body or used to produce heat or allow the body to move. So energy in nutrition is focused on chemical energy and the kinetic energy of motion.

Energy is a precisely defined property of chemical compounds and other physical systems. The carbohydrate, lipid, protein and alcohol in the diet are responsible for its energy content. Water, vitamins and minerals provide no energy although they are essential for other reasons. The energy of carbohydrates, lipids, proteins and alcohol is made available to the body when these compounds are oxidised in the energy-releasing reaction of respiration.

Combustions in living beings was first described by Lavoisier (1793–94). He discovered that in the body, oxygen in union with carbon and hydrogen formed carbon dioxide and water during the production of heat. In human experiments he observed that oxidation was increased by food, by cold environment and by muscular work.

In 1842 Liebig announced that the substances burned in the body were carbohydrate, fat and protein. Later Voit found that muscular exercise did not increase protein metabolism. Rubner, a pupil of Voit, determined the fuel values of the foodstuffs. By means of a respirometer, he showed that the heat production as calculated from the respiratory exchange was the same as that obtained by the direct measurement of the heat given off by the body.

In 1883, Rubner demonstrated the relationship between the surface area of the body and the heat production, thus providing a basis for comparison of the metabolism of different individuals. In 1915 DuBois devised the most satisfactory method for estimating the surface area of the body and later published normal standards of heat production for males and females.

Atwater, Armby, Benedict, Lusk and Dubois have contributed significantly to the knowledge of normal metabolism. Benedict and those associated with him in the Carnegie Nutrition Laboratory have perfected respiration apparatus.

UNITS

All forms of energy are interconvertible. The energy value of food is expressed in kilocalories. Kilocalories of energy is defined in terms of the amount of heat energy to which it corresponds. One kilocalorie is defined as the amount of heat energy required to raise the temperature of 1 kg of water by 1°C from 14.5°C to 15.5°C at normal atmosphere pressure.

The unit of energy which has been used in nutrition for a long time is the kilocalorie. However, recently the International Union of Science and the International Union of Nutritional Science (IUNS) have adapted 'Joule' as the unit of energy in place of kcal.

A joule is defined as the energy required to move 1 kg mass by 1 metre by force of 1 newton acting on it. One newton is the force needed to accelerate 1 kg mass by 1 m per sec.

The interconversion factors are:

1	kcal = 4.184 kJ		1	kJ = 0.239 kcal
1000	kcal = 4184 kJ		1	mJ = 239 kcal
1000	kcal = 4.184 mJ		100	mJ = 23900 kcal

DIRECT AND INDIRECT CALORIMETRY

The amount of energy released from foods and the amount of energy expended by an individual can be obtained by direct and indirect calorimetry.

The chemical changes that occur when carbohydrate or fat oxidised during respiration in the body are identical overall to the chemical changes, when these chemicals are burnt in air. This is the principle of direct calorimetry. The amount of energy released or expended is measured by the heat produced.

Indirect claorimetry is based on the principle that when an organic substance is completely combusted either in calorimeter or in the human body, oxygen is consumed in amounts directly related to the energy liberated as heat.

Table 5.1: Equipment used in direct and indirect calorimetry

Principle	Equipment	Purpose
I. Direct calorimetry	Bomb Calorimeter	Energy value of food
Direct calorimetry	At water Rose respiration calorimeter	Energy expenditure during BMR/REE of at light activity
II. Indirect calorimetry	Benedicts oxy calorimeter	Energy value of food
Indirect calorimetry	Eenedict-Roth respiration	Determination of BMR
Indirect calorimetry	*Douglas bag	energy expenditure during work
	* Max Planck respirometer	
	* Kofranyi Michaelis respirometer	

DETERMINATION OF ENERGY VALUE OF FOOD

The amount of energy released from foods can be obtained by measurements of heat produced when food is burnt in air. Bomb calorimeter works on the principle of direct calorimetry.

Bomb Calorimeter

It consists of a heavy steel bomb, with a platinum or gold-plated copper lining and cover held tightly in place by means of a strong screw collar. A weighted amount of sample is placed in a capsule, within the bomb, which is then closed except for the oxygen valve, charged with oxygen to a pressure of at least 20 atmospheres (300 pounds or more to the square inch), oxygen valve closed, and the bomb is immersed in a weighted amount of water. The water is constantly stirred and its temperature taken at intervals of one minute by means of differential thermometer, capable of being read to one thousand of a degree. After the rate at which the temperature of the water rises or falls has been determined, the sample is ignited by means of an electric fuse and on account of the large amount of oxygen present, undergoes rapid and complete combustion. Figure 5a gives in detail parts of Bomb calorimeter.

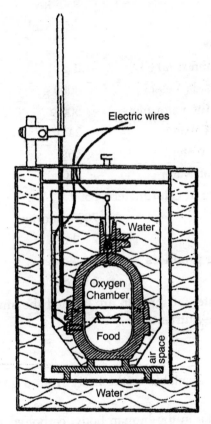

Figure 5a. The Bomb calorimeter. The bomb is placed inside a vessel of water, the temperature of which can be accurately measured. The foodstuff is placed in a small crucible. The bomb is filled with oxygen at high pressure and the foodstuff ignited by means of electric leads. The material in the bomb burns and the heat produced leads to a rise of temperature in the surrounding water.

The heat liberated is communicated to the water in which the bomb is immersed, and the resulting rise in the temperature is accurately determined. The thermometer readings are also continued through an "after period" in order that the "radiation correction" may be calculated and the observed rise of temperature corrected accordingly. This corrected rise, multiplied by the total heat capacity of the apparatus and the water in which it is immersed, shows the total heat liberated in the bomb. From this, must be deducted the heat arising from accessory combustions (the oxidation of the iron wire used as a fuse, etc.) to obtain the number of kilocalories arising from the combustion of the sample.

By using the definition of kilocalorie and from the amount of heat liberated, energy value of food can be calculated.

The energy value derived from bomb calorimeter is as follows:

1 g of carbohydrate	— 4.10 kcal
1 g of fat	— 9.45 kcal
1 g of protein	— 5.65 kcal

Calculations

Weight of food substance taken	— 2 g
Weight of water outside vessel	— 3000 g
Water equivalent of the calorimeter	— 500 g
Initial temperature of water	— 24° C
Final temperature of water	— 26°C
Rise in temperature of water	— 2°C
Heat gained by water in calorimeter	= 3500 × 2
	= 7000 calories
	= 7 kcal
2 g of food substance produces	= 7 kcal
1 g of food produces	= 3.5 kcal

When samples of carbohydrate, fat, protein are burned the amount of heat produced is always the same for each of the nutrients.

Physiological Fuel Value

The amount of energy actually available to the body from a given amount of nutrient is called physiological fuel value.

In the bomb calorimeter, unlike in the human body, carbohydrates, fats and proteins are completely oxidized. In the human body the process of digestion does not proceed with 100 per cent efficiency and so the entire amount of any ingested nutrient does not eventually become available to the body. The efficiency with which nutrient is digested must be taken into account. The coefficient of digestibility is used to express the proportion of an ingested nutrient that ultimately becomes available to the body's cells. For carbohydrate, fat and for protein the coefficient of digestibility is 0.98, 0.95 and 0.92 respectively.

In bomb calorimeter, the fibre present in vegetable foods is burnt and yields energy which is not utilized by human beings.

There is no loss in metabolism of carbohydrate and fat. But in the case of protein, a part of the energy is lost as urea due to incomplete oxidation. This loss has been estimated as 1.3 kcal per gram of protein oxidized. The physiological energy values of carbohydrate, fat and protein are 4, 9 and 4 after making allowances for losses of food energy in digestion and metabolism. These values are known as Atwater Bryant factors or physiological fuel values.

Table 5.2 gives the calculation of physiological fuel values.

Table 5.2: Calculated physiological fuel value of nutrients allowing for losses kcal/g

	Carbohydrate	Fat	Protein
Heat of combustion	4.15	9.45	5.65
Energy from combustion of nitrogen unavailable to the body	–	–	1.30
Net heat of combustion	4.15	9.45	4.35
Coefficient of digestibility	0.98	0.95	0.92
Physiological fuel value (kcal)	4.00	9.00	4.00
Physiological fuel value (kJ)	17.00	38.00	17.00

Source: Guthrie Helen A. and Picciano Mary Frances, 1995, Human Nutrition, McGraw–Hill, Boston.

Benedict's Oxy-Calorimeter

This is based on indirect calorimetry and on the principle that when an organic substance is completely combusted either in calorimeter or in the human body oxygen is consumed in amounts directly related to the energy liberated as heat.

Another apparatus for determination of the energy value of foods is the oxy-calorimeter, devised by Benedict and coworkers This measures the volume of oxygen required to burn a known weight of the food. From this, by means of factors established by use of the bomb calorimeter, the calorific value of the food is calculated. Figure 5b shows Benedict's Oxy-calorimeter. The apparatus, consists of a combustion chamber, A, in which the weighed sample is burnt, a soda lime container for absorption of carbon dioxide, B, a spirometer for measuring the oxygen used, S, and a motor-blower unit for circulating the gas mixture, C. Using this instrument, the amount of oxygen consumed in burning 1 g of pure carbohydrate, fat or protein can be determined. The factors for converting litres of oxygen consumed to calories are given by Benedict and Fox.

Relation between Oxygen required and Calorimeter value

It is of importance to know the amount of heat produced when 1 litre of oxygen is used for the oxidation of carbohydrates, fats or proteins. This can be calculated from the data obtained by the oxy-calorimeter as explained below:

1 g of carbohydrate requires 0.8 litres of oxygen for complete oxidation and yields 4.1 kcal.

1 g of fat requires 2.2 litres of oxygen for complete oxidation and yields 9.5 kcal.

1 g of protein requires 1.2 litres of oxygen for complete oxidation and yield 5.5 kcal.

1 litre of oxygen oxidises 1.25 g of carbohydrate and produces 5 kcal heat.

1 litre of oxygen oxidises 0.49 g of fat and produces 4.5 kcal heat.

1 litre of oxygen oxidises 0.83 g protein and produces 4.6 kcal heat.

One litre of oxygen oxidising carbohydrate, fat or protein produces the same amount of heat that is, 4.5 to 5 kcal. This is an important conclusion as this is the basis for indirect determination of energy requirements from the oxygen consumed.

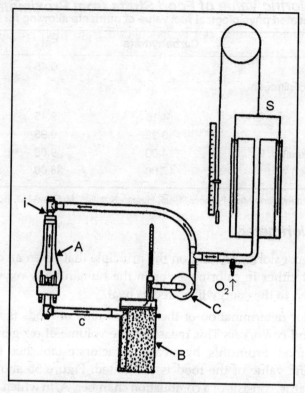

Figure 5b. Diagram of Benedict's oxy-calorimeter.
A-Combustion Chamber B – sodalime container
C-Circulating gas mixture S-Spirometer.

Source: Sherman Henry, C., 1945, Chemistry of food and nutrition, the Macmillan company, New York.

Table 5.3: Differences between physiological fuel value and gross fuel value

PHYSIOLOGICAL FUEL VALUE	GROSS FUEL VALUE
• Amount of energy actually available in the body from a given amount of nutrient	Amount of energy released from the nutrient in bomb calorimeter or oxy-calorimeter
• In the human body the process of digestion does not proceed with 100% efficiency	Here the carbohydrates, proteins and fats are completely oxidized
• In human body the fibre content is not digested and its energy is not utilized	In calorimeters the fibre present in vegetable foods is burnt and its energy yield is calculated
• In protein a part of energy is lost as urea due to incomplete oxidation	Protein is also completely oxidized
• The physiological fuel value of Carbohydrate 4 kcal Fat 9 kcal Protein 4 kcal	The gross energy value of Carbohydrate 4.10 kcal Fat 9.45 kcal Protein 5.65 kcal

Calculation of Calorific Value of Food Stuffs from Proximate Composition

The calorific values of food stuffs can be calculated from their contents of carbohydrates, fats and proteins using the physiological fuel values.

TOTAL ENERGY REQUIREMENT

The energy requirement of an individual is the level of energy intake from food that will balance energy expenditure. Estimates of energy requirements could be based on measurements of either energy intake or energy expenditure. In practice, measurements of energy intake are usually less reliable than measurement of energy expenditure. This when the individual has a body size and composition and level of physical activity, consistent with long term good health and that will allow for maintenance of economically necessary and socially desirable activity. In children, pregnant and lactating women the energy requirement includes the energy needs associated with the deposition of tissues or the secretion of milk at rates consistent with good health.

The human body's total energy needs can be subdivided into three separate categories:

—The energy required to maintain basal metabolism; the basic essential metabolic processes required to keep the body alive and healthy and where applicable growing at an appropriate rate.

—There energy required to power physical activity, meaning, all of the muscle movements.

—The energy that is released as a result of the thermic effect of food. It is a process of increased energy expenditure and therefore heat release that inevitably occurs between 1 to 3 hours after a meal due to the stimulating effect that the nutrients of food have on metabolism in general.

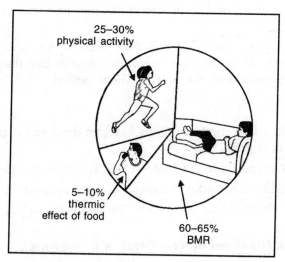

Figure 5c. Components of energy expenditure.

Generally, basal metabolism, represents a person's largest expenditure of energy, followed by exercise and the thermic effect of foods. Of these categories, energy spent in physical activity is most responsive to voluntary control .

BASAL METABOLIC RATE

The amount of energy required to carry on the involuntary work of the body is known as basal metabolic rate.

It includes the functional activities of the various organs such as brain, heart, liver, kidney and lungs. The secretory activities of glands, peristaltic movement of gastro intestinal tract, oxidation occurring in resting tissue, maintenance of muscle tone and body temperature. The brain and nervous tissue account for 1/8 of the energy utilized at the basal state and the lungs, liver and heart and kidney for additional 3/5th.

MEASUREMENT OF BASAL METABOLISM

Direct calorimetry

The direct calorimetric methods require the subjects to be in a human calorimeter or respiration chamber, to measure the amount of heat evolved.

To determine energy expenditure during BMR or at activity, Atwater and Rosa respiration calorimeter is used. Figure 5d shows Atwater Rosa respiration calorimeter. The subject is placed in a calorimeter a small room with heavily insulated walls. The heat generated by the subject is taken up by water, pumped through a series of finned pipes which pass through the calorimeter. Multiplying the difference in temperature between the incoming and outgoing water, by the volume of water flowing, heat output can be obtained. Atwater showed that measurements by direct calorimetry agreed well with measurements by indirect calorimetry which is more convenient and relatively cheap and very nearly as accurate.

A modified version of the respiration chamber is the metabolic chamber in which the heat given off by the subject is measured using thermocouples and heat exchange discs attached to the skin.

One disadvantage of direct calorimetry is that measurements can only be made over periods of several hours or more since the technique assumes that there is no net increase or decrease in body temperature over the measurement period.

Indirect calorimetry

Indirect calorimetry is based on the fact that the oxygen used and carbon dioxide produced is in proportion to the heat generated.

The basal metabolic rate is measured by indirect calorimetry under the following conditions:

Post absorptive stage: 12–16 hrs after the meal, usually performed in the morning.

Reclining but awake: 1½ hrs –1 hr rest before the test is necessary if there has been any activity in the morning.

Relaxed and free from emotional upsets or fear of the test itself.

Normal body temperature.

Comfortable room temperature and humidity of about 21°C-24°C.

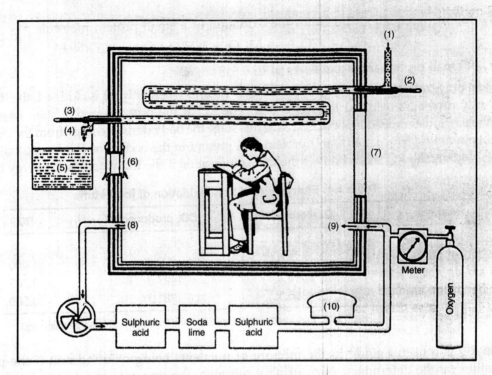

Figure 5d. The Atwater and Rosa respiration calorimeter. The walls of this chamber are insulated. Heat produced in it is absorbed by water passing in at (1) and out at (4), its temperature on entering and leaving being recorded on the thermometers (2) and (3). The volume of water that has flowed through the cooling system is measured in the vessel (5). The subject may be observed through the window (7), while food may be introduced and excreta removed through the porthole (6). Air leaves the chamber at (8) and passes through a blower and over sulphuric acid and soda-lime to absorb water and carbon dioxide. Oxygen measured by a gas meter is added to the system before the air passes into the chamber at (9). (10) is a tension equaliser.

Source: Passmore, R. and M.A. Eastwood, 1987, Davidson and Passmore, Human Nutrition and Dietetics, ELBS, Churchill, Livingstone.

Respiratory quotient: Respiratory quotient is defined as the ratio of the volume of CO_2 produced to the volume of O_2 used on oxidation of a given amount of the nutrient.

$$RQ = \frac{\text{Carbon dioxide exhaled}}{\text{Oxygen consumed}}$$

Respiratory quotient varies with the type of food being oxidised.

For example for pure glucose

$$C_6 H_{12} O_6 + 6O_2 = 6\ CO_2 + 6\ H_2O$$

$$RQ = \frac{6CO_2}{6O_2} = 1.0$$

For a fatty acid, such as palmitic acid

$$CH_3 (CH_2)_{14} COOH + 23O_2 = 16\ CO_2 + 16H_2O$$

$$RQ = \frac{16CO_2}{23O_2} = 0.7$$

The following equation illustrates the oxidation of a small protein molecule

$$C_{72}H_{112}N_{18}S + 77O_2 \longrightarrow 63CO_2 + 38H_2O + SO_3 + 9CO(NH_2)_2$$

RQ of small protein molecule is equal to 0.818.

When only carbohydrate is oxidized the RQ is 1.0 and when only fat is oxidised, the RQ is 0.7 and only protein is oxidised the RQ is 0.82. The RQ at the post absorptive state when basal metabolism is determined is about 0.82 as at this stage the body derives energy from the oxidation of carbohydrates, 50%, fat 40% and protein 10% present in the body. The RQ for alcohol is 0.66. Over 24 hours the RQ should reflect the diet composition if the individual is in energy balance.

Table 5.4: Energy yields from oxidation of food stuffs

Nutrient	O₂ required ml	CO₂ produced ml	RQ
1 g of			
Starch	828.8	828.8	1.000
Animal fat	2019.2	1427.3	0.707
Protein	966.1	781.7	0.809

Source: Passmore, R and M.A. Eastwood, 1987, Davidson and Passmore, Human Nutrition and Dietetics, ELBS, Churchill, Livingstone.

The RQ is a useful guide to the mixture of nutrients being oxidised and if the protein oxidation can be determined from urinary nitrogen, the amounts of fat and carbohydrate oxidised can be calculated. It is known that 1g of urinary nitrogen arises from the metabolism of 6.25 g of protein.

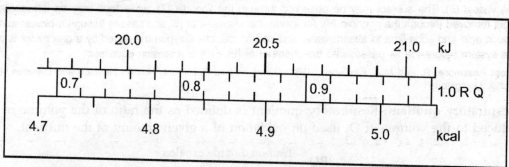

Figure 5e. Relationship between RQ and energy value.

Nomogram from which may be read off the energy value of a litre of oxygen (at s.t.p.) in kJ and kcal at non-protein R.Q. from 0.7 to 1.0.

Source: Bell H. George et al., 1972, Text book of physiology and biochemistry, ELBS, Churchill, Livingstone.

Some of the important findings, from studies of respiratory quotient are the following:

—Immediately after a meal almost all the food metabolized is carbohydrates so that the respiratory quotient at that time approaches 1.0.

—Approximately 8-10 hrs after a meal the body has already used up most of its readily available carbohydrate and the respiratory quotient approaches that for fat metabolism approximately 0.70.

—In diabetes mellitus very little carbohydrate can be utilized by the body cells under any conditions because insulin is required for this. Therefore when diabetes is very severe the respiratory quotient remains most of the time, very near to that for fat metabolism, 0.70.

Basal metabolism is usually determined using the apparatus of Benedict and Roth (Figures 5f and 5g). The subject wears a nose-clip and breathes through a mouthpiece which is connected to the apparatus by two tubes. The subject breathes in oxygen through the respiratory valve and breathes out into the carbon dioxide absorber and then through the expiratory valve, into the spirometer bell. The amount of oxygen used is recorded on the revolving drum by the pen attached. Since the subject is in the post-absorptive state, RQ is assumed to be 0.82 and the calorific value of one litre of O_2 consumed is taken as 4.8 kcal. Example

Oxygen consumed in 6 mtrs = 1,100 ml

Heat produced in 6 mts   = 4.8 x 1.1 litres

1 g of protein   = 5.28 kcal

Heat produced in 24 hours $= \dfrac{5.2}{6} \times 60 \times 24 = 1247$

The basal metabolism of the individual for 24 hours = 1247 kcal.

Closed-circuit Indirect Calorimetry: This is a closed-circuit system in which the subject receives oxygen only from a measured source of oxygen rich air and exhales into a container in which the carbon dioxide and water are removed while the remaining oxygen and nitrogen are recirculated. The amount of oxygen in the air mixture is measured before and after each standard 6-minute test, allowing the amount of oxygen consumed to be determined. The use of 1 litre of oxygen under normal conditions of temperature and pressures corresponds to the release of 4.82 kcal of energy when the RQ is 0.82 under basal conditions. Thus the kilocalories released during the consumption of any volume of oxygen can be readily calculated under these conditions.

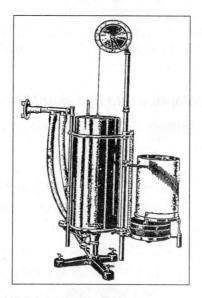

Figure 5f. Benedict-Roth respiration apparatus with kymograph.
Source: Hawk's Physiological Chemistry 1954.

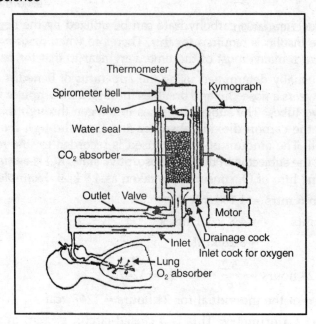

Figure 5g. Benedict Roth Apparatus in operation.
Source: Bell H. George et al, 1972, Textbook of physiology and biochemistry, ELBS, Churchill, Livingstone.

Open-circuit Indirect Calorimetry: In this method, normal room air is breathed in and the exhaled carbon dioxide generated from it is collected and measured. Knowing the amount of carbon dioxide produced in a given time allows calculation of the amount of oxygen consumed to generate that carbon dioxide and thus the amount of energy released can be calculated. The open circuit indirect method is even less expensive than either direct calorimetry or closed circuit indirect calorimetry. It also reduces the possibility of errors as a result of stimulation of metabolism caused by the use of oxygen rich air in the closed circuit method.

Determination of Basal metabolic rate by calculations

Basal metabolic rate can be calculated not only by direct and indirect calorimetry but also by using the following formulae.

1. Body weight

   For Female   — Weight in kg × 0.9 kcal × 24 hours

   For Male   — Weight in kg × 1 kcal × 24 hours

2. Harris-Benedict equation

   For Female   — 655.5 + (9.56 × W) + (1.85 × H) – (4.68 × A)

   For Male   — 66.5 + (13.75 × W) + (5.0 × H) – (6.75 × A)

3. Metabolic body size   — 70 × wt in kg¾.

4. FAO/WHO/UNU equation

For Female	— $8.7 \times W + 829$
For Male	— $11.6 \times W + 879$

A=Age in years, W = Weight in kg, H = Height in cm.

5. BMR for Indians can be predicted using the Table 5.5. For example to calculate the BMR for an Indian male aged 45 years the following formula is used.

$$BMR = 10.9 \times B.W. \ (kg) + 833$$
$$= 10.9 \times 60 + 833 = 654 + 833 = 1487$$

Table 5.5: Equations for predicting BMR (kcal/24hr) from body weight in kilograms

Sex	Age	Prediction equation proposed by ICMR expert group for Indians* from body weight in kilograms
Male	18–30	$14.5 \times W. + 645$
	30–60	$10.9 \times W. + 833$
	>60	$12.8 \times W. + 463$
Female	18–30	$14.0 \times W. + 471$
	30–60	$8.3 \times W. + 788$
	>60	$10.0 \times W. + 565$

*5% lower than that proposed by FAO/WHO/UNU (1985).

Source: A report of the Expert Group of the Indian Council of Medical Research, 2000, Nutrient requirements and recommended dietary allowances for Indians, ICMR, National Institute of Nutrition, Hyderabad, 500 007.

Table 5.6: FAO/WHO/UNU equations for predicting basal metabolic rate from body weight in kilograms (W)*

Age range (years) Males	kcal/day	Age range (years) Females	kcal/day
0–3	$60.9 \times W - 54$	0–3	$61.0 \times W - 51$
3–10	$22.7 \times W + 495$	3–10	$22.5 \times W + 499$
10–18	$17.5 \times W + 651$	10–18	$12.2 \times W + 746$
18–30	$15.3 \times W + 679$	18–30	$14.7 \times W + 496$
30–60	$11.6 \times W + 879$	30–60	$8.7 \times W + 829$
>60	$13.5 \times W + 487$	>60	$10.5 \times W + 596$

*Used for resting energy expenditure in developing recommended dietary allowances (National Research Council/Institute of Medicine: Recommended dietary allowances, ed. 10, Washington, DC, 1989, National Academy of Sciences)

Source: Report of a Joint FAO/WHO/UNU Expert consultation:1985. Energy and Protein requirements, Technical Report Series, Geneva, Switzerland, WHO.

Table 5.7: Comparision of energy cost of some common activities in terms of BMR units

Activity	Energy cost of activities in BMR units (Indian Data)
Sitting quietly	1.20
Standing quietly	1.40
Sitting at desk	1.30
Standing and doing lab work	2.0
Harvesting	3.6
Hand saw	7.4
Typing (Sitting)	1.58
Walking 3 MPH	3.71

Source: A report of the Expert Group of the Indian Council of Medical Research, 2000, Nutrient requirements and Recommended Dietary Allowances for Indians, ICMR, National Institute of Nutrition, Hyderabad 500 007.

ENERGY REQUIREMENTS DURING WORK

Physical activity, includes both the cost and quantum of the activity as well as the type of activity namely.

(a)   essential; economic or occupational activities and

(b)   discretionary activities; household tasks, social activities and activities aimed at maintenance of physical fitness.

Factorial method: Using the factorial method, the FAO/WHO/UNU Expert consultation has derived the BMR factors for computing the daily energy requirements of men and women engaged in sedentary, moderate and heavy activity. The BMR factors for Indian men and women are 1.6, 1.9 and 2.5 respectively for the three categories of activities. Details are given in Tables 5.7, 5.8 and 5.9.

Table 5.8: Recommended BMR factors for computing energy requirements of Indians

Recommending Body	Sex	Activity Category		
		Sedentary	Moderate	Heavy
ICMR 1989	Man	1.6	1.9	2.5
	Woman			
FAO/WHO/UNU 1985	Man	1.55	1.78	2.10
	Woman	1.56	1.64	1.82

Source: A report of the Expert Group of the Indian Council of Medical Research, 2000, Nutrient requirements and Recommended Dietary Allowances for Indians, ICMR, National Institute of Nutrition, Hyderabad 500 007.

Table 5.9: Computation of energy requirements of Indian adults in terms of BMR units

Activity	Duration (hr)	Rate of energy expenditure in terms of BMR units		
		Sedentary activity	Moderate activity	Heavy activity
Sleep	8	1.0	1.0	1.0
Occupational activity	8	1.7	2.8	4.5
Non-occupational activity	8	2.2	2.0	2.0
Average for 24 hr.		1.6	1.9	2.5
Computed 24 hr. energy expenditure				
Reference Man, 60 kg		2424	2882	3788
Reference Woman, 50 kg		1872	2223	2925

Source: A report of the Expert Group of the Indian Council of Medical Research, 2000, Nutrient requirements and Recommended Dietary Allowances for Indians, ICMR, National Institute of Nutrition, Hyderabad 500 007.

There is a wide variation in the energy cost of any activity both within and between individuals, due to differences in body size and the speed and dexterity with which an activity is performed. To compensate for differences in body size, it is now common to express the energy costs of activities as multiples of BMR Indians have 10 percent less BMR for the same age, height and weight for height.

Physical activity accounts for 20–40% of total daily expenditure in most individuals. The energy expended in activity depends on the type of activity and the time spent in different activities. Energy costs of activities are expressed as multiples of BMR or RMR.

Indirect calorimetry: The energy metabolism during work can be determined by using the following equipment.

Douglas bag (Figure 5h) and Max — Planck respirometer

The general principles underlying the above methods are:

1. Measuring the volume of expired air during work for fixed periods of 5-10 mts.
2. Collection of sample of expired air for the analysis of oxygen and carbon dioxide contents.
3. Calculation of oxygen consumption, carbon dioxide output and respiratory quotient and
4. Calculation of the energy output from the respiratory quotient and oxygen consumption.

Although the Douglas bag has been used for many short term measurements of energy expenditure at rest and during exercise. It is not ideal for use during heavy exercise as the bag may fill in a few minutes and may physically interfere with the exercise.

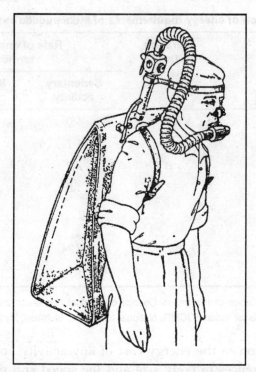

Figure 5h. Douglas bag used for determining energy expenditure during work. The subject is wearing a 100 litre capacity Douglas bag which is partly filled with expired air. The cylindrical box attached to the mouth-piece contains valves so arranged that the subject breathes atmospheric air in and breathes out through the corrugated tubing into the bag.

Source: Bell H. George *et al*, 1972, Textbook of physiology and biochemistry, ELBS, Churchill, Livingstone.

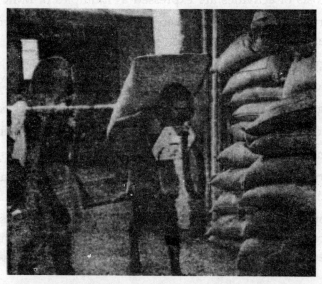

Figure 5i. Measuring energy expenditure in Hamalis

Several portable respirometers have been designed to overcome these problems by measuring expired volume at the time of collection, thereby removing the need to store all the expired air. The first portable respirometer to be developed for exercise was the Kofrani – Michaelis (Max – Planck respirometer) in which a small sample of expired air was stored for subsequent analysis in the laboratory. This has been replaced by instruments which incorporate oxygen analysers as well as gas volume meters and electronic components to calculate energy expenditure instantaneously. The oxylog developed in the 1970s weighs 2.2 kg and is powered by rechargeable batteries.

Cosmed K2 weighs only 400g and incorporates both an oxygen sensor and a radio transmitter to relay the data to a receiver at a base remote from the subject.

Whole-body indirect calorimeters operate on the same principle but provide a small ventilated room for the subject in which he/she can carry out some of the activities of a normal day. A number of indirect calorimeter chambers have been constructed with volumes ranging from 5-25 m^3. In the majority of these systems both O_2 and CO_2 are monitored continuously and the subjects follow a fixed routine of meals, exercise, recreation and sleep. In this way a value for 24h energy expenditure with a reproducible activity pattern may be obtained.

THERMIC EFFECT OF FOOD

The third category of energy requirement to be taken into account in estimating total energy needs is the energy needed to provide for thermic effect of food. Earlier this was known as Specific Dynamic Action (SDA).

The energy corresponding to the thermic effect of food includes the energy cost of absorption, metabolism and storage of nutrients within the body. In this as a result of the stimulation of metabolism increased heat production occurs from 1-3 hours after a meal. Processing of food in the stomach and intestine and of all nutrients in the blood and body cells causes heat production. The magnitude of thermic effect of food overall is that of 10 per cent of needs for basal metabolism and activity.

MEASORING TOTAL ENERGY REQUIREMENT
Energy balance method

Total energy needs are based on comparison of total energy intake over several days with the amount of energy required for any observed change in body composition. If the person is neither gaining nor losing weight, that calorie intake would be the requirement. The accuracy of this procedure obviously depends on the accuracy of the food intake record and the accuracy of measurements of change in body composition.

Heart Rate Monitoring Method

Estimating total energy needs by constantly monitoring the heart rate is based on the strong positive correlation that exists between heart rate and oxygen consumption and therefore energy release from food or energy stores. The relationship between heart rate and oxygen consumption can be explained by the fact that the oxygen needed to release energy from food is transported through the blood. Increased oxygen consumption requires increased blood flow powered by an increase in heart rate. During the preliminary study, heart rate and oxygen are both directly monitored while the subject undertakes a series of activities. A mathematical equation describing the relationship between heart rate and oxygen consumption can then be derived that is unique to the individual subject. This equation allows an approximate level to be predicted for any heart rate across the entire range.

Doubly Labelled Water Technique

This method provides information on the total energy expended by a free-living subject for periods of 10-20 days, which is likely to reflect the normal energy requirement of the subject. The subject takes an oral dose of water containing a known amount of stable (non-radioactive) isotopes of both hydrogen and oxygen. The isotopes, ^2H (deuterium) and ^{18}O mix with the normal hydrogen and oxygen in body water within a few hours. As energy is expended in the body, CO_2 and water are produced. The CO_2 is lost from the body in breath, while the water is lost in breath, urine, sweat and other evaporation. As ^{18}O is contained in both CO_2 and water, it is lost from the body more rapidly than ^2H, which is contained in water but not CO_2. The difference between the rate of loss of ^{18}O and ^2H reflects the rate at which CO_2 is produced, which in turn can be used to estimate energy expenditure using indirect calorimetry formulae.

FACTORIAL METHOD

A factorial method of measuring total energy expenditure involves calculation of each of the three categories of energy need.

Method I :

—Calculate the basal metabolism using any given method.
—Calculate the activity costs over a 24 hours period.
—Add 1+2 and calculate 10 per cent allowance as thermic effect of food.
—Calculate total energy expenditure by adding basal energy needs + activity needs + thermic effect.

Method II :

Total energy cost can be calculated using Tables 5.3, 5.4 and 5.6
Example:

Sex	: Male
Age	: 25
Weight Kg	: 60
BMR	: 14.5 × 60 + 645
	: 1515 kcal

BMR Unit for sedentary work = 1.6 (includes thermic effect of food)
Total energy requirements = 1515 × 1.6 = 2424.

RESTING ENERGY EXPENDITURE

The REE is basically a combination of basal energy needs, plus the thermic effect of food, plus a small amount of energy needed to perform the most sedentary activities such as sitting quietly.

Total energy needs = REE + Needs of activity

Multiply REE by an activity factor of 1.5 for women and 1.6 for men for light activity to estimate daily caloric need. REE is usually considered to be 10% above basal energy needs. Equation predicted by Mifflin and St. Jeor is as follows :

Adult males: REE = (10 × weight in kg) + (6.25 × ht in cm) – (5 × age in yrs) + 5
Adult females: REE = (10 × weight in kg) + (6.25 × ht in cm) – (5 × age in yrs) – 161

DETERMINANTS OF BASAL METABOLIC RATE

There are many factors that determine basal metabolic rate of an individual.

Body Composition: All body tissues are metabolically active and being constantly maintained. Their components are degraded and resynthesised with an accompanying requirement of energy. Muscle, brain and various glands and organs such as liver are relatively more active and metabolically consume large amounts of oxygen/unit of weight and produce more heat than the less active tissue. Bone tissues and adipose tissue are relatively inactive metabolically and require less oxygen per unit weight. Total basal energy requirement per unit of body weight is higher when muscle tissue is in higher proportion in the total body weight.

Gender: The BMR of a 65 kg adult man is around 1 mJ/day higher than a woman of the same age and weight. Women have more adipose tissue and less muscle tissue compared to the men of the same height and weight. Young adult male contains 14 per cent of fat and young adult female contains 23–32 per cent of fat. The BMR for women is 10–12 per cent lower than those of men of the same age, height and weight. Figure 5i shows distinctly that after the age of ten years, females have lower BMR than males. In women there is premenstrual rise and postmenstrual fall in the basal metabolic rate.

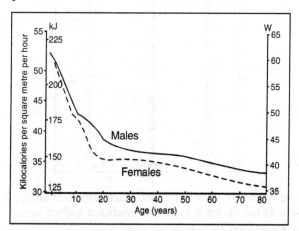

Figure 5j. Basal metabolic rate in kJ or kcal/m²/h from one year onwards.
Source: Bell H. George *et al.*, 1972, Textbook of Physiology and Biochemistry, Churchill, Livingstone.

Age: Figure 5j shows that per unit of surface area, the BMR is at its highest during the first two years of life. It declines gradually throughout childhood and accelerates slightly in adolescence. Thereafter the decline continues throughout life, with an average of about 2 per cent per decade after the age of 21 years. The rapid growth rate explains the high metabolic rate in early childhood. Whenever there is growth there is increase in the BMR. In the later years muscle tone decreases and there is reduction in muscle mass and hence the BMR is low.

Body size and Surface area: It is one of the major determinants of energy expenditure in mass, accounting for more than half of the variability in BMR between normal individuals. About 80 per cent of energy is from glucose and fat which is lost as heat, 15 per cent of the heat loss being from skin. The remaining heat loss occurs from the lungs and through the excreta. Since the heat loss is proportional to the surface area, BMR is directly proportional to surface area. Basal metabolism is most closely related to the body surface area and less directly related to either weight or height of an individual. A tall thin person has a greater surface area than an individual of the same weight who is short and fat. The former will have higher basal metabolism. The body surface area can be calculated according to the formula of DuBois and DuBois given below.

$A = W^{0.425} \times H^{0.725} \times 71.84$ where

A = Body surface area in square centimeters

H = Height in centimeters

W = Weight in kilograms

From the height and weight of the individual, surface area can be calculated with the help of a nomogram given in Figure 5k. The more the surface area, the higher the basal metabolic rate. A difference of weight of 10 Kg would account for a difference of around 500 kJ/day in BMR in adult men and women.

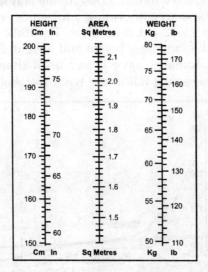

A line joining the height on the left-hand scale with nude weight on the right-hand scale cuts the centre scale at the predicted surface area.

Figure 5k. Nomogram for calculating surface area.

Source: Bell H. George *et al*, 1972, Text book of physiology and biochemistry, Churchill, Livingstone.

Sleep: During the sleeping hours the basal metabolism is about 10 per cent lower than the waking state. It also depends on the amount of motion during sleep of an individual.

Body temperature: An elevation in the body temperature above 37°C or 98.4°F increase the basal metabolism by 13 per cent for each degree celsius, 7 per cent for each degree of Fahrenheit. Increase in chemical reaction increases the temperature hence increase in BMR. Calorie requirement increases during fever.

Endocrine glands: The hormone thyroxin, containing iodine, is secreted by the thyroid gland and is a powerful stimulator of metabolism. Deviation in basal metabolism of more than 20 per cent from the normal predicted levels almost always indicates some problem in the thyroid function. In hypothyroidism BMR may be depressed as much as 30 per cent as a result of under secretion of thyroxin. People with hypothyroidism have low total energy needs and so they gain weight easily. In hyperthyroidism basal metabolism is elevated to 50–70 per cent above the normal level due to over secretion of thyroxin.

The growth hormone that stimulates new tissue formation is responsible for enhanced metabolism that is observed in children, infants, and teenagers. An increased secretion of epinephrine during excitement or fear temporarily raises the metabolic rate. Disturbances of the pituitary gland may also modify the metabolic rate. Just prior to the onset of menstrual period, the metabolism is increased slightly.

Pregnancy: BMR increases by about 5 per cent during the first and second trimesters. During the last trimester the BMR increases by 12 per cent. This increase can be accounted for by the high rate of metabolism of foetus and placenta, the increased activity of maternal tissue and increase in weight of the mother.

State of nutrition: After prolonged calorie under nutrition the BMR may fall to atleast 20–30 per cent below normal. This reflects the body's adaptive efforts to conserve energy when there is a deficiency.

The luxus consumption theory says that when a person takes more calories than needed the body tries to adapt using more calories and thereby avoids the deposition of fat.

BMR is affected by food consumption. Over feeding increases BMR by 5–10 per cent while underfeeding reduces BMR by similar amount under most dietary condition.

Environment temperature: The lowest metabolic rate is observed at an environment temperature of 26°C or 78°F. Higher metabolic rates are observed at temperatures both above and below this figure. A sudden decrease in environmental temperature causes shivering and a temporary process of heat production with the result there is an increase in BMR. This adaptive response of the body to lowered environmental temperature is called "Cold Induced Thermogenesis". BMR is also increased at temperatures above 30°C due to the energy cost of sweating.

Smoking: Research indicates that habitual smokers when they stop smoking have a tendency to gain weight. This may be caused by the fact that the nicotine taken in increases BMR by 10 per cent.

Genetic differences: BMR varies by up to ±10% between individuals of the same age, sex, body weight and fat free mass and there is growing evidence that some of this variation is determined by genetic factors.

Psychological state: Psychological state may affect energy expenditure as acute anxiety is a potent stimulant of epinephrine secretion and this increases energy expenditure .

Pharmacological agents: Nicotine and caffeine increase energy expenditure by small but measurable amounts. Beta-blockers commonly used to treat hypertension may lead to a slight decrease in energy expenditure and hence a tendency to gain weight.

Disease processes: This may increase metabolic rate like in fevers, tumors and burns to the skin. The mechanisms by which these processes influence energy expenditure are likely to involve intracellular signaling agents such as the cytokines.

FACTORS AFFECTING THE THERMIC EFFECT OF FOOD

The thermic effect of food varies with the composition of the diet, being greater after carbohydrate and protein consumption than after fat. This is attributable to the metabolic inefficiency of metabolizing carbohydrate and protein in comparison with fat. Fat is stored very efficiently with only 4 per cent wastage compared with 25 per cent wastage when carbohydrate is converted to fat for storage. These factors are thought to contribute to the obesity promoting characteristics of fat.

Spicy foods both enhance and prolong the effect of the thermic effect of food. Meals with added chillie and mustard increase the metabolic rate significantly, more than unspiced meals. This effect may be prolonged for more than 3 hours. Cold, caffeine and nicotine also stimulate the thermic effect of food. The amount of caffeine in one cup of coffee if ingested every 2 hours for 12 hours has been shown to increase the thermic effect of food by 8 per cent to 11 per cent. Nicotine has a similar effect. Table 5.10 summarises the factors affecting total energy requirement.

Table 5.10: Factors affecting total energy requirement

Factors Increasing TER	Factors Decreasing TER
Increase in muscle mass	Increase in body fat
Males	Females
Growth, Infancy, puberty	Hypothyroidism
More surface area	Less surface area
Hyperthyroidism	Sleep
Fever	Ageing
Pregnancy, lactation	Under nutrition
Good physical condition	
Extreme environmental temperature	
Smoking	
Psychological state	
Pharmacological agents	
Disease processes	
Thermic effect of food	

RECOMMENDED DIETARY ALLOWANCES

The level of intake of the individual at which he remains in steady state or in energy balance, maintaining the predetermined levels of body weight and physical activity is considered to be the individuals' energy requirement. In the case of energy, RDA represents only the average daily requirements corresponding to daily average energy expenditure. The energy requirements are based on energy expenditure and not on energy intake.

The RDA for proteins and energy were revised by a Joint Expert Consultation group of the Food and Agriculture Organisation, World Health Organization and United Nations University (UNU) in 1985. The expert group constituted by the Indian Council of Medical Research, ICMR, along with several resource persons met in 1988 and discussed RDAs for Indians.

RDA is based on Indian reference man and reference woman.

Reference Man: Reference man is between 20–39 years of age and weighs 60 kg. He is free from disease and physically fit for active work. On each working day he is employed for 8 hours in occupation that usually involves moderate activity. While not at work he spends 8 hours in bed, 4–6 hours sitting and moving about and 2 hours in walking and in active recreation or household duties.

Reference Woman: Reference woman is between 20–39 years of age and weighs 50 kg. She is engaged in 8 hours in general household work or in light industry or in any other moderate active work. Apart from 8 hours in bed, she spends 4–6 hours sitting or moving around in light activity and 2 hours walking or in active recreation or household chores.

Employing the factorial approach and the computed BMR from body weights and the recommended BMR factors for Indians for different levels of physical activity the suggested energy requirements of adult man and woman are given in Table 5.11.

In an average Indian diet 60–70 per cent energy comes from carbohydrate, 10–12 per cent from protein and the rest from fat.

Table 5.11: ICMR Recommended Dietary Allowances of energy

Group	Energy kcal
Man	
Sedentary Work	2425
Moderate Work	2875
Heavy Work	3800
Woman	
Sedentary Work	1875
Moderate Work	2225
Heavy Work	2925
Pregnant Woman	+300
Lactation	
0–6 months	+550
6–12 months	+400

Contd...

Group	Energy kcal
Infants	
0–6 months	108/kg
6–12 months	98/kg
Children	
1–3 years	1240
4–6 years	1690
7–9 years	1950
Boys	
10–12 years	2190
13–15 years	2450
16–18 years	2640
Girls	
10–12 years	1970
13–15 years	2060
16–18 years	2060

SOURCES

Oils and fats are concentrated sources of energy. Butter which contains 20 per cent moisture comparatively yields less energy. Nuts and oil seeds contain high amount of energy. Soyabean, being rich in oil is a fairly good source of energy. Sugar is also a good source of energy. Cereals and pulses contain good amount of carbohydrate and contribute substantially for the total energy requirement. Fruits and vegetables, rich in moisture are poor sources of energy.

Table 5.12 Energy value of foods

Name of the foodstuff	Energy kcal/100g
Ghee, Oil	900
Butter	729
Walnut	687
Coconut dry	662
Groundnut, roasted	570
Soyabean	432
Sugar	400
Rice, Wheat	345
Read gram dal	335
Egg	173

QUESTIONS

1. Define the units of energy and give the interconversions.
2. How do you determine the energy value of food? Explain the principle and draw the diagram.
3. What is physiological fuel value? How is it different from gross fuel values?

4. Draw the diagram and explain the principle of Benedict oxy-calorimeter.

5. Define total energy requirement and factors determining it.

6. How do you measure basal metabolic rate in direct calorimetry and indirect calorimetry?

7. Calculate total energy requirement for an adult man aged 30 weighing 60 kg.

8. Give the RDA for energy for pregnant and lactating woman.

9. What is respiratory quotient?

10. How do you estimate Basal Metabolic Rate by calculation?

11. Explain the steps involved in calculating total energy requirement by factorial method.

12. How do you estimate energy requirement during work?

13. Define thermic effect of food and explain the factors affecting it.

14. Define reference man and reference woman.

15. What is direct calorimetry and how will you find the energy value of a food substance?

16. Give the relation between oxygen required and calorific value.

17. Give the percentage of kilocalories that should come from carbohydrate, fat and protein in a balanced diet.

18. Explain the non-caloric methods used to determine total energy requirement.

19. In which conditions energy requirements are increased?

SUGGESTED REFERENCES

- Wimberly M.G. et al, 2001, Effects of habitual physical activity on resting metabolic rates and body composition of women aged 35–50 years. J. Amer. Diet. Assoc. **101**

- Energy requirements of men engaged in moderate work, Annual Report, 1991-92, National Institute of Nutrition, Hyderabad.

- Nutrition and Physical activity : www.cdc.gov/nccdphp/dnpa/

- Owen OE et al, 1987, A reappraisal of the calorie requirements of men. Am J clin Nutr, 46.

CHAPTER 6

UNDERNUTRITION

Nutrition is a major factor in bringing out the maximum potentiality that one is endowed with both physically and mentally. Good nutrition depends on an adequate food supply and this in turn on sound agricultural policy and a good system of food distribution. The social, cultural, economic and agricultural factors are the basic etiological factors causing nutritional disease and they are closely linked with excessive increase in the population. Undernutrition is the condition which results when insufficient food is eaten over an extended period of time. Undernutrition is a type of malnutrition.

Though undernutrition can occur at any age, the main victims are children. Kwashiorkor, marasmus and keratomalacia which used to be a major public health problem till the 1960s have declined since. However, population at large is affected by "hidden" undernutrition which may not be easy to diagnose.

The direct effects of undernutrition are occurrence of frank and subclinical nutritional deficiency diseases. The indirect effects are a high morbidity and mortality among young children, retarded physical and mental growth, lowered vitality leading to lowered productivity and reduced life expectancy. Undernutrition predisposes to infection and infection predisposes to undernutrition. The high rate of maternal mortality, still births and low birth weight are all associated with undernutrition.

The Human Development Index:

Human Development Index is being widely used for measuring the health inequality and standards of living of countries.

The Human Development Index is calculated from

* Life expectancy—to measure longevity
* Educational attainment—to represent knowledge
* Real Gross Domestic Product—GDP—representing the basic needs.

India's Human Development Index—HDI—rank for nutrition is 132, reflecting a major deficiency in the quality of life of a vast majority of the population. The high levels of malnutrition in the country particularly among children and women are directly or indirectly associated with high morbidity and mortality rates such as infant mortality rate, mortality under 5 years, material mortality rate, life expectancy at birth—the indicators used for measuring the development of a country in the present age.

According to NNMB survey, 2000–2001, the proportion of individuals in any age group, meeting 100 per cent the RDA for all the nutrients was less than 1 per cent. With respect to energy and protein about third of males and females (non pregnant and non lactating women) meet 100 per cent RDA, as compared to 7–14 per cent in children. Vitamin A and riboflavin consumption were much below the RDA. Severe grade undernutrition reduced from 30 per cent in 90–91 to 21 per cent in the year 2000-2001.

PREVALENCE

According to the surveys conducted by UNICEF, malnutrition is prevalent throughout India in different degrees as shown in Figure 6a (Appendix 10).

Malnutrition in Children

The NNMB survey (1998–90) of rural children has shown that only about 10 per cent are normal with weight above 90 per cent of the standard National Center for Health Statistics, USA (NCHS). A majority of them exhibit mild or moderate malnutrition, while 8.7 per cent are "severely" malnourished. The malnutrition was similar among boys and girls.

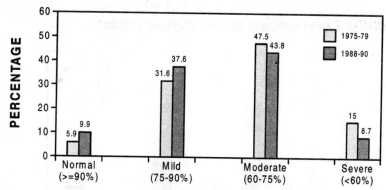

Figure 6b. Prevalence of malnutrition among children—1 to 5 years (using Weight /Age Gomez grades).

Source: NNMB Report of Repeat Surveys 1988–90.

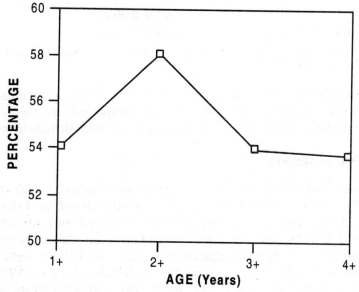

Figure 6c. Malnutrition among preschool children—1 to 5 years.
Source: NNMB Survey 1991–92.

This is contrary to the general belief that girls have poorer status than boys. Figure 6c shows incidence of malnutrition is maximum among preschool children of 2 years.

Nutrient Deficiencies among Pre-school Children

The major nutritional deficiency signs among pre-school children are protein energy malnutrition, vitamin A deficiency and vitamin B-complex deficiency. The prevalence of figures indicate a greater degree of vitamin deficiencies than of PEM. The prevalence of severe PEM is less than one percent. A survey showed that 0.04 per cent of blindness is due to nutritional cause. Figure 6e shows prevalence of nutritional deficiency signs in children—1 to 5 years (88–90).

ICMR Multicentric Longitudinal Study Report (1996)

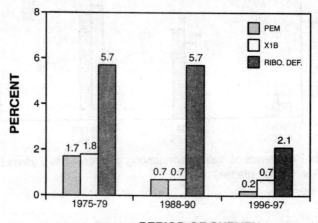

Figure 6d. Nutritional deficiencies in India NNMB 1999

Source: Vijayaraghavan, 2001. National Nutrition Programmes–Current status, Proc Nutr. Soc. India, *49*

The study on Indian children showed those stunted by 5–7 year of age maintain lower stature throughout adolescence as the growth spurt did not compensate for the early life growth retardation. 33 per cent births being low weight for gestation also contribute to later life stunting.

Nutritional Status of Adults

The Body Mass Index (BMI) defined as weight (kg)/height^{2}m, is used to assess the nutritional status of adults. Persons with BMI less than 18.5 are considered to suffer from Chronic Energy Deficiency (CED). The CED group is further classified into different degrees first (17 to 18.5), second (16 to 17) and third (below 16) Figure 6d shows according to NNMB data that only about half the adult population had normal nutritional status while the rest suffered from different degrees of CED. According to NFHS survey in 1998-99, in India 33 per cent were underweight with BMI < 18.5 and 11 per cent were overweight in the age group 15–49 years. The National Family Health Survey (1999) revealed that as many as 10.6 per cent of women had BMI > 25, the problem being greater in urban areas.

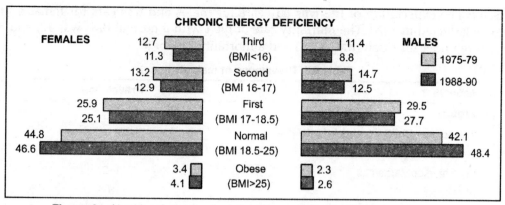

Figure 6e. Nutritional status of adults. (Percentage Distribution).
Source: National Nutrition Monitoring Bureau 1991.

VITAL HEALTH STATISTICS

Low Birth Weight: About 30 per cent of infants born in the country are of low birth weight (< 2.5 kg). The NNMB surveys showed (Figure 6f.) that the birth weights increased with increasing BMI status of mothers. The incidence of low birth weight deliveries was highest (53%) in women with Grade III Chronic Energy Deficiency (CED) and gradually declined as the BMI status of mothers improved.

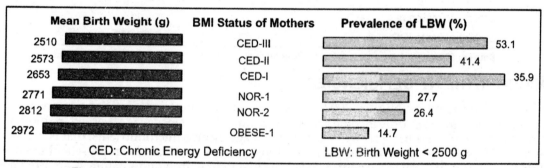

Figure 6f. Birth weight of infants and maternal nutrition.
Source: Nutrition News 1991.

Child Mortality Rate: The Infant Mortality Rate (IMR) and the under 5 Mortality Rate (U5MR) are valuable indicators of the socio-economic development and nutritional status of the society. The IMR was 80 per 1000 live births in 1991 and the U5MR was 35 per 1000 in 1987. In rural areas the mortality rates were higher than those in urban areas. The IMR is lowest in Kerala and highest in Orissa. The neonatal mortality was 56 in 1989.

States with higher levels of malnutrition among preschool children also had higher levels of under 5 child mortality. A reduction in the levels of severe degree of malnutrition would thus reduce child mortality levels.

Maternal Mortality Rate: The Maternal Mortality Rate in the country is estimated at 3.5 per 1000 live births as compared to 0.24 for industrialised countries. About one-sixth of these deaths are due to anaemia.

Life Span: The expectation of life was 60 years for males and 62 years for females by the surveys conducted in 1990. The mortality rate of men with a normal BMI was 12, and those with severe under nutrition (BMI < 16) had a mortality rate of 32.

Table 6.1: Prevalence of malnutrition

Aspects	Prevalence
Groups	
Pre-school Children and Infants (%)	
Low birth weight	30
Kwashiorkor/Marasmus	1–2
Bitot spots	3
Iron deficiency anaemia	50
Underweight (weight for age)	53
Stunting (height for age)	65
Adults (%)	
Chronic Energy Deficiency (BMI < 18.5)	50
Anaemia in pregnant women	70–90
General Population	
Anaemia (%)	50
Goitre (millions)	40
Cretinism (millions)	2.2
Stillbirths due to IDD	90,000

Source: Dietary guidelines for Indians 1998—a manual, National Institute of Nutrition, Hyderabad.

MICRONUTRIENT DEFICIENCIES

A study conducted by NIN in 2002, revealed that micronutrient deficiencies are widely prevalent even in the middle income groups. Subclinical deficiency was observed in riboflavin, folate and calcium. From figure 6g, it is clear in all age groups micronutrients, that is, minerals and vitamins are deficient in the diets of all age groups particularly in preschool children. Table 6.2 shows that micronutrient deficiencies like iodine, iron and vitamin A are prevalent and with preventive measures the incidence can be reduced.

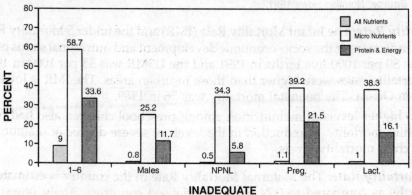

Figure 6g. Proportion of individuals not meeting (< 70% RDA) multiple nutrients.
Source: NNMB survey NIN, Annual report 2001–2002.

Table 6.2: Micronutrient malnutrition in developing countries, 1995 and 2025

Disorder	Number of affected persons (millions)	
	1995	2025
Goitre	834	350
Iron deficiency	3580	2750
Vitamin A deficiency	2.85	0.17

* Projected.
Source: World Health Organisation (1998).

Anaemia in General Population

Haemoglobin surveys among pregnant women revealed that as many as 87.5 per cent were anaemic (Hb<11 g per cent). About 13 per cent were severely anaemic (Hb<7 g per cent) and 33.6 per cent were moderately anaemic (Hb 7 to 9 g per cent).

Multicentric studies conducted by the ICMR showed that anaemia is not confined to pregnant women alone but affects other segments of the population as well. Prevalence of anaemia was higher in rural than in urban areas. According to NNMB surveys 24.4 per cent of males and 21.8 per cent of females suffer from anaemia.

Iodine Deficiency Disorders

Sample surveys conducted by the Directorate General of Health Services in 216 districts of 25 states in India have identified 186 districts as IDD endemic with a goitre rate of over 10 per cent.

As per the results of these surveys, no state in India is free from iodine deficiency; 167 million people are considered to be at risk of IDD, of whom 54 million have goitre. With continuous depletion of iodine from natural resources, the situation is expected to worsen in the coming years unless intensive efforts are made to ensure universal consumption of iodized salt.

Cost of Micronutrient Malnutrition: The cost of ill health due to micronutrient malnutrition is difficult to quantify, as it is a "hidden hunger". Only in recent years, sophisticated mathematical models have been developed to measure economic losses due to disability and premature death. One of them is the indicator created by the WHO and the World Bank for the 1993 World Development Report, measured in DALYs (Disability, Adjusted Life Years). By connecting the number of years of healthy life lost due to disability and premature death and adjusting for a variety of parameters (age, sex, demographic region etc.) experts were able to estimate the global burden of disease.

By this calculation, 1.36 billion DALYs were lost world wide in 1990 the equivalent of 42 million deaths of newborn children or of 80 million deaths at age 50. In the developing word, two thirds DALY losses were due to premature death.

The cost of malnutrition has been estimated to be much higher than the investment of public expenditure required for its prevention. As per the studies conducted by the Administrative Staff College of India, Hyderabad, 1997, malnutrition reduced India's Gross Domestic Product by 3 to 9% in 1996 or approximately 10–28 billion US dollars.

AETIOLOGY OF UNDERNUTRITION

Malnutrition is a man made disease. The great advantage of looking at malnutrition as a problem in human ecology is that it allows for variety of approaches towards prevention. The main causes of undernutrition can be categorised under the headings host, environment and agent.

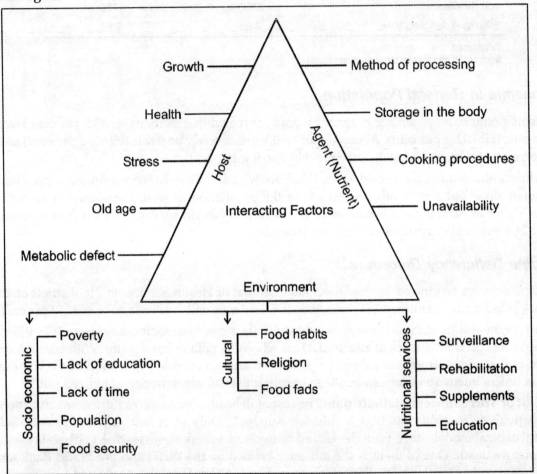

Figure 6h. Summary of factors contributing to undernutrition–Host, Environment and Agent. The causes of malnutrition are complex. They include conditions that preexist within the individual– the host, the quality of the environment and the specific agents that provide. Each element of this triad interacts with others.

HOST

Incidence of malnutrition is high when rate of growth increases. For example, growing children and pregnant women require high amount nutrients. If not satisfied in the diet, they may suffer from undernutrition. Infections and infestations also increase the requirement of nutrients. Psychological stress may affect the intake of food. During oldage the nutrient requirements may affect due to degerative diseases or consumption of drugs. Metabolic defects like insulin deficiency may affect utilisation of glucose. Sometimes children are born with deficiency of lactase resulting in lactose intolerance. A child deprived of milk may not be well nourished.

ENVIRONMENTAL FACTORS

Socio-economic Factors

Malnutrition is largely the byproduct of poverty, ignorance, insufficient education, lack of knowledge regarding the nutritive value of foods, poor sanitation and large family size. Increase in population has made the solution of malnutrition problem more difficult.

Poverty: Poverty is responsible for underfeeding and malnutrition, especially in children.

Food is a problem for the poor at all levels—availability, affordability, access and absorption.

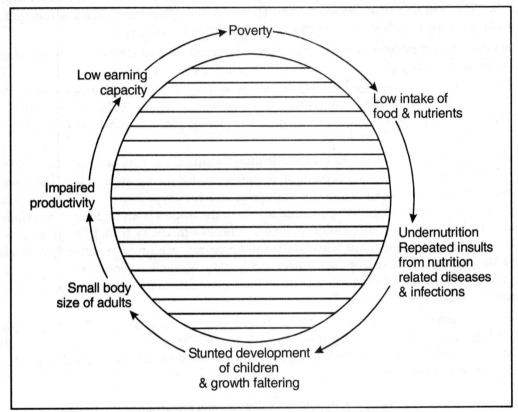

Figure 6i. The Vicious cycle of Poverty.

Source: National Nutrition Policy, Government of India, Department of Women and Child Development, Ministry of Human Resource Development, New Delhi, 1993.

In poverty, enough food is not available as they cannot afford hence the family members may suffer from undernutrition. During the time of famine or failure of crops, the farmers families may be deprived of food. In urban areas, unemployment of the family members can lead to poverty. Tribals who live in remote areas where there is no access, may suffer from underfeeding and undernutrition.

Poor families who live on locally available staple cereal and who cannot afford to include pulses, animal foods and fruits and vegetables will definitely suffer from undernutrition.

The nature of the foods eaten and the quality of diets is related to income. Even if there is enough to eat in the poorest countries which is unlikely the supplies of vitamin A and C are almost certainly insufficient. If most of the protein comes from a single vegetable source, the supply of one or more amino acids, probably is insufficient to meet the needs of young children. Milk tends to show sharp differences in quantity between the income groups.

Figure 6i shows how poverty leads to poverty underfeeding causes undernutrition and stunted development which inturn leads to low earning capacity and more poverty.

Lack of education: People of all income classes and at all educational levels lack knowledge regarding the essentials of an adequate diet. Those who are ignorant concerning nutrition are particularly to food faddism, superstitions and nutritional quackery.

The cause of their poverty is as much as people with minimal education and technical skills are unable to secure employment to earn a satisfactory living wage. Somehow, the poor must use each rupee more carefully but they have too little consumer information to help them. Moreover, in as much as the amount and quality of food available to them are limited, they need to employ the best techniques in food preparation to preserve nutritive values but they lack the facilities and skills to do so.

Lack of time: A secondary cause of inadequate nutrition may be lack of leisure. Proper nutrition demands time for the preparation of meals and for their consumption. The working mother may not have enough time for shopping and for preparing meals. The increasing employment of women in industry in large towns in the tropics is an important contributory cause of malnutrition in young children. People who live far away from their place of work may leave home at an early hour without a proper breakfast. Children are often sent to school with a hastily prepared lunch of poor nutritional quality. Many workers are still not provided with adequate breaks for their meals and no suitable place for eating. There may not be enough restaurants and proper canteens.

Population growth: The population has increased from 548 million in 1971 to 844 million in 1991. At this rate of increase the population will touch 1200 millions by 2020. Agricultural production should increase correspondingly and it should be available at affordable price to all to prevent malnutrition.

Table 6.3: Population estimates and projections

Year	Population in millions
1990	841
2000	1,002
2010	1,155
2020	1,296

Source: BUCEN-IDB

At present the food supply in the developing countries is just about keeping pass with the growth in population. Half of the world's population live in the fareast but only one fourth of the world's food supply is produced here. Control of population growth is especially difficult to achieve in countries where infant and child mortality is high and each couple wants survivors who can care for them in old age.

Food security: Increased food production should lead to increased food consumption. Given the best technology known at present, most developing countries could increase their food production several fold. But increased food production will not cure the basic problem of hunger and malnutrition in much of the developing world. Uneven distribution between the countries and within the countries is the problem. It is said that there will be very little malnutrition in India today, if all the food available can be equitably distributed in accordance with physiological needs.

Household food security is defined as sustainable access to safe food of sufficient quantity to ensure adequate intake and healthy life for all members of the family. Household food security depends on access to food as distinct from its availability. There may be abundant food available in the market but poor families that cannot afford it are not food secure. Food prices and economic status of the population are important determinants of food security.

Even in households where adults consume adequate dietary energy, it is observed that nearly 50 per cent of the children have inadequate intake. This would suggest that food security at the household level alone is not enough to ensure adequate intake among the children. Efforts are needed to educate the parents about the child's nutritional needs.

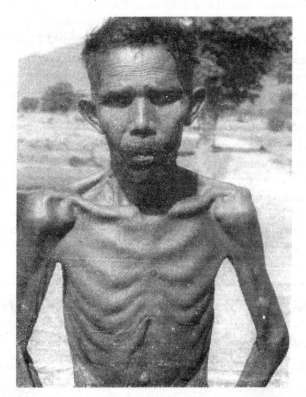

Figure 6j: Adult marasmus—deprivation of food due to famine.

The dependence of a satisfactory food supply upon a flourishing agriculture is self-evident. The world wars with their interference first with food distribution and then with food production gradually awakened the people of most countries to the importance of the relationships between food, agriculture and population.

In those countries where the majority of the poor and malnourished live, agriculture is barely keeping up with the growth of population. Though agricultural production has risen, since birth rates are high, amount of food available per head is less. Undernutrition remains widespread.

The prices of agricultural products are in general less well maintained than those of industrial goods. This leads to a series of economic crisis adversely affecting health and nutrition. In many poor countries these can only be improved by a great increase in agricultural production and slowing down of the growth of population. Both depend on higher standards of education.

There is no doubt that agricultural development has helped in achieving national food security, but without a significant impact on nutrition. The availability of cereals today is around 570 g/capita/day, which is almost 25 per cent more than the suggested level in the "balanced diet". Yet the surveys show that about 40 per cent of our population consume less than 80 per cent of energy required. Low purchasing capacity and limited access to food are the major constraints. Food and nutrition policies should address themselves to these issues and aim at achieving food security at the household level to improve nutritional status.

Cultural Influences

Lack of food is not the only cause of malnutrition. Too often there is starvation in the midst of plenty. People choose poor diets when good ones are available because of cultural influences which vary widely from country to country and from region to region.

Food habits, customs, beliefs, traditions and attitudes: Food habits are among the oldest and most deeply entrenched aspects of any culture. They have deep psychological roots and are associated with love, affection, warmth, self-image and social prestige. The family plays an important role in shaping the food habits and the habits are passed from one generation to another. Rice eaters may not include ragi or wheat in their diet as partial substitute for staple food.

Many customs and beliefs apply most often to vulnerable groups—infants, toddlers, expectant and lactating women. Papaya is avoided during pregnancy because it is believed to cause abortion. In some communities fresh fruits and vegetables are avoided during a certain period. Sometimes nursing mothers are given diet restricted in dals, greens and fruits. There is a wide spread belief that if a pregnant woman eats more, her baby will be big and delivery would be difficult. Certain foods are forbidden as being harmful to the child. There are certain beliefs about hot and cold foods, light or heavy foods. Some families avoid certain combinations of foods due to superstitious beliefs.

CAUSES OF NUTRITIONAL DEFICIENCY

- Inadequate ingestion,
- Inadequate absorption,
- Inadequate utilization,
- Increased excretion,
- Increased requirement,
- Increased destruction.

Any one or combination of these may result in nutritional deficiency.

Religion: It has a powerful influence on the food habits of the people. Hindus do not eat beef and Muslims pork. Some orthodox Hindus and Jains do not eat meat, fish, eggs and certain vegetables like onion. These are known as food taboos which prevent people from consuming nutritious foods even when, these are easily available. Fasts do not harm healthy individual. They may be of benefit to the richer members of a community but impair the health of people whose day to day food consumption is limited by inadequate supplies or low purchasing power.

In Ethiopia, there are over 100 fast days during the year in which the intake of energy, protein and other nutrients are restricted among vulnerable groups.

Food Fads: Irrational views and prejudices about food are not confined only to developing countries. Food myths, fads and fallacies are held tenaciously in all communities.

The food fads may stand in the way of correcting nutritional deficiencies.

SOME FADS AND FALLACIES

Green leafy vegetable should not be bought during night.
Non-vegetarian foods should not be taken on Saturday/Friday.
Bitter gourd should not be consumed on Friday.
Curd should not be eaten in the nights.
Juice is not be given during cold.
During fever curds should not be taken.
Fish and curd in combination should not be taken.
Snake gourd and egg taken together can lead to instataneous death.
Onion and garlic should not be eaten on puja days.
Papaya and sesame balls should not be given to pregnant ladies.

Miscellaneous: Draining away the rice water at the end of cooking, prolonged boiling in open pans, peeling of vegetables, all influence the nutritive value of foods.

The nutritional status of the child is influenced by premature curtailment of breast feeding, the adoption of bottle feeding and adoption of commercially produced refined foods.

In some communities men eat first and women eat last and poorly. When resources are limited, priority is given to boys than girls. Consequently the health of women and girls is affected. Chronic alcoholism may lead to serious malnutrition not only in the concerned person but also indirectly in the whole family. Most Indian women continue the same nutritional intake during pregnancy as before thus affecting both their health and their child's health.

Nutritional Services

The health sector if properly not organised and not given adequate resources the community may suffer from malnutrition. Some of the aspects that can be taken up by health sector are:

Nutritional surveillance: It implies the continuous monitoring in a community or area of factors or conditions which indicate the nutritional status of individuals or groups of people (WHO, 1976). The first task is to identify the groups and individuals affected — through clinical examination and simple body measurements of persons attending health centers and hospitals. A further step is to carry out surveys in the villages. The data will give a more realistic picture of the nutritional status of the community.

Nutritional rehabilitation: Children suffering from severe PEM with complications need urgent care, may be in a hospital. Less severely affected children can be treated on a domiciliary basis or in special nutrition rehabilitation centres. These centres should be linked with health centers.

Nutrition supplementation: The target groups are mothers and children. Supplementary feeding is normally regarded as a stop-gap measure for the rehabilitation of malnourished children.

In the case of the distribution of folic acid and iron tablets in the last 100 days of pregnancy, it has been found that there is only 20 per cent coverage of the scheme. Thus most women receive half or not even half of what they are expected to consume. Food and medicines supply is erratic and insufficient besides being of poor quality.

Under Bal Parivar Mitra the following nutritional services are given:

+ Concentrating on 'at risk' families
+ Improving registration of pregnancy
+ Encouraging cousumption of IFA tablets and colostrum
+ Feeding vitamin A supplementation
+ Use of ORS in diarrhoea and
+ Use of iodised salt

Health and nutrition education: It is opined that by appropriate educational action, about 50 per cent of nutritional problems can be solved. Health education programme in nutrition is often a weak component. Its reinforcement is a key element in all health services development.

Experience of what constitutes a good diet is passed from one generation to another. The situation is very different when a family moves into a city. Many customary foods are not available. New and strange foods are present in the markets and shops. The housewife may receive false or misleading information from advertisements and shopkeepers. Ignorance of the nutritional value of foods is widespread, especially in the rapidly growing urban population in developing countries. This is responsible for much nutritional disease especially in young children.

Important points on which education is frequently needed include proper choice of foods and methods of cooking vegetables, the nutritional value of fish, the deleterious effects of overmilled cereals, the value of vegetable gardens and the special needs of children for milk, fruit juices and sunlight.

In prosperous countries, ignorance leads to faulty food habits which certainly contribute to the onset of obesity and diabetes and probably to degenerative disorders.

AGENT

The nutrient, due to its natural properties may cause malnutrition in some individuals. Due to improper processing or refining nutrients like thiamin may be lost. Water soluble vitamin cannot be stored and need to be replenished constantly. Loss of nutrient may take place during cooking due to oxidation or leaching. Micro nutrients like iodine and fluorine if not present in the water endemic deficiency diseases can occur.

Public Distribution System (PDS) designed to make food accessible to the poorer groups must be further reinforced so that its benefits percolate to the lower economic brackets, ensuring a more equitable distribution and restricting it to the really needy groups. Fortification of food with micro nutrients can prevent malnutrition.

Initiatives to improve Nutritional status of the population during the last five decades.

- Increasing food production – building up buffer stocks.
- Improving food distribution – building up PDS.
- Improving household food security through
  - * improving purchasing power
  - * food for work programme
  - * direct and indirect food subsidy
- Food supplementation to address special needs of vulnerable groups – ICDS, midday meals
- Nutrition education through ICDS
- Efforts of the health sector to tackle
  - * adverse health consequences of undernutrition
  - * adverse effects of infection on nutritional status
  - * micro nutrient deficiencies and their health consequences.

INDICES RELATED TO UNDER NUTRITION OF ADULTS

Index of ill-health

- Adults with BMI < 18.5 have reduced VO_2 max, reduced capacity for sustained heavy work and a lower productivity.
- Pregnant women show a proportional increase in the risk of an underweight baby born in relation to post partum BMI as BMI range from 25 to 16 or less.
- Progressively greater proportions of time are spent off work or in bed ill when BMI levels are below 17 in men and women.
- There is a progressive curvilinear increase in mortality in groups of men with BMI ranging from 18.5 to below 16.0.
- Immunological deficits are seen particularly in men with low BMI concomitant micro nutrient deficiencies are present.

State of Chronic Energy Deficiency

- Low BMI signifies low body energy stores.
- BMI falls seasonally in relation to energy imbalances induced by food shortages and/or increased seasonal demands of agricultural work.

The unequal division of labour and resources in families and communities jeopardise the well being of both children and women.

Action against malnutrition is both imperative and possible. Policies for combating micronutrient malnutrition must be firmly rooted in food based rather than drug based approaches.

WORLD DECLARATION AND PLAN OF ACTION FOR NUTRITION

The International Conference of Nutrition (ICN) adopted World Declaration and Plan of Action for Nutrition and this has proven to be a global instrument for guiding the countries and international communities in evolving strategies to combat malnutrition.

The Declaration points to poverty and lack of education as root causes of malnutrition in the least developed countries and emphasises the need for major universal policy change, if malnutrition is to be radically reduced. The nine decade goals and nine action oriented strategies of the World Declaration and Plan of Action for Nutrition are summarised as follows:

World Declaration on Nutrition

As a basis for the Plan of Action for Nutrition and guidance for formulation of national plans of action, including the development of measurable goals and objectives within time frames, the Ministers and Plenipotentiaries pledge to make all efforts to eliminate before the end of this decade:

- famine and famine-related deaths;
- starvation and nutritional deficiency diseases in communities affected by natural and man-made disasters;
- iodine and vitamin A deficiencies;

They also pledged to reduce substantially within this decade:

- starvation and widespread chronic hunger;
- under nutrition, especially among children, women and the aged;
- other important micronutrient deficiencies, including iron;
- diet related, communicable and non-communicable diseases;
- social and other impediments to optimal breastfeeding;
- inadequate sanitation and poor hygiene, including unsafe drinking water.

Plan of Action for Nutrition

- incorporating nutritional objectives, considerations and components into development policies and programmes;
- improving household food security;
- protecting consumers through improved food quality and safety;
- preventing and managing infectious diseases;
- promoting breastfeeding;
- caring for the socio-economically deprived and nutritionally vulnerable
- preventing and controlling specific micronutrient deficiencies;
- promoting appropriate diets and healthy lifestyles;
- assessing, analysing and monitoring nutrition situations.

India is a signatory to this World Declaration. The genesis of the National Nutrition Policy (promulgated by Government of India in 1993) lies in this Rome Declaration.

According to NNMB (Technical report no.18) data from all the states indicated that the intake of cereals and millets has declined from 505 g in 1975–1979 to 450 g /cu/day in 1996–97. While the reduction of cereal intake with better socio-economic status has been observed earlier, an improvement in the intakes of protective foods also occur simultaneously. There was improvement only in intake of green leafy and other vegetables.

Inspite of no positive changes in the dietary status, there was an improvement in the nutritional status of pre-school children (1–5 years). In most of the states, there was an increase in percentage of normal children and a decrease in the severe grade under nutrition. The prevalence of CED decreased over the period with concomitant increase in the prevalence of over weight among adult males and females. There was also reduction in the prevalence of clinical malnutrition like oedema, marasmus, vitamin A deficiency and B-complex deficiency signs among pre-school children.

The improvement in nutritional status despite no change in overall food intakes at the household level may be due to changes in non-nutritional factors such as improved water supply, reduction in infections, nutrition interventions and better health care.

World Food Day is celebrated on 16th October.

QUESTIONS

1. Explain the prevalence of malnutrition among preschool children.
2. Discuss the ecological factors of malnutrition.
3. Explain how nutrient (agent) itself is responsible for malnutrition.
4. Explain the policies of world declaration and plan of action for nutrition.
5. What type of nutrition education would you give to mothers "who are in Poverty amongst plenty"?
6. Enumerate the superstitious beliefs practiced in our community.
7. What is vicious cycle of poverty?
8. What is food security? Explain at national, community and household level.
9. One of the reasons for malnutrition is poor health services. What kind of services should we have to improve the nutritional status?
10. How is population growth related to malnutrition?
11. Write notes on the interrelationship between nutrition and health.

SUGGESTED READINGS

- Rajagopalan, S, 2001, Perspective plan of Human Development, Proc. Nutr. Soc. India, **49**.
- Bellamy Carol, 2003, The state of the world's children UNICEF.

CHAPTER 7

PROTEINS

Dietary protein performs all three functions of nutrients. It is needed for growth, maintenance and repair of body tissue; it regulates key processes within the body and any excess protein can be used as source of energy.

The term protein, meaning "to take first place" was introduced by the Dutch chemist Mulder in 1838. He defined protein as a nitrogen-containing constituent of food and felt life was impossible without it.

About 50 per cent of protein is present in muscle, 20 per cent in bone, 10 per cent in skin and the rest is present in other parts of the body.

CHEMICAL COMPOSITION

All proteins are synthesised from amino acid molecules and 20 different amino acids are used in protein synthesis, although a protein can contain many hundreds of aminoacid units (or residues) over all. All the amino acids used in protein synthesis contain carbon, hydrogen, oxygen and nitrogen atoms and cysteine and methionine contain sulphur atom. Unlike carbohydrates and lipids proteins contain nitrogen. The percentage composition of protein in general falls between the following limits:

$$C = 50 - 55; \quad H = 6.0 - 7.3; \quad O = 19 - 24; \quad N = 15 - 19; \quad S = 0 - 4$$

All amino acids contain an amino group (NH_2) a carboxyl group (COOH) and a hydrogen atom (H) attached to central carbon atom, which is also bonded to the side chain or side group of the amino acid. Figure 7a shows general structure of amino acid.

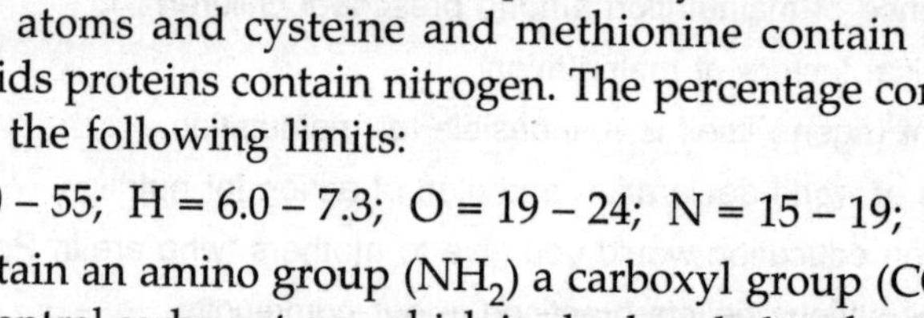

Figure 7a. General structure of amino acid.

PROPERTIES

Amphoteric nature: Like amino acids, proteins are ampholites, that is, they act on both acids and bases. Since proteins have electric charges, they migrate in an electric field, the direction of migration depending on the net charge on the molecule. For each protein, there is a pH at which the positive and negative charges will be equal and protein will not move in an electric field. The pH is known as the isoelectric point of the protein.

Solubility: Each protein has a definite and characteristic solubility in a solution of known salt concentration and pH. Albumins are soluble in water. Globulins are soluble in neutral sodium chloride solutions but are almost insoluble in water.

Some proteins like casein are soluble in alkaline pH. The differences in the solubility are made use of in the separation of proteins from a mixture.

Colloidal nature of protein solutions: Proteins have large molecular weights and protein solutions are colloids. They do not pass through semi-permeable membranes. This property of proteins is of great physiological importance.

CLASSIFICATION

Depending on the chemical composition proteins are classified as given in Table 7.1.

Table 7.1: Classification of proteins

Protein	Characteristics	Example or Occurrence
Globular		
Albumins	Soluble in water, dilute salt solutions, dilute acids, and bases. Coagulated by heat.	Lactalbumin, egg albumin, serum albumin
Globulins	Soluble in salt solutions, insoluble in water.	Serum albumin, arachin and conarchin of peanuts, myosin
Histones	Basic proteins. Soluble in most common solvents, fairly small molecules.	Nucleoprotein
Fibrous (scleroproteins)		
Collagens	Resistant to digestive enzymes; insoluble, converted to digestible proteins and gelatins on boiling; contain large amount of hydroxyproline; lack sulfur containing amino acids.	Skin, tendons, bones
Elastins	Partially resistant to digestive enzymes; contain little hydroxyproline	Arteries, tendons, elastic tissues
Keratin	Highly insoluble and resistant to digestive enzymes; high cystine content	Skin, hair, nails.
Proteids - Conjugated Proteins		
Nucleoproteins	Salts or basic protein or polypeptide and nucleic acids	Chromosomes, nucleoli
Mucoproteins	Protein or small polypeptide containing mucopolysaccharide; hexosamine less than 4%	Glycoid of serum alpha globulin; submaxillary and gastric mucoids.
and Glycoproteins	Protein or small polypeptide containing mucopolysaccharide; hexosamine less than 4%	Serum alpha, beta, and gamma globulins

Contd...

Protein	Characteristics	Example or Occurrence
Lipoproteins and	Complexes of protein and lipids having solubility properties of proteins.	Cell and organelle membranes
Proteolipids	Complexes of protein and lipids having solubility properties of lipids.	Myelin
Chromoproteins	Compounds consisting of proteins and a nonprotein pigment	Flavoproteins, hemoglobin cytochromes
Metalloproteins	Metals attached to protein; metals not part of a non-protein prosthetic group	Ferritin, Hemosiderin, Transferrin, Carbonic anhydrase
Phosphoproteins	Phosphoric acid joined in ester linkage to protein	Casein of milk

Source: Pike Ruth L and Myrtle L. Brown, 1975, Nutrition-an integrated approach, John Wiley and Sons, Inc., New York.

NUTRITIONAL CLASSIFICATION OF PROTEINS

Nutritional classification of proteins depending on the quality are classified as follows :

Table 7.2: Nutritional classification of Proteins

Group	Limiting essential amino acids
● **Complete proteins** e.g., egg proteins promote good growth in rats and other animals	Nil
● **Partially complete** proteins wheat proteins: promote moderate growth	Partially lacking in one or more essential amino acids
● **Incomplete proteins** e.g., gelatin or zein. Do not promote growth.	Completely lacking in one or more essential amino acids.

Higher quality protein produces a faster growth rate. Such growth rate measurements evaluate the actual factors important in a protein. Pattern and abundance of essential amino acids, relative amounts of non-essential and essential amino acids, digestibility and presence of trypsin inhibitors – all affect the quality of proteins and in turn affect the growth rate.

NUTRITIONAL CLASSIFICATION OF AMINO ACIDS

Essential amino acids

Essential amino acids are ones that cannot be synthesised by the body at a rate sufficient to meet the needs for growth and maintenance.

The human body has certain limited powers of converting one amino acid into another. This is achieved in the liver by the process of transamination, whereby an amino group is shifted from one molecule across to another under the influence of amino transferases, the co-enzyme of which is pyridoxal phosphate. Inability to synthesise the carbon skeleton of these amino acids is the probable reason why they are dietary essentials. Table 7.3 shows 9 out of 20 amino acids are classified as essential amino acids.

Non-essential amino acids

Non-essential amino acids are ones that the body can make in adequate amounts if nitrogen is available in the diet. They are nonessential only in the sense that they are not essential components of the diet.

Conditionally essential amino acids

These are needed in the diet unless abundant amounts of their precursors are available for their synthesis. The new born may not have enzymes in adequate amounts to synthesise nonessential amino acid. Or in intestinal metabolic dysfunction arginine may not be synthesised. Hence it becomes conditionally essential amino acid. Amino nitrogen is not freely interchanged between all amino acids. The precursors of conditionally essential amino acids are given in Table 7.4.

Classified list of amino acids is given in Table 7.3.

Table 7.3: List of essential and non-essential amino acids

Essential amino acids	Conditionally essential amino acids	Nonessential amino acids
Histidine	Arginine	Alanine
Isoleucine	Cysteine	Asparagine
Leucine	Glycine	Aspartic acid
Lysine	Proline	Glutamic acid
Methionine	Tyrosine	Glutamine
Phenylalanine		Glutamine
Threonine		Serine
Tryptophan		
Valine		

Table 7.4: Precursors of conditionally essential amino acids

Amino acid	Precursors
Cysteine	Methionine, serine
Tyrosine	Phenylalanine
Arginine	Glutamine/glutamate, aspartate
Proline	Glutamate
Glycine	Serine, Choline

FUNCTIONS

Virtually every biochemical reaction within the body is catalysed by a protein enzyme. All structural tissues of the body contain protein, so the importance of proteins to all aspects of life cannot be overemphasised.

Growth and Maintenance of Tissue

New growth, including the building of muscles, can occur only when an appropriate mixture of amino acids is available over and above the amount needed for the maintenance and repair of existing tissue. The vital process of cell division is also dependent on proteins. Specific proteins form the intracellular scaffolding or cytoskeleton that is involved in moving the contents of the dividing cell, especially the chromosomes containing the genes and distributing them properly between the two new cells being formed. One sixth of the wet cell mass is contributed by proteins.

The structural matrix or frame work, within bones and teeth is composed of protein molecules, particularly the protein known as collagen. Collagen is also the main protein within tendons and ligaments and it is the intercellular material that binds cells together.

The contractile fibres of muscles are composed of two kinds of protein, actin and myosin, which slide past one another in a process powered by the hydrolysis of adenosine triphosphate to allow muscle to contract.

Proteins are continually degraded and then resynthesised in a process known as protein turnover which is 0.3 to 0.4 per cent of body protein. Body reuses most of the amino acids released by the break down of proteins. Protein is lost from the skin, hair and nails which are constantly shed from the body's surface. Protein is also lost from the continuously shed intestinal wall cells that are excreted in faeces. In addition to the need to replace proteins during turnover, proteins must also be synthesized for the repair of damaged tissue.

Formation of Essential Body Compounds

Enzymes, including those responsible for digestion are proteins. Many of the hormones such as insulin, gastrin and growth hormone produced by various glands in the body are proteins or peptides. Hormones regulate metabolic functions of a cell. They also control very important biological functions like reproduction. Epinephrine a hormone secreted by the adrenal gland is derived from the amino acid tyrosine. Glycoproteins have specific binding function for thyroxine and cortisol .

The oxygen molecules needed to oxidise food molecules during respiration are transported through the blood by the protein haemoglobin. Almost all of the substances responsible for clotting of blood are proteins. The photoreceptors in the eye, which initiate the nerve signals responsible for the sense of vision when they absorb light are proteins. The amino acid tryptophan serves as the precursor for the vitamin niacin and for serotonin, a vital neurotransmitter that is involved in transmitting nerve signals from one nerve cell to another.

Contractile proteins, myosin and actin regulate muscle contraction.

Transport of Nutrients

Proteins play an essential role in the transport of nutrients from the intestine across the intestinal wall to the blood, from the blood to the tissues of the body and across the membranes of the cells of the tissues. These transport and membrane bound carrier proteins are usually specific to one nutrient. Retinol binding protein, for example, binds to and transports only retinol. But some like metallothione, transports both copper and zinc ions. Lipoproteins can transport many different lipid molecules.

Regulation of Water Balance

Fluid in the body is distributed in intracellular and extracellular compartments. The extracellular is divided into the intercellular (between the cells) and intravascular (within the blood vessels) compartments. The balance between the compartments is achieved by dissolved proteins and dissolved ions (electrolytes) primarily sodium and potassium ions. Protein molecules in the blood that are too large to pass out of the blood into the intercellular space exert an oncotic pressure, drawing water from the intercellular space back into the blood. A hydrostatic pressure, pushing fluid in the opposite direction out of the blood and into the intercellular space is also always present because of the pumping action of the heart. When the level of protein in the blood is low, the hydrostatic pressure dominates and pushes fluid out of the blood. This causes accumulation of fluid within the tissues resulting in oedema.

Maintenance of Appropriate pH

Normal processes of the body continually produce acids and bases that must be carried by the blood to the organs of excretion. Acidosis or alkalosis can cause death.

Proteins in the blood serve as buffers. They can combine with both hydrogen ions and hydroxide ions if the concentration of either of these determinants of the pH should rise.

Defense and Detoxification

The body's ability to fight off infection depends on its immune system which has defensive proteins known as antibodies. Specific antibody is required for specific antigen. Whenever required, the body produces antibodies quickly.

The toxins present in foods are detoxified by enzymes found mainly in liver which convert them into harmless substances.

Source of Energy

Though proteins can also provide 4 kcal energy per gram like carbohydrates, they are used for energy purpose only when the diet has inadequate carbohydrate and fat.

SPECIFIC FUNCTIONS OF AMINO ACIDS

Glycine: It is needed during periods of rapid growth. Biological systems incorporate glycine molecule into purines, glutathione, creatine and creatinine, bile acids, hippuric acid and serine. It is also essential for biosynthesis of porphyrin ring of haemoglobin. Many aromatic substances whether produced endogenously or consumed as drugs or food additives are conjugated in the liver with glycine and excreted in the bile or urine.

Glutamic acid: Glutamic acid, cysteine and glycine are components of glutathione, which functions in cellular oxidation reduction reactions. It plays an important role in the metabolism of ammonia. It is a precursor of the neurotransmitter, γ-amino butyric acid in brain.

Arginine: Cleavage of arginine results in the formation of urea in the liver. It is a precursor amino acid for neurotransmitters.

Lysine: It is the parent substance of carnitine, which transports fatty acids within the mito-chondria.

Methionine and Cysteine: Present in the keratin of hair and in insulin.

- Involved in transmethylation.
- Cysteine is a component of glutathione.
- Fatty liver can be cured by methionine or choline which is formed from it.
- Methionine protects the liver from damage by poisons such as carbon tetrachloride, arsenic and chloroform.
- Taurine conjugated with bile acids, is derived from the metabolism of cysteine.

Phenylalanine and Tyrosine: For foetal and childhood brain development, these amino acids are required.

- Epinephrine and thyroxine are synthesised from tyrosine.
- This helps in the synthesis of melanin pigment in hair, choroid lining of the eye and in the skin.

Histidine: It is found in the muscle constituent carnosine.

- It is probably a precursor of the red blood cell constituent ergothioneine. It is present to the extent of 8 per cent in haemoglobin.
- Converted to histamine; it is a stimulus for acid secretion in the stomach. Histamine is also involved in allergic reaction.

Tryptophan: Milk is a good source of tryptophan.

- Nicotinic acid is synthesised from tryptophan.
- Precursor of serotonin (5-hydroxytryptamine) which causes vaso constriction. When blood clot occurs, platelets, release 5-hydroxy tryptamine which prevents bleeding by causing vasoconstriction. 5-hydroxytryptamine is also a neurotransmitter.

Proline and Hydroxy Proline: It has same ring structure is found in porphyrin.

- It is present in haemoglobin and cytochromes.
- Prevalent in the collagen of connective tissue.

Leucine, isoleucine and valine: These are branched-chain amino acids.

- In the muscle they are oxidized and the nitrogen is used for the formation of alanine.

DIGESTION AND ABSORPTION

The hydrolysis of proteins in the gastro-intestinal tract is accomplished by proteases secreted in gastric juice and pancreatic juice and also by proteases present in the intestinal mucosa.

Gastric digestion: Proteins are denatured by the acid in the stomach. The proteolytic enzyme present in gastric juice is pepsin. The optimum pH is about 2.0. Pepsin is an endopeptidase and it can hydrolyse peptide bonds in the interior of the protein molecule. It hydrolyses mainly peptide bonds containing phenylalanine, tyrosine or tryptophan and also peptide bonds containing leucine and acidic amino acids. Since food remains in the stomach for a limited time, pepsin hydrolyses dietary proteins mainly into a mixture of polypeptides.

If gastric HCl production is low and not adequate to maintain the pH of the stomach contents between 2 and 3, protein digestion in the stomach may be negligible.

Proteolysis in the Intestines: The main digestion of polypeptides produced in the stomach takes place in the intestines. The proteases involved in the digestion are trypsin, chymotrypsin and carboxy peptidase secreted in pancreatic juice and amino peptidases present in the intestinal mucosa. Trypsin and chymotrypsin act at pH 7.4 to 8.0. Trypsin hydrolyses mainly peptide linkages containing arginine or lysine and chymotrypsin hydrolyses, peptide linkages containing tyrosine or phenylalanine.

Carboxy peptidase A: It hydrolyses the end group in peptides containing aromatic or aliphatic amino acid, thus releasing free amino acids. Carboxy peptidase B hydrolyses peptides containing arginine and lysine residues. The intestinal mucosa contains a group of amino peptides which complete the hydrolysis of peptides to amino acids. The intestinal mucosa also contains tripeptidase, dipeptidase etc., which hydrolyse tri and dipeptides.

Absorption of amino acids: Absorption of amino acids takes place in the small intestines. This process requires energy.

The basic amino acids lysine, arginine and histidine share a carrier system with cystine. The dependence of amino acid transport on Na ion suggests a direct interaction between the carrier and Na ion. This is similar to that observed in the absorption of glucose.

According to the available information, the amino acid associates with the carrier and Na ion in the microville and the complex travels to the inner side of the membrane where it dissociates, releasing the amino acid and Na ion into the cytoplasm. The carrier returns back and functions repeatedly. The Na ion is then actively transported out of the cell.

Digestibility of protein: The digestibility of protein varies from food to food and affects protein quality profoundly. The protein of oats, for example, is less digestible than that of eggs. Generally, animal proteins are most easily digested and absorbed over 90 per cent. Those from legumes are digested about 80 percent. Those from grains and other plant foods vary from 60–90 per cent. Cooking with moist heat generally improves protein digestibility, whereas dry heat methods can impair it.

Factors Affecting Protein Utilisation

Amino Acid Balance: An excess of one amino acid may in certain circumstances, reduce the total nutritive value. It is now recognized that relative amino acid requirements vary with age. Therefore the value of the pattern of amino acids in a specific food or diet towards promoting growth will vary considerably depending on a person's age. It is the ratio of the amino acid to nitrogen in a food relative to the ratio of the need for that amino acid to nitrogen that determine how useful a particular protein is in meeting the protein requirement. Therefore a protein may have an amino acid pattern that meets the needs of one age group, while it may be relatively limited in meeting the needs of another age group.

Calorie intake: The protein content of the diet cannot be evaluated without consideration of the adequacy of the calorie intake. When the calorie intake drops below a certain critical point, protein will be deaminated and used as a source of energy and cannot be used for the synthesis of tissues.

Immobility: The ability to synthesise protein is greatly reduced among people who are immobile. Elderly who are bedridden lose protein mass even when dietary protein and energy seem adequate. There has been a similar problem among astronauts, who lose protein as a result of both weightlessness and immobility in space flight.

Injury: An increase in nitrogen loss after injury is well documented. High protein intakes either before or after injury do not prevent this loss. However, losses are recovered more rapidly once healing begins.

Emotional stability: Emotional stresses such as fear, anxiety or anger increase the secretion of epinephrine from the adrenal gland, which in turn causes a series of changes that result in the loss of nitrogen. Students lose nitrogen under the stress of exams. Other stresses that can result in nitrogen loss are severe pain, emotional anxiety, reversal of biological rhythms caused by night shift work, extreme cold and jet travel across time zones.

QUALITY OF PROTEINS

The nutritive value of a protein depends to an important degree on the relation of amino acids in its molecule to those required for building new tissues. If the amino acid composition of a food substance meets the amino acid composition of a tissue, the food protein is of a high quality.

Quality of protein is affected by the amino acid content, amino acid imbalance, interference of non-available carbohydrates and trypsin inhibitors and influence of heating and processing.

In 1915, American nutritionist Mendel divided proteins into two classes; those which when fed to rats "allowed growth" and those with which there was "failure of growth". A relative lack of a particular amino acid can cause failure in synthesis of tissues. In any protein the amino acid which is furthest below the standard is known as the limiting amino acid. Inadequacy of even a single essential amino acid will grossly interfere with body protein synthesis. Tryptophan is the limiting amino acid in maize protein, lysine in wheat protein and the sulphur containing amino acids methionine and cysteine in beef and legume protein.

BIOLOGICAL ASSAYS

Digestibility coefficient: The term digestibility coefficient of protein refers to the percentage of the ingested protein absorbed into the blood stream after the process of digestion is complete.

$$\text{Digestibility coefficient} = 100 \times \frac{\text{N intake} - (\text{N in faeces} - \text{endogenous faecal N})}{\text{Nitrogen intake}}$$

$$= 100 \times \frac{I - (F - Fm)}{I}$$

Where F—Fm is the food nitrogen lost in digestion.

Biological Value

This was developed by Mitchell in 1925. Biological value of a protein is measured as the percentage of absorbed nitrogen that is retained for use in growth or maintenance.

$$\text{Biological value} = \frac{\text{Retained nitrogen}}{\text{Absorbed nitrogen}} \times 100$$

Two groups of 28 days old albino rats are used. One group is fed on non protein diet while the other group is fed on test diet containing 10 per cent protein for 10 days.

The protein to be tested is fed to the animal as the sole source of nitrogen in the diet and below the level needed for maintenance.

The diet, urine, faeces are analysed for nitrogen.

$$\text{Biological value} = \frac{\text{Nitrogen digested} - \text{Nitrogen lost in metabolism}}{\text{Nitrogen digested}} \times 100$$

$$= \frac{I - (F - F_m) - (U - U_e)}{I - (F - F_m)} \times 100$$

where, I, F, U are dietary, faecal and urinary nitrogen on the test diet F_m and U_e are faecal and urinary nitrogen on a protein free diet.

This indicator is based on the assumption that more nitrogen is retained when the essential amino acids are present in sufficient amounts to meet the needs for growth. A food with a biological value of 70 or more is considered capable of supporting growth. The higher the biological value the better is the quality of the dietary protein.

The determination of biological value ascertains the differences on proteins due to processing alterations. Biological value determinations can be conducted with animals in various physiological states such as pregnancy, lactation and growth in order to examine the effectiveness of a protein to meet demands during these altered conditions.

Animals on protein-free diet often do not consume sufficient feed to maintain their body weight. Endogenous nitrogen losses may thus be over estimated due to the catabolism of tissue protein of these animals. It has been suggested that this error may be overcome by feeding diets containing 4 to 5 per cent protein from a source assumed to be totally utilised by the control animals.

Oreyer noted that the amount of nitrogen retained by an animal on the absolute basis is proportional to the amount needed for maintenance and growth and that excess of dietary nitrogen are excreted reducing the apparent B.V. This method is laborious.

Net Protein Utilisation

The biological value makes no allowance for losses of nitrogen in digestion. This is included in the net protein utilisation.

$$\text{Net protein utilisation} = \frac{\text{Retained nitrogen}}{\text{Intake of nitrogen}} \times 100$$

Miller and Bender (1955) developed a direct method of estimating NPU. Groups of 28 day old albino rats are used. One group is fed on non-protein diet while other groups are fed on the test diets containing 10 per cent proteins for 10 days. The animals are killed at the end of 10 days. Body nitrogen is estimated by Kjeldahl method.

$$NPU = \frac{\text{Body nitrogen of the test group} - \text{Body nitrogen of the non-protein group} + \text{nitrogen consumed by non-protein group}}{\text{Nitrogen consumed by test group}}.$$

This is equal to BV x availability. NPU can be calculated from nitrogen balance data in man.

NPU standard or NPU[st] refers to determinations of NPU when proteins are fed at minimum requirements or on below requirements. NPU operative, or NPUop refers to the utilisation of a protein under those conditions in which it is actually eaten. The efficiency and concentration of a protein may be combined in a single index, called the Net Dietary Protein Value, NDpV.

The expression is the product of protein concentration and NPU.

To measure both the quantity and quality of the protein in a diet the net dietary protein value NDpV in used.

$$NDpV = \text{Intake of Nitrogen} \times 6.25 \times \text{NPUop}.$$

Net Dietary Protein Energy Ratio

It is often convenient to express the protein content of a food in terms of the percentage of the energy content provided by protein. The protein content of a diet can be similarly expressed and an additional factor given for the quality of the mixed protein.

$$\text{Net dietary protein energy ratio} = \frac{\text{Protein energy}}{\text{Net dietary intake}} \times \text{NPUop}.$$

The NPU of different protein sources ranges from approximately 40 to 94 with the animal protein sources near the top and that from vegetable protein sources near the lower end. The average Indian diet has NPU of 65.

NPU measurements like BV which consider only one intake level and zero, tend to overestimate the nutritional quality of some proteins. The best biological estimates of protein quality are provided by the slope of the intake response line from several points in the range of intakes where the line is linear, it should not include zero protein intake. If carcass N retentions in animals are used in this way, the index is the relative nutritive value and the line of the test protein is related to a standard.

Protein Efficiency Ratio

Protein efficiency ratio is defined as the weight gain per gram of protein intake.

This method was developed by Osborne, Mendel and Ferry in 1919 and is based on the growth of young rats. Groups of Albino rats are fed for a period of 4 weeks on different protein diets at 10 per cent protein. Records of the gain in body weight and protein intake of rats are maintained.

$$PER = \frac{\text{Gain in weight (g)}}{\text{Protein intake (g)}}$$

= gain in weight per g protein consumed.

Table 7.5 shows PER of different proteins.

Table 7.5: PER of different proteins

Diet	Protein intake in 4 Weeks g	Gain in body weight in 4 weeks g	PER
Egg hen	28	132	4.7
Wheat flour	26	40	1.5
Gelatin	20	−4	−0.2

Source : Swaminathan, M., 1989, Essentials of Food and Nutrition, BAPCO, Bangalore.

This method has been very useful in comparing a new protein source against reference protein such as egg protein and does evaluate other factors such as relative digestibility.

The test has some serious limitations.

- The PER is not a true efficiency ratio because not all the protein is used for growth only that consumed above maintenance.
- It varies with the food intake.
- The calorie intake must be adequate. Proteins should not be at excessive level since at high levels of dietary protein, weight gain does not increase proportionately with the protein intake.
- The greatest source of error in the PER method lies in the use of weight gain as the sole criterion of protein value. Weight gain cannot be assumed to represent proportional gain in body protein under all conditions.

In terms of speed of operation and expenses, however, the PER method is advantageous.

Net Protein Ratio

This method was introduced by Bender and Doell (1957). It is a modification of PER method. In this method, an allowance is made for the protein requirements for maintenance.

The method consists in feeding a group of weanling rats on a diet containing 10 per cent of the test protein and another comparable control group on a nonprotein diet for a period of 10 days. The NPR is calculated by adding the loss in weight of the control group to the gain in weight of the test group and dividing the total weight (g) by the quantity of protein consumed by the test group.

$$NPR = \frac{\text{Gain in weight (g) of the test group + loss in weight (g) of the nonprotein group}}{\text{Protein intake (g) of test group}}$$

Table 7.6 compares the biological value, NPU and PER values of proteins from different food stuffs.

Table 7.6: Nutritive value of proteins of some food stuffs

Food	B.V.	NPU	PER	Limiting amino acid*
Egg	96	96	3.8	Nil
Milk	90	85	2.8	SAA
Meat	74	76	3.2	SAA
Fish	80	74	3.5	Tryp
Rice	80	77	1.7	Lys, Thr
Wheat	66	61	1.3	Lys, Thr,
Maize	50	48	1.0	Lys, Thr, Tryp
Bengalgram	74	61	1.1	SAA
Redgram	72	54	1.7	SAA, Tryp
Groundnut	55	-	-	Lys, SAA and Thr
Gingelly seeds	62	-	-	Lys

Source: Gopalan, C., B.V. Rama Sastri and S.C. Balasubramanian, 1999, Nutritive Value of Indian Foods, National Institute of Nutrition, ICMR, Hyderabad.
*Swaminathan M., 1988. Essentials of food and nutrition, Bappco. Bangalore.

SCORING SYSTEMS

Amino Acid Scores

A chemical grading of the quality of a protein can be made by comparing its amino acid content with that of a reference protein. The FAO/WHO (1973) suggested 'Amino acid pattern of reference' based on needs for each amino acid. Hen's egg protein is also recommended as reference protein because egg proteins contain all essential amino acids in adequate amounts. Chromatographic, chemical and microbiological methods are used for estimating the amino acid content of proteins.

$$\text{Amino acid score} = \frac{\text{mg of amino acid in 1 g test protein}}{\text{mg of amino acid in 1 g reference protein}}$$

The score should be calculated for all the essential amino acids using the above formula and the lowest score is taken. In practice, the scores need to be calculated only for lysine, the sulphur-containing amino acids and tryptophan, as one or other of these, is the limiting amino acid in common foods. The chemical score is the ratio between the content of the most limiting amino acid in the test protein to the content of the same amino acid in egg protein expressed as a percentage.

Although there is a good correlation between amino acid score and biological value for a protein with a BV > 0.4, the relationship varies with the limiting amino acid below the level.

Chemical scores of foods are as follows: eggs-100; meat-70; liver-66; milk cow-65; fish-60; rice-60; soyabean-57; Bengal gram-44; groundnuts-44; wheat-42; sesame-40; and gelatin-0.

PDCAAS

The WHO and the US FDA adopted Protein Digestibility Corrected Amino Acid Score (PDCAAS) as the official assay for evaluating protein quality.

The PDCAAS is based on amino acid requirements of children aged 2–5 years estimated by FAO. This represents the amino acid score after correcting for digestibility. Proteins that after correcting for digestibility, provide amino acids equal to or in excess of requirements receive a PDCAAS of 1.0. Soya protein has PDCAAS of 1.0 and meets protein needs of human adults when consumed as a sole source of protein at the rate of 0.6 g per kg body weight.

Table 7.7: PDCAAS of selected foods

Food	PDCAAS value
Soya protein	1.0
Milk powder	1.0
Casein and whey	1.0
Egg white	1.0
Beef protein	0.92
Pea protein	0.73
Rolled oats	0.57
Peanut meal	0.52
Lentils	0.52
Rice	0.47
Whole wheat	0.40

Chemical methods are the simplest and fastest and least expensive of all methods for determination of protein quality. The limiting amino acid for a protein can readily be identified by the use of scoring procedures. For the identification of limiting amino acid, an amino acid score of 1973 FAO/WHO pattern has been used.

Chemical scores are highly correlated to NPU. The amino acids may be biologically unavailable and the chemical analysis may be misleading. There is also the problem of interaction between nutrients and amino acids which may affect the quality of protein.

COMPLEMENTARY VALUE OF PROTEINS

If the protein of the diet is seriously deficient in one or more of the essential amino acids, nitrogen equilibrium cannot be sustained, no matter how complete and excellent the diet may be in other respects. If, however, another protein containing the missing amino acid in adequate amounts is added to the diet, nitrogen equilibrium and normal nutrition can be established. This capacity of proteins to make good one another's deficiencies is known as their complementary or supplementary value.

Lappe, 1971, described methods to ensure that vegetable proteins with different chemical scores complement each other to provide complete proteins. Table 7.8 gives the combinations to improve the quality of protein.

Table 7.8: Combinations of foods to improve quality of protein

Excellent combination	Example
Cereals + legumes	Idli, dosa, kichidi, chapathi channa
Cereals + milk and milk products	Payasam, paneer pulao, cheese sandwich, curd rice, pasta and cheese.
Legumes + nuts and oil seeds	Gingelly seeds or groundnut or coconut chutney with roasted bengal gram dal

Other combinations like dairy product and oil seeds or cereals and oil seeds are less effective because the chemical scores are similar and do not effectively complement each other.

Quality of dietary protein can also be improved by the addition of the limiting amino acid (fortification of wheat flour with lysine) or by developing strains with high amount of limiting amino acids. Addition of good quality proteins like meat, egg or milk or concentrated protein like fish protein concentrate can also improve the quality of protein.

Table 7.9 gives amino acid composition of foods.

Table 7.9: Amino acid composition of some foods

Food	Methion-ine	Isoleu-cine	Luecine	Lysine	Pheny-lalanine	Threo-nine	Trypto-phan	Valine
Cheese, Egg, Milk, Meat	–	√	√	√	–	√	–	√
Corn	–	–	–	–	–	–	–	–
Cereal	√	–	–	–	–	–	–	–
Legumes	–	–	–	√	–	√	–	–
Whole grains with germ	√	–	–	√	–	–	–	–
Nuts seed oils and soyabean	√	–	–	×	–	×	–	–
Seasame and Sunflower seeds	√	–	–	×	–	–	√	–
Peanuts	×	–	–	×	–	×	–	–
Gelatin	×	–	–	×	–	–	×	–

√ indicates high amount of amino acids, × indicates low amount of amino acid, – indicates general good balance of amino acids.

Source: Mahan Kathleen L, Sylvia Escott Stump, 2000, Krause's Food, Nutrition and Diet Therapy, W.B. Saunders Company, Philadelphia.

Lappe in 1991, has found that it is not necessary to consume complementary proteins at the same meal. They should be eaten within 3 to 4 hours to ensure that all amino acids are available when needed.

Ethnic cuisine with complementary protein dishes	
Rice and soyabean	– Oriental
Rice and peas	– Caribbean
Rice and dal	– Indian
Beans and tortillas	– Mexicans
Pasta and beans	– Mediterranean
Pizza	– Italian
Rice and milk	– Indian
Chickpeas with bulgar wheat	– Middleeasterners
Tofu with rice	– Asians
Blackeyed peas and rice	– Americans
Blackeyed peas and rice	– Americans
Peanut butter and bread	– Americans
Cheese and Wheat bread	– Americans
Cereal and Milk	– Americans
Wheat and bengal gram dal	– Indian

A mixed diet even solely based on plant proteins can meet the protein requirement of adults and older children, provided they consume enough of the diet to meet their energy needs.

REQUIREMENTS

For Infants: The need for protein and amino acids is estimated in there different ways for infants, children and adults. For young infants growing at a satisfactory rate, the amount of protein and the pattern of amino acids in human milk are considered appropriate for optimal growth. Therefore, recommendations for infants are based on the total protein content and amino acid pattern of the average daily intake of human milk.

For Children: Factorial method is used for children. This method involves an estimate of all the endogenous/obligatory nitrogen losses through urine, faeces and skin plus an allowance for growth.

The subject is put on a protein free diet adequate in calories and the minimum level is found at which the urinary nitrogen will fall, before the body will be depleted of nitrogen. At this point nitrogen through urine is called basal or endogenous excretion.

$$R = U + F + S + G.$$

R = Nitrogen requirements

U = Loss of endogenous nitrogen in urine

F = Loss of endogenous nitrogen in faeces

S = Loss of endogenous nitrogen in skin

G = Nitrogen requirements for growth.

For adults: For adults, nitrogen balance method is used, in which adequate energy is provided to find the requirements of protein.

The primary functions of dietary proteins are to make up the endogenous losses of nitrogen from the body and to meet the protein needs for growth, convalescence, pregnancy or lactation. Nitrogen balance is calculated by subtracting the nitrogen lost in urine, faeces and sweat from nitrogen intake.

It is estimated that the total obligatory nitrogen losses through faeces, urine and skin is 3.2 mg nitrogen/basal kilocalorie

Faeces – 0.4 mg/basal kilocalorie

Urine – 2.0 mg/basal kilocalorie

$$\left.\begin{matrix} \text{Skin/nails} \\ \text{Sweat/hair} \end{matrix}\right\} - 0.8 \text{ mg/basal kilocalorie}$$

Total – 3.2 mg/basal kilocalorie

N balance = N intake − (N in urine + N in faeces + N in sweat).

If the nitrogen lost from the body in urine, faeces and sweat is less than the nitrogen intake, the body is in positive N balance.

When the nitrogen intake equals the nitrogen lost in urine, faeces and sweat, the body is in a state of nitrogen equilibrium.

If the nitrogen lost from the body in urine, faeces, and sweat is greater than nitrogen intake, the body is in negative nitrogen balance.

Negative nitrogen balance is observed in persons suffering from under nutrition, burns, fever, injury, after surgery and in starvation and also on inadequate protein intake.

The need for protein has always been considered to be just below the lowest level of intake that results in nitrogen equilibrium and just above the highest level of intake that results in negative nitrogen balance. The nitrogen equilibrium point can be carefully determined by a series of nitrogen balance studies in which the amount of dietary protein is reduced step by step until a negative balance occurs. The intake is then increased in another series of experiments, each of which usually takes 1 to 3 weeks, until positive balance is restored. The real required intake lies between these two levels of intake. This conforms to the definition proposed by the FAO/WHO/UNU Committee on Protein and Energy requirements.

The FAO/WHO/UNU definition states that the "requirement for protein is the intake needed to prevent loss of body protein and to allow for adequate deposition or production of protein during growth, pregnancy or lactation."

There is now evidence that protein requirements should be set slightly higher to allow for the fact that even when high quality protein is being consumed, some is used as a source of energy. So not all of the amino acids absorbed are available for the synthesis of protein and other vital nitrogen containing compounds in the body.

RECOMMENDED DIETARY ALLOWANCES

An important factor in relation to defining protein needs is the quality of protein. The relative biological quality of the mixture of vegetable proteins which are present in Indian diets that are based on cereals and pulses is only about 65 compared to the 100 of egg protein.

The average daily protein requirement of an Indian adult in terms of a high quality protein like milk/egg at the physiological level is estimated to be 0.5 g/kg. When adjusted for the lower quality of dietary proteins with 65 NPU, the safe level of intake in terms of dietary proteins will be 1.0 g/kg.

During pregnancy, the safe level of intake in terms of a high quality protein during three trimesters will be 1.2, 6.0 and 10.5 respectively. After adjusting for dietary protein quality of NPU 65, the safe intake during the latter half of pregnancy recommended by the committee is 15 g/day.

During lactation, protein requirement has been computed on the basis of secretion in milk of 9.4 g protein per day during 0–6 months and 6.6 g during 6–24 months, which correspond to 820 ml and 600 ml of milk respectively with protein content of 1.15 g/100 ml. Assuming a 70 per cent efficiency of conversion of dietary protein into milk protein and a 25 per cent for individual variation with dietary protein NPU 65, the committee recommended 25 g during the first six months, 18 g during 6–12 months of lactation.

Infant protein requirement at various periods during the first year of life are derived from the breast milk intake. Protein requirements for children have been computed based on per kilogram body weight and expected gain in weight. Protein energy percent between 8 and 12 would meet the protein requirement of any group provided its energy needs are met.

ICMR Recommended Dietary Allowances of Proteins are given in Table 7.10.

Table 7.10: ICMR Recommended Dietary Allowances of Proteins

Group	Protein g/day
Man	60
Woman	50
Pregnant woman	50 + 15
Lactation	
0–6 months	50 + 25
6–12 months	50 + 18
Infancy	
0–6 months	2.05/kg
6–12 months	1.65/kg
Children	
1–3 years	22
4–6 years	30
7–9 years	41
Boys	
10–12 years	54
13–15 years	70
16–18 years	78
Girls	
10–12 years	57
13–15 years	65
16–18 years	63

SOURCES

Animal foods like meat, fish and egg and plant foods like pulses, oil seeds and nuts are good sources of protein. Milk can also be classified (though it contains 3–4 per cent) under this category as it has good quality protein and due to high content of water it can be consumed in large quantities.

Table 7.11: Protein content of foods

Animal sources	Protein g/l00g	Plant Sources	Protein g/l00g
Skimmed milk powder (Cow's milk)	38	Soyabean	43
Whole milk powder (Cow's milk)	26	Watermelon seeds	34
Fowl	26	Wheat germ	29
Cheese	24	Groundnut	25
Herring, India	20	Green gram dhal	24
Liver Goat	20	Peas, dry	20
Prawn	19	Bengal gram whole	17
Mutton	18	Wheat whole	12
Egg, Hen	13	Agathi	8
Milk Buffalo's	4	Rice	7

Soyabean is the richest source containing 40 per cent protein. Defatted oil seed cakes contain 50–60 per cent protein. Cereals and millets are moderate sources of protein as they contain about 10 per cent protein. Rice contains less protein than wheat but its quality is better. However, the cereals as they are consumed in large amounts daily contribute a considerable amount of protein to the daily intake. Leafy vegetables, fruits, roots and tubers are generally poor sources of protein as they contain less than 2 per cent protein.

QUESTIONS

1. Give the classification of proteins.
2. Give the nutritional classification of amino acids.
3. Discuss the functions of proteins.
4. Explain the specific function of the following amino acids.
    (a) Glutamic acid
    (b) Methionine
    (c) Phenylalanine
    (d) Tryptophan.
5. Explain the term 'Quality of proteins'. Discuss any four methods.
6. What is complementary value of proteins? How can you achieve this through diet?
7. Give the ICMR Recommended Dietary Allowances for proteins for different age groups.
8. Give 5 good quality of proteins.
9. List and describe the factors affecting protein requirement.
10. Define limiting amino acid.
11. What are the limitations of biological value method and protein efficiency ratio method?
12. How does animal protein differ from vegetable protein?
13. Explain the properties of proteins.

SUGGESTED READINGS

- Raghuramulu, N. *et al* (editors) 2003, A manual of laboratory techniques, National Institute of Nutrition, Hyderabad, 500 007.
- Information on 'protein' in foods : www.eatright.org.
- Laid law SA and Kopple JD, 1987, Newer concepts of the indispensable amino acids. Am J chin Nutr **46**.

CHAPTER 8

PROTEIN ENERGY MALNUTRITION

The term protein energy malnutrition covers a wide spectrum of clinical stages ranging from the severe forms like kwashiorkor and marasmus to the milder forms in which the main detectable manifestation is growth retardation. Protein energy malnutrition is due to 'food gap' between the intake and requirement. The average energy deficit in Indian children is 300 kcal/day.

The term kwashiorkor was first introduced by Cicely Williams in 1935. This is a local name used by the Ga tribe in Accra, West Africa and means "disease of the displaced child".

PREVALENCE

The prevalence rate of severe degree of PEM in our community is 3–5 per cent. For every 3–5 cases of severe PEM, we can detect 80–90 cases of mild to moderate PEM and about 10 per cent of well nourished children.

According to National Nutrition Monitoring Bureau (1988-90) the prevalence of malnutrition among 1-5 years is high. The underweight children are 68.6 per cent, while stunting is at 65.1 per cent and wasting 19.9 per cent (Figure 8a).

In more than 50 per cent of deaths in children, malnutrition is the direct or indirect cause. PEM is a silent killer in many children.

AETIOLOGY

Different combinations of many aetiological factors can lead to PEM in children.

Social and Economic Factors

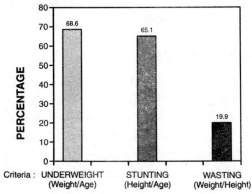

Figure 8a. Prevalence of malnutrition among children (1 to 5 years).
Source: NNMB Report of Repeat surveys (1988–90).

Poverty that results in low food availability, over crowded and unsanitary living conditions and improper child care is a frequent cause of PEM. Ignorance by itself or associated with poverty leads to poor infant and child rearing practices, misconceptions about the use of certain foods, inadequate feeding during illness and improper food distribution within the family members.

A decline in the practice and duration of breast feeding, combined with inadequate weaning practices are the important causes of PEM.

Most women in these communities work whole day and young children are looked after by older siblings. Thus the children are deprived of maternal care and attention at a critical time. High incidence of kwashiorkor has been reported in children belonging to larger families and high birth orders.

Cultural and social practices that impose food taboos and food fads are powerful social factors which influence nutritional status.

Migration from traditional rural settings to urban slums can contribute to or precipitate PEM.

Biological Factors

Maternal malnutrition prior to and/or during pregnancy is more likely to produce an underweight newborn baby. This intrauterine malnutrition can be compounded after birth by insufficient food to satisfy the infant's needs. Malnutrition can result in less enzyme synthesis and less appetite leading to less consumption of food. Diets with low concentration of proteins and energy occur with over diluted milk formulas or bulky vegetable foods that have low nutrient density. Though the child's stomach gets filled, its calorie and protein requirement cannot be met due to low density of food.

Infectious diseases are major contributing and precipitating factors of PEM. Diarrhoeal diseases, measles and respiratory and other infections result in negative protein and energy balance. This is due to anorexia, vomiting, decreased absorption and increased catabolic processes.

Intestinal parasites when extensively affected cause anemia and diarrhoea.

Environmental Factors

Over crowded and/or unsanitary living conditions lead to frequent infections like diarrhoea. Agricultural patterns, droughts, floods, earthquakes, wars and forced migrations lead to cyclic, sudden or prolonged food scarcities. Post harvest losses of food can occur due to bad storage conditions and inadequate food distribution.

Role of Free Radicals and Aflatoxins

Two new theories have been postulated recently to explain the pathogenesis of kwashiorkor. These include "free radical damage" and aflatoxin poisoning. Free oxygen radicals potentially toxic to cell membranes, are produced during various infections. These oxides are normally buffered by protein and neutralized by antioxidants such as vitamins A, C and E and selenium. In the malnourished child, deficiency of these nutrients in the presence of infection or aflatoxin may result in the accumulation of toxic free oxygen radicals. These may damage liver cells giving rise to kwashiorkor.

Age of the Host

PEM can affect all age groups but it is more frequent among infants and young children whose rapid growth increases nutritional requirement. The long term intake of insufficient food can result in marasmus before one year. Kwashiorkor is common after 18 months.

PEM in pregnant and lactating women can affect the growth, nutritional status and survival rates of their foetuses, new born and infants. Elderly can also suffer from PEM due to alteration in gastrointestinal system.

CLINICAL FEATURES

The clinical presentation depends on the type, severity and duration of the dietary deficiencies. The five forms of PEM are given in Table 8.1.

Table 8.1: Classification of PEM (FAO/WHO)

Type of PEM	Body weight as percentage of standard	Oedema	Deficit in weight for height
*Kwashiorkor	80–60	+	+
*Marasmic Kwashiorkor	<60	+	++
*Marasmus	<60	0	++
*Nutritional dwarfing	<60	0	Minimal
*Under weight child	80–60	0	+

Theory of Adaptation

Gopalan (1971) did systematic diet surveys and found that kwashiorkor and marasmic children consume similar diets. He brought out the "theory of adaptation." Marasmic child is able to adapt itself to low calorie and protein diet by producing more cortisol. Kwashiorkor child is not able to adapt itself to low calorie and protein diet because of an acute infective episode or significant quantitative reduction in the already low food intake or a qualitative change in the food consumed. Figure 8b explains the metabolic differences that lead to marasmus and kwashiorkor.

Marasmus

Child reacts to the stress of PEM and secretes cortisol, which mobilises protein from muscle and subcutaneous tissue to amino acid pool resulting in wasting with no oedema and no hepatomegaly. Raised cortisol level lowers growth hormone and so the child is stunted. Maramus is said to be well adapted to the stress of deficit in protein and calories. The signs and symptoms observed in marasmic child are the following :

- Severe growth retardation
- Loss of subcutaneous fat
- Severe muscle wasting
- The child looks appallingly thin and limbs appear as skin and bones
- Shrivelled body

- Wrinkled skin
- Bony prominence
- Associated vitamin deficiencies
- Failure to thrive
- Irritability, fretfulness and apathy
- Frequent watery diarrhoea and acid stools
- Mostly hungry but some are anorectic
- Dehydration
- Temperature is subnormal
- Muscles are weak
- Oedema and fatty infiltration are absent.

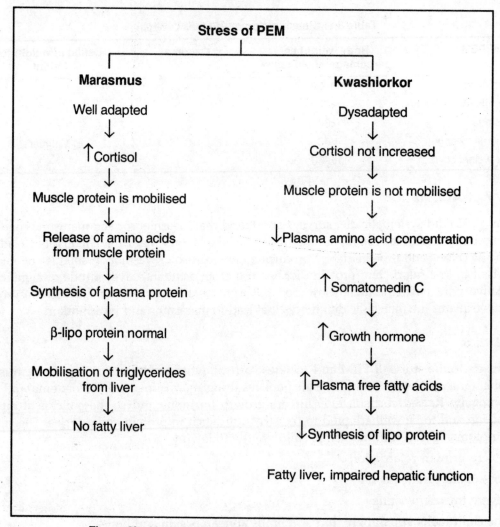

Figure 8b: Metabolic changes in marasmus and Kwashiorkor.

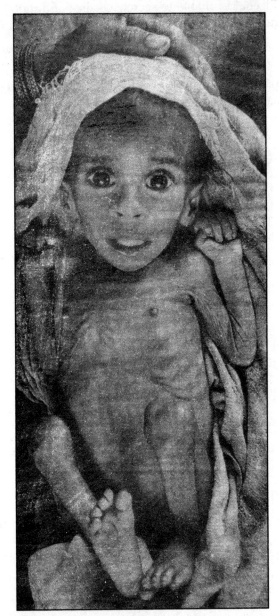

Figure 8c. Marasmic child

This child was found in Nandurbar district of Maharashtra in July, 2004. Poor accessibility, healthcare and the complete failure of the Integrated Child Development Services in the district account of severe undernutrition.

Kwashiorkor

Sometimes the child is not able to adapt to the stress of inadequate diet, infection and separation from mother due to subsequent pregnancy. (In African language 'Kwashiorkor' means the disease the elder child gets when the younger child is born).

In dysadaptation the adrenal is unable to secrete cortisol and mobilisation of protein from muscle is not possible and liver cannot synthesise β-lipo protein and fatty liver occurs.

Dysadaptation occurs and the child ultimately land up as kwashiorkor and the following symptoms appear.

- Low body weight inspite of oedema showing growth failure, and some degree of muscle wasting which is masked by oedema.

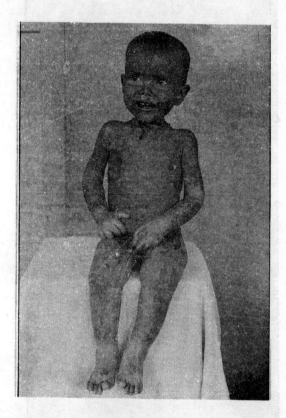

Figure 8e. Kwashiorkor child. Note irritability, changes in pigmentation of skin and oedema.

Source: *Courtesy:* National Institute of Nutrition, Hyderabad, 500 007.

- Pitting oedema appears first on the feet and legs and later spreads to the whole body. The face looks puffy with sagging cheeks and swollen eye lids. Puffyness of oedema is known as moon face.

Oedema, in kwashiorkor is attributed to hypoalbuminmia and increased blood cortisol. Increased free radical generation has also been suggested since levels of antioxidant nutrients in protein energy malnutrition have been reported to be low. Copper could play an important role in the aetiology of oedema in kwashiorkor. Plasma copper and its carrier protein ceruloplasmin and RBC superoxide dismutase are significantly decreased. This suggests that oedema formation could be due to lower levels of copper and its metalloenzyme superoxide dismutase. Recurrent infections and diarrhoeal episodes and inadequate dietary intake could have contributed to diminished copper status.

- Mental changes like apathy and irritability are common.
- Mental development is affected.
- Scaly pigmentation of the skin is common and in severe cases the epithelium peels off leaving behind depigmented patches with oozing fluid which is described as "crazy pavement dermatosis". There is hypo as well as hyper pigmentation with flaky paint appearance.

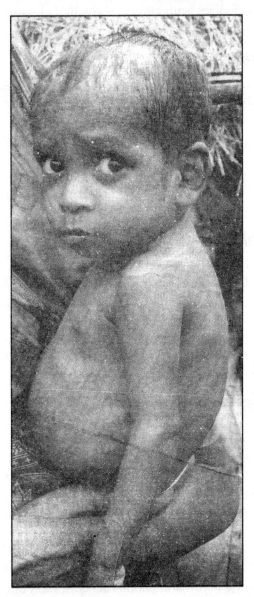

Figure 8f. Observe hepatomegaly and sparse hair of PEM child.

- Bulb and root of the hair are distorted unlike marasmus. The hair becomes thin, dry and can be pulled out easily without causing pain. Loss of hair results in diffuse or patchy alopecia. The changes in colour which include brownish or reddish discolouration may be generated or localised with alternate bands of pigmentation and depigmentation described as 'flag sign'. It is record of the nutritional history of the child.
- Anorexia is common making it difficult to feed the child.
- Diarrhoea may occur due to defective digestion and absorption or as a result of secondary infection.
- Other nutritional deficiencies particularly vitamin A deficiency leading to xerophthalmia and B-Complex deficiencies with clinical signs like glossitis and angular stomatitis are observed in PEM.

Marasmic Kwashiorkor

The child shows a mixture of some of the features of marasmus and kwashiorkor. This is due to the varying nature of the dietary deficiency and the social factors responsible for the disease and presence or absence of infections.

Nutritional Dwarfing or Stunting

Some children adapt to prolonged insufficiency of food-energy and protein by a marked retardation of growth. Weight and height are both reduced and in the same proportion so they appear superficially normal.

The Underweight Child

Children with subclinical PEM can be detected by their weight for age or weight for height which are significantly below normal. They may have reduced plasma albumin. These children grow smaller than their genetic potential and they are at risk of gastroenteritis, respiratory and other infections which can precipitate frank malnutrition.

Mild to moderate PEM is probably the major reason why the mortality in children from 1 to 4 years of age in some parts of Africa, Asia and Latin America is 30 to 40 times higher than in those of Europe or North America.

CHANGES IN THE ORGANS AND SYSTEM

Digestive organs: Cells of the pancreas and intestinal mucosa are atrophied. The activity of amylase, trypsin, lipase and disaccharases are reduced. Mucosal atrophy is associated with impaired absorption of nutrient. With treatment it comes back to normal.

Liver: Fat first accumulates in small droplets within liver cells, situated at the periphery of the lobules. Droplets increase in size and extend from the periphery to the centre of the lobules. Severe liver failure is unusual. Plasma bilirubin is normal. Prothrombin is reduced.

Cardiovascular system: Atrophy of the heart reduces cardiac output and a poor circulation. Extremities are cold and cyanosed (too much CO_2 in blood) and the pulse is small and impalpable.

Kidneys: Mild albuminuria is present. Glomerular filtration rate is low due to dehydration and reduced cardiac output.

Immunological system: In kwashiorkor and marasmnus thymus, tonsils, spleen and other lymphoid tissues are atrophied. Reduced complement activity in the serum specially the C_3 component, reduced T cells in the blood and lymphocytes. These signs of reduced cell-mediated immunity are in contrast to a usually unimpaired humoral immunity. Depression of cell-mediated immunity–mainly due to protein deficiency but lack of zinc, folate and other nutrients are sometimes in part the cause. Reduced immunity is responsible for high mortality from measles, gastrointestinal diseases and other infections. Once the immunological system has reached maturity, it is much less susceptible to malnutrition.

Mental development: Reduction in glial cells, DNA, RNA, protein, total lipid cholesterol, phosphohipid and myelin content of brain have been reported in PEM.

Maximum insult occurs, during the period of maximum brain growth. The 'critical period' of brain growth extends from mid gestation through the early pre-school years. It is the period of neurological proliferation. During the critical period, the brain has biosynthetic abilities that do not persist into later life. The germinal cell population for neurons becomes inactive after early development, making it impossible to generate new neurons, even substrate becomes available after the critical period.

PEM during preschool stage can have a permanent damage on the brain.

BIOCHEMICAL AND METABOLIC CHANGES

These changes vary with the severity of malnutrition as well as type of malnutrition. The basal metabolic rate is reduced. Severe protein deficiency in diet leads to intestinal villus atrophy. Nutritional injury is reversible.

Protein Metabolism

Plasma concentrations of essential amino acids, especially branched chain amino acid, tyrosine are low but those of some nonessential amino acids may be higher than normal.

The plasma albumin concentration is low, owing to a failure of synthesis in the liver. In patients with severe kwashiorkor it is usually below 20 g/1. In marasmus the concentration is also lowered but not to the same extent and values around 25 g/1 are common. A low albumin concentration certainly is in part responsible for the oedema which is often present.

Plasma IgG is often raised if infections are present, but other immunoglobulins are usually normal. Plasma transferrin and ceruloplasmin are lowered. Plasma retinol-binding protein is also lowered and this may be a contributory cause of keratomalacia.

Concentrations of some plasma enzymes are reduced reflecting depletion of these enzymes in the tissues and organs. Cholinesterase, amylase and lipase are lowered in kwashiorkor but not altered in marasmus.

These differences suggest that hepatic and pancreatic functions are better maintained in marasmus. The blood urea is usually low and may fall to 1 mmol/1 (6 mg/100 ml) Urinary creatinine is also reduced, reflecting decreased muscle mass. Urinary excretion of hydroxy-proline is also reduced due to a reduction in body collagen.

Lipid Metabolism

A fatty liver is characteristic of kwashiorkor but is unusual in marasmus. The excess fat in the liver is triglyceride. In kwashiorkor but not in marasmus plasma triglyceride and plasma cholesterol are low, due to a decreased ability of the liver cells to mobilise lipid in the form of lipoproteins.

In all forms of PEM, concentrations of free fatty acids in the plasma tend to be high. This probably is a result of the state of partial starvation.

Carbohydrate Metabolism

Blood glucose is usually normal. Glucose tolerance is also usually normal but may be impaired.

Electrolyte and Water Metabolism

A deficiency of potassium arises as a result of diarrhoea. Losses in the stools can amount to 20 to 30 mmol/day. Plasma K^+ is often below normal and very low values, less than 2.5 mmol/l may be found.

A deficiency of magnesium also arises from increased losses in the stools and plasma magnesium concentrations are generally low.

Plasma Na^+ is usually normal. Low values are found if there have been large losses in sweat or stools and when intake of salt is diminished but intake of water is large.

Effect on Vitamin A status

Protein malnutrition influences vitamin A metabolism by interfering with intestinal absorption of vitamin A and the conversion of β-carotene to vitamin A. Protein malnutrition also affects hepatic storage of vitamin A and its utilisation and transport from the liver to the tissues and utilization at the tissue level. Vitamin A levels in children suffering from kwashiorkor are lower than normal levels. Mortality in children with PEM increases fourfold when they have xerophthalmia as well. This is due to the irreversible damage cause by vitamin A deficiency to the epithelial cells which may lead to infections.

Drug Metabolism

Malnourished children suffer from infections. Drugs may interfere with nutrition. Streptomycin, chloramphenical and tetracyclins inhibit protein synthesis by interfering with the action of messenger RNA.

Antimalarial trimethoprim is a folate antagonist. They should be used with caution in PEM. Low plasma albumin has a reduced binding capacity for salicylates, digoxin and barbiturate thiopentone. Detoxification in the liver by the microsomal enzyme, oxidising system and its function may be impaired in PEM. Their half-life of the drug is prolonged and a standard dose may be toxic.

NUTRITIONAL REQUIREMENT

The rationale behind the dietary management is to provide levels of protein and energy which will not only meet immediate demands but will also promote 'catch-up' growth. Foods specially rich in protein or protein concentrates are unnecessary. The protein calorie ratio of the most commonly used foods is adequate, when employed in judicious combinations. Foods of animal origin are not essential. Foods of vegetable origin are almost as good. The response of children with kwashiorkor is more dramatic and more rapid than is that of children with marasmus who take a much longer time to respond as far as weight gains are concerned.

Table 8.2: Differences between kwashiorkor and marasmus

Characteristic lesion	Kwashiorkor	Marasmus
General		
Deficient nutrient involved	Calories and protein but more protein	Calories and protein but more calories
Biochemical		
Adaptation	Not able to adapt	Able to adapt
Cartisol production	Not increased	Increased
Mobilisation of muscle protein	Not mobilised	Release of amino acids from muscle protein
Plasma amino acid concentration	Low	Normal
Mobilisation of triglycerides from liver	Not mobilised and fatty liver occurs	Normal mobilisation, no fatty liver
Growth hormone	Normal	Decreased
Cell division	Slightly below normal	Decreased
Enzymes: Cholinesterase, amylase and lipase	Low	Normal
Ratio of Essentional to Nonessentional amino acids in serum	Decreased ratio	Normal ratio
Serum cholesterol triglycerides and phospholipids	Low	Normal
GT T	Impaired	Normal
Signs and Symptoms		
On set	1-3 years'	Any age
Weight	60-80%	<60%
		Appalingly thin, shrivelled body
Oedema	Present	Absent
Muscle wasting	Less	More
Mental changes	More affected	Usually normal
Hair changes	Thin, dry, can be pulled out easily. Patchy alopecia, reddish discolouration, alternate bands of pigmentation and depigmentation, flag sign	Hair changes are infrequent
Hair Morphology	Bulb and root of the hair are distorted	Bulb and root of the hair is not altered
Skin changes	Scaly pigmentation, crazy pavement, dermatosis	wrinkled skin due to loss of muscle and subcutaneous fat
Growth retardation	Not so severe	Severe
Diarrhoea due to defective digestion	Present	Not common
Complications	Severe	Moderate
Response to treatment	Dramatic	Takes longer time
Mortality	High	Not so high

Energy

The child should be given 150 to 200 kcal/kg body weight/day for the existing weight. For children less than 2 years 200 kcal/kg body weight and for older children 150 to 175 kcal/kg body weight should be given. It is very important that there should be enough calories in the diet, otherwise proteins will be utilised for energy purposes and not for building the tissues. Malted cereals can also be given to increase calorie density. Fifty per cent of total calories can be from carbohydrate.

Protein

For the existing weight 5 g of protein/kg body weight/day should be given. The calories derived from protein should be 10 per cent of the total calculated calories per day if the main source is animal protein. If the main and the only source is from cereal and pulse, then the calories derived from protein can be 13 to 14 per cent of the total calories. This is because the net protein utilisation of cereal and pulses is around 60 whereas for milk or egg it is around 90. Though vegetable proteins are as good as milk protein in reversing the acute manifestations of kwashiorkor, they are inferior in their ability to promote regeneration of serum albumin. This can be overcome by giving 3 parts of vegetable protein to one part of animal protein like skimmed milk.

Fats

Forty per cent of total calories can be from fat which can be tolerated by children. Saturated fats such as butter, milk and coconut oil are preferred because unsaturated fatty acids worsen diarrhoea.

Electrolytes

Potassium chloride (2.4 g) and magnesium chloride (0.5 g) should be added daily to the diet for a period of 2 weeks.

Vitamins

If vitamin A deficiency is present, oral administration of a single dose of 50,000 IU. of fat soluble vitamin A should be given immediately, followed by 5000 units daily. The deficiency symptoms disappear in about two weeks.

TREATMENT

Treatment strategy can be divided into three stages.
- Resolving life-threatening conditions.
- Restoring nutritional status without disrupting homeostasis.
- Ensuring nutritional rehabilitation.

Criteria for improvement:
- Disappearance of mental apathy in 4 to 5 days.
- Disappearance of oedema in 7 to 10 days.

- Weight gain in 3 to 4 weeks.
- Rise in serum albumin level in about 2 weeks time.

The management scheme described in WHO guidelines when applied results in lowering death rates to less than 5% in severely malnourished children.

Severe cases of malnutrition, especially those with complications like severe infection or dehydration require intensive care and should therefore be referred to a hospital for initial treatment. Once the life threatening conditions are controlled the treatment can be continued outside the hospital. Noncomplicated cases can be managed on an outpatient basis in a hospital or primary health care facility.

Dehydration: Patients with mild to moderate dehydration can be treated by oral or nasogastric administration of fluids. The oral rehydration solution (NaCl 3.5 g; NaH CO$_3$ 2.5 g ; KC1 1.5 g and glucose 20 g dissolved in 1 litre of water) recommended by the WHO can be safely used for correcting dehydration even in malnourished children. Depending on the dehydration 70–100 ml ORS/kg body weight can be give. This amount should be given in small quantities at frequent intervals over a period of 4–6 hours.

For patients with severe dehydration, intravenous fluid therapy is required to improve the circulation and expand plasma volume rapidly.About 70–100 ml of fluid can be given in the first 3–4 hours. In a majority of cases, after correcting the deficit of body fluid, maintenance therapy can be instituted with oral rehydration solution. As soon as urine flow is established, potassium supplements can be given orally (1-2 g/kg/day).

Infections: Diarrhoea and measles are often the immediate cause of death in PEM. When the causative agent of the infection is known or suspected, appropriate antibiotic therapy can be given. For the most frequent infections such as pneumonia, otitis and skin infections, penicillin is the drug of choice. If the infection does not respond to penicillin, broad spectrum antibiotics must be used. Giardiasis and ascariasis must be treated with appropriate deworming agents.

Hypoglycaemia: In mild cases, giving milk feed or glucose in water may be sufficient. If a child develops convulsions or becomes unconscious, glucose should be given intravenously (1 mg of 50% dextrose solution/kg).

Hypothermia: Marasmic children are prone to have low body temperature. If the room is cold, the child should be properly covered with a blanket. The state of shock should be treated with intravenous injection of glucose - saline or blood transfusion. The mother should sleep with the child.

Anaemia: Severe anaemia is dangerous as it can result in heart failure. If the haemoglobin falls below 5 g/dl, blood transfusion should be given. Ten ml of packed cells per kg body weight should be given slowly over 3 hours.

Congestive heart failure: This can occur as a result of severe anaemia or as a complication of IV fluid therapy. The main symptoms are rapid pulse and respiratory distress, cold extremities and cyanosis. Treatment must be started urgently with diuretics and digitalis.

Dietary management: Dietary management is the same for all clinical types of PEM. The child should be given a diet providing sufficient quantities of calories and protein in gradually increasing amounts, without provoking vomiting or diarrhoea.

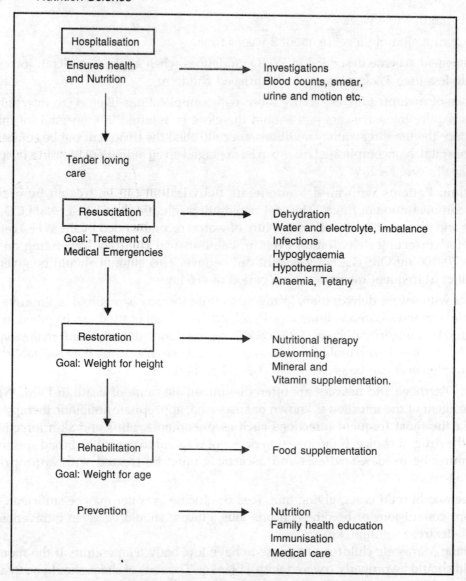

Figure 8f. Sequence in management of PEM

Initially the child may refuse the feeds due to lack of appetite. If necessary nasogastric tube feeding can be given for a day or two. It is best to begin with a liquid formula with diluted milk. When this is accepted the strength can be increased and vegetable oil can be added to increase energy content. Most hospitals use milk-based formulae for feeding malnourished children. A formula containing 90 g skimmed milk powder + 70 g sugar + 50 g vegetable oil in 1000 ml water will provide approximately 100 kcal and 3g protein/100 ml. The children can be fed 100–150 ml/kg of this formula and the amount can be increased to as much as they can take. If there is milk intolerance, milk formulas can be substituted by buttermilk or cereal foods. In elder children with malnutrition, easily digestible solid foods like bread + milk + sugar can be given. A mixed cereal based diet can be given with added oil to increase energy density.

There will be improvement in mental apathy in 3 to 4 days. There will be increase in appetite and the child gains weight for age. Oedema disappears by 7–10 days. Diarrhoea and respiratory infection disappear in about 2 weeks. After clinically and bio-chemically improving in 3 to 4 weeks the child is discharged from the hospital. Figure 8g shows recovery of kwashiorkor child after the treatment.

Suggested diet during Convalescence

- Increasing the quantity of existing food (like idlis, rice, chapathies).
- Increasing the number of meals to satisfy calorie and protein requirement.
- Addition of oil or ghee 1 to 2 tsp to increase calories without increasing bulk.
- Consumption of sugar and banana can be increased to increase calories in the diet.
- The child can be given cereal and pulse mixture in 5:1 proportion.
- If the patient can afford, milk, egg and skimmed milk can be included in the diet.
- The diet should be locally available, inexpensive and easily digestible.

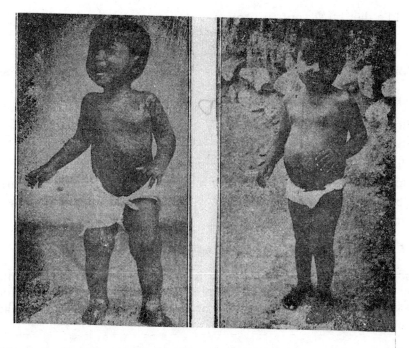

Figure 8g. Kwashiorkor child before and after treatment.
Source: *Courtesy:* National Institute of Nutrition, Hyderabad.

PREVENTION

PEM is a consequence not only of inadequate food intake, but also of poor living conditions, unhygienic environment and lack of health care. It is primarily a disease of socio-economic inequalities and maldistribution of food and health.

There is no simple solution to the problem of PEM. The following steps are suggested by FAO /WHO Nutrition Expert Committee:

Health Promotion

- Measures directed to pregnant and lactating women (education, distribution of supplements).
- Promotion of breast feeding.
- Development of low cost weaning foods. The child should be made to eat more food at frequent intervals.
- Measures to improve family diet.
- Nutrition education, promotion of correct feeding practices.
- Home economics.
- Family planning and spacing of births.
- Improving family environment.

Specific Protection

- The child's diet must contain protein and energy rich foods. Milk, eggs, fresh fruits should be given if possible.
- Immunisation schedule should be followed.
- Food fortification may help the child in meeting micronutrient requirements.

Early diagnosis and treatment

- Periodic surveillance.
- Early diagnosis of any lag in growth.
- Early diagnosis and treatment of infections and diarrhoea.
- Development of programmes for early rehydration of children with diarrhoea.
- Development of supplementary feeding programmes during epidemics.
- Deworming of heavily infested children.

Integrated Child Development Services

Isolated feeding programs will not be effective unless efforts are made simultaneously to improve the environment and to control infections. Supplementary nutrition is therefore integrated with other health activities like immunisation, treatment of minor illnesses, growth monitoring and health education under the ICDS.

Nutrition Education

Education programmes to improve child nutrition should stress the importance of breastfeeding and timely introduction of supplements. Mothers should be advised to give supplements based on the household foods like cereals and pulses. Addition of oil/sugar increase calorie density. Amylase rich food prepared from wheat or maize can be used to reduce the bulk of the cereal mixture.

UNICEF's inexpensive measures to prevent PEM is by GOBI, Growth monitoring, Oral rehydration, Breast feeding and Immunisation.

QUESTIONS

1. Give the classification of PEM.
2. What is the difference between underweight and stunting?
3. Explain the aetiological factors of PEM.
4. Explain the theory of adaptation.
5. Discuss the differentiating factors leading to marasmus and kwashiorkor.
6. Distinguish the clinical and biochemical features of marasmus and kwashiorkor.
7. Why does oedema occur in kwashiorkor?
8. Describe the treatment of kwashiorkor.
9. How do you prevent PEM?
10. Explain the changes that occur in hair and skin in PEM.

SUGGESTED READINGS

- Molecular mechanisms of immunosuppression in severe protein energy malnutrition, 2000–2001, Annual Report, NIN, Hyderabad.
- Information on 'Protein energy malnutrition' : www.who.org.

CHAPTER 9

MACRO MINERALS

The minerals present at levels more than 0.05 per cent in the human body are defined as macro minerals. Calcium, phosphorus, magnesium, sodium and potassium belong to this category.

CALCIUM

Calcium makes up between 1.5–2 per cent of body weight accounting for 1200–1600 g of the typical adult male body. Almost 99 per cent of this calcium is found in the hard tissues of the body-namely the bones and teeth. The rest is distributed in blood and soft tissues, such as muscles, the liver and the heart. In the blood half the calcium exists in the form of free dissolved calcium ions, about 40 per cent is loosely bound to protein molecules and the remaining 7–10 per cent is within low-molecular weight ionic compounds such as calcium citrate and calcium phosphate.

Calcium content of the blood plasma is maintained within a narrow range of 9-11 mg /dl rarely varying by more than 3 per cent. When levels in the plasma begin to fall bone calcium is mobilised.

FUNCTIONS

Bone Formation

The important minerals within bone are calcium, phosphate and magnesium. There is about 1kg of calcium in the adult skeleton as a complex crystalline material with phosphate in the form of hydroxyapatite, $Ca_{10}(PO_4)_6(OH)_2$. Calcium comprises 39.9 per cent of the weight of bone mineral. This mineral is laid down in an organised manner on an organic matrix, the main constituent of which is collagen. There are also important noncollagen proteins within the skeleton.

Skeleton contains more than half of the body's collagen. There is a wide variety of noncollagen substances within the organic matrix sialoprotein, proteins which contain γ-carboxy glutamic acid, phospho proteins including osteonection and bone proteoglycans.

The turnover of bone is controlled by the activities of its bone cells: osteoblasts, osteoclasts, and osteocytes. The osteoblasts and osteoclasts appear to act in remodelling units, whose activities are closely coupled by locally acting cell messangers known as cytokines.

Osteoclasts are derived from haemopoietic cells and are responsible for the resorption of bone. Osteoblasts belong to the stromal cell systems and are responsible for bone formation. Osteocytes derived from osteoblasts lie within the mineralised bone matrix, communicating with each other through the canaliculi of bone. At any given time only a minor percentage of bone cells are active.

Skeleton is constantly being resorbed and replaced. The osteoblast responds to a large number of endocrine and mechanical signals. It also appears to control mineralisation and to modify the activity of the major bone resorbing cell, the osteoclast.

Radio isotopes are used to study the turnover of calcium in the body. In adult man calcium turn over is normally from 400 to 600 mg daily (about 0.05 per cent of the total calcium).

The bone calcium pool turns over every 5 to 6 years on an average, the lumbar vertebral bone turning over most rapidly. Dental calcium turnover is negligible. Remodelling of bone continues throughout life. Bone resorbing osteoclasts begin this process by extruding packets of citric and lactic acids to dissolve bone and proteolytic enzymes to digest organic matrix. Bone forming osteoblasts then synthesise new bone to replace resorbed bone. Usually these processes are coupled. Bone formation exceeds resorption during growth. Bone resorption exceeds formation during development of osteoporosis.

The bone shaft which is the main and most rigid part of the bone contains hydroxyapatite, calcium phosphate and ions of magnesium, zinc, sodium, carbonate and fluoride. This part of the bone is reshaped throughout life as the body grows or its weight distribution shifts putting different stresses on the bones. At the end of a long bone is the epiphysis, a region that regulates bone growth. Beneath the epiphysis is a more porous region of bone known as the trabeculae. The porosity of the trabeculae permits access to the blood supply, allowing this part of a bone to act as a reservoir of calcium, ready to supply calcium to the blood if plasma calcium levels begin to fall. Trabeculae bone tissue also predominates in the vertebrae.

Figure 9a shows the bone remodelling cycle and 9b shows bone structure.

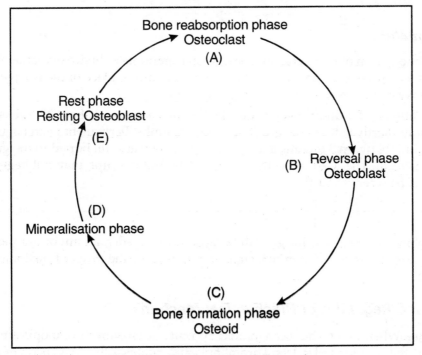

Figure 9a. The bone remodelling cycle.

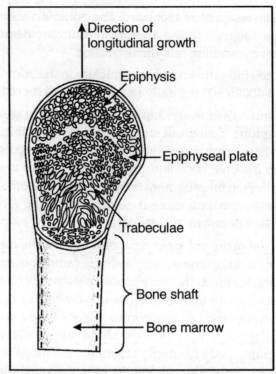

Figure 9b. Diagrammatic representation of bone structure.
Source: Guthri Helen A and Mary Frances Picciane, 1999, Human Nutrition, WCB McGraw Hill, Boston.

Tooth Formation

The enamel and dentin of tooth contain considerable amounts of hydroxyapatite. In teeth the hydroxyapatite is present alongside a protein called keratin in place of the collagen found in bones. Hydroxyapatite crystals in teeth are more dense.

The calcification of deciduous teeth begins by the time a foetus is about 20 weeks old and is completed only shortly before they erupt at about 6 months. Permanent teeth begin to calcify when the child is between 3 months and 3 years while they are still buried in the gums below the deciduous teeth. The wisdom teeth, which are the last to erupt, may not begin to calcify until a child is between 8 and 10 years.

Growth

Calcium is obviously required for growth because it forms such an important part of bones and teeth and is also required in much smaller amounts for the proper functioning of every cell in the body.

Cofactor and Regulator of Biochemical reactions

Blood clotting: When a tissue has been injured by a cut, the enzyme thromboplastin is released from affected cells or blood platelets. Thromboplastin, catalyses the conversion of the protein prothrombin (present in the blood) into thrombin, a process that requires the presence of calcium ions. Thrombin is an enzyme that converts a soluble blood protein called fibrinogen into fibrin, which forms the insoluble network of fibrous protein that composes the basic structure of a blood clot. Figure 9c illustrates the role of calcium in blood clotting.

Contraction of muscle: Calcium ions are readily bound by electrostatic forces to proteins inside and outside the cells and to cell membranes. Proteins which bind calcium include albumin, myosin, troponin C, modulator and transport proteins, extracellular hydrolytic enzymes and prothrombin. The binding alters the shape and configuration of the protein molecules and this determines their biological activity. Thus change at a neuromuscular junction, initiated by the arrival of nerve impulses cause calcium bound to the sarcoplasmic reticulation to be liberated. The resultant free Ca^{++} ions are then bound to troponin molecules and this is the internal trigger which leads to shortening of myofibrils and so to contraction of muscle.

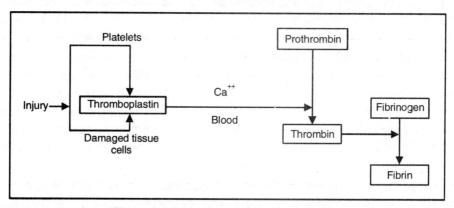

Figure 9c: Role of calcium in blood clotting.

Several hormones may stimulate metabolic changes by increasing the uptake of Ca^{2+} by cells. Within the cell, Ca^{2+} is bound to enzymic proteins, changes their configuration and so activates them. For example, adrenaline promotes glycolysis by activating phosphorylases in this way.

Calcium is essential in initiating neurotransmitter release in the nervous system. Calcium is involved in the absorption of vitamin B_{12}, in the action of the fat-digesting enzyme, pancreatic lipase and in the secretion of insulin from the pancreas.

ABSORPTION

Calcium is absorbed by two distinct mechanisms, passive diffusion and active transport. The active process requires the expenditure of energy stored within adenosine triphosphate (ATP). It is mediated by a carrier protein, calbindin and is saturable. It means it can occur no faster than at a maximal rate corresponding to the rate when all of the carrier molecules are carrying calcium all of the time. The active process also requires the presence of vitamin D. The passive process relies on simple nonsaturable diffusion of calcium down its concentration gradient with no requirement for energy expenditure to make it happen. In normal adult, 95 per cent of calcium from a low calcium diet is absorbed by the active process.

Active absorption is more efficient in the duodenum and proximal jejunum where the pH is more acid (6.0) where calbindin is present. However, absorption is greater in the ileum where the residual time is greatest. Absorption from the colon accounts for about 5 per cent of food intake.

On an average 30–40 per cent of the dietary calcium is absorbed in adults. Growing children, pregnant and lactating women absorb 50–60 per cent of calcium. The efficiency of calcium absorption decreases to 20–30 percent after 45 years of age in women and 60 years in men. Estrogen enhances calcium absorption and hence absorption declines after menopause. Calcium absorption decreases to about 10 per cent in elderly.

Factors Favouring Absorption

Vitamin D: The active form of vitamin D, the 1–25 dihydroxy cholecalciferol, regulates the synthesis of a calcium binding protein that serves as a calcium carrier in the intestinal cell, transporting calcium across the intestinal cells for it to be released into the blood. The presence of the active form of vitamin D can result in a 10-30 per cent increase in calcium absorption.

Acidity of the digestive mass: Calcium is more soluble and absorbed in acidic conditions. Most calcium absorption occurs in the small intestine, in which the acidity of the digestive mass released from the stomach is soon neutralised. Anything that increases the acidity of the digestive mass before it enters the small intestine prolongs the time taken for this neutralisation to occur and so increases the efficiency of calcium absorption. The normal decline in the efficiency of calcium absorption with age is at least partly caused by an associated decline in hydrochloric acid secretions into the stomach.

Lactose: Lactose favours absorption of calcium in infants. This is due to the effect of lactose on intestinal flora and the consequent lowering of the pH or on calcium per se that maintained it in the form available for transport. The lactose in breast milk and formula improves calcium absorption in human infants. In infants, for example, lactose can raise the proportion of dietary calcium absorbed from 33 per cent to 48 per cent. A relatively high ratio of lactose to calcium is required to promote calcium absorption. Lactose increases the diffusional component of calcium and perhaps of phosphorus, especially in the ileum and probably acts osmotically to alter the junctions between the epithelial cells. Beyond infancy it is doubtful whether lactose improves the absorbability of calcium from dairy products.

Protein and phosphorus : The extent to which protein intake affects calcium absorption may depend on the amount of calcium in the diet. If the calcium intake is 800 to 1400 mg/day increased dietary protein is associated with increased calcium absorption Protein has no effect when calcium intake reduces to 500mg/day.

Increased protein is reported to increase the excretion of calcium in urine. Increase in protein intake could lead to a 50 per cent increase in urinary calcium excretion. An increase in the amount of phosphate in the diet has the opposite effect on calcium excretion, causing a reduction in the amount excreted. Fortunately, foods with a high protein content are also rich in phosphate, so the net effect of increased protein intake on calcium losses via urine is considerably less than is expected from the effect of the protein alone. Protein supplements composed of purified protein practically devoid of phosphate, however, may have an adverse effect on calcium balance if consumed in large amounts.

There is an inverse relationship between the dietary phosphorus intake and urinary calcium. Neither dietary phosphorus level nor the calcium/phosphorus ratio affect calcium absorption in adults or low-birth-weight infants. In contrast, prolonged, continuous feeding of high-phosphorus diet results in hyperparathyroidism and secondary bone reabsorption.

Need for calcium: The efficiency with which calcium is absorbed may be influenced by the body's need for calcium. During pregnancy, lactation and adolescence when calcium needs are greatest, absorption efficiency is as high as 50 per cent. Also when calcium intakes are low the body adapts, by absorbing a greater proportion of the dietary calcium available and excreting less.

Factors Depressing Absorption or Increasing losses

Oxalic acid: Oxalic acid present in spinach, combines with calcium to form an insoluble complex of calcium oxalate which cannot be absorbed. Approximately 55 per cent of the oxalic acid in spinach, for example, is in the form of free and soluble oxalic acid, rather than insoluble form, calcium oxalate. Free oxalic acid in such foods as spinach can reduce absorption of calcium in other foods. The amount of oxalic acid present in cocoa is insufficient to depress calcium absorption.

Phytic acid: In 1925 Mellanby showed that puppies developed rickets when fed a diet poor in vitamin D and calcium and containing large amounts of bread. Whole wheat flour was more rachitogenic than white flour and oatmeal worse than either. Later it was found that phytic acid present in cereals prevents calcium absorption. Chapathies made from whole wheat flour may affect calcium absorption since phytic acid is found primarily in the outer most layers of whole grain cereals.

The phytic acid content of seeds, which depends on the phosphorus content of the soil, influences calcium absorption. Fermentation, as occurs during bread making, reduces phytic acid because of the phytase present in yeast.

Steatorrhoea: When high fat diets result in steatorrhoea (large foul smelling stools containing unabsorbed fat) calcium absorption is certainly reduced. Malabsorbed fat promotes the formation of insoluble salts of fatty acids combined with calcium (soaps)resulting in reduction of calcium absorption.

Emotional instability: Stress, tension, anxiety, grief and boredom can all interfere with calcium absorption. Studies revealed that decreased efficiency of absorption and increased excretion of calcium occur under conditions of stress, such as during examination.

Increased gastrointestinal motility: Laxatives increase the rate of passage of food through the intestinal tract. This decreases calcium absorption by reducing the time available for the absorption to occur.

Fibre reduces the absorption of calcium and other minerals by increasing gastrointestinal motility. Fibre binds minerals within the structure. Dietary Fibre binds calcium in proportion to its uronic acid content. Pectin does not affect calcium absorption in humans, probably because 80 percent of its uronic acids are methylated and cannot bind calcium.

Lack of exercise: People who do not engage in weight-bearing exercise, such as walking, and bed ridden people who are essentially immobile, can lose as much as 0.5 per cent of bone in a month and have a reduced ability to replace it. This may be an important cause of decalcification of bone found in many old people. It is the lack of weight on the bones, rather than actual immobility that causes the loss of calcium during bed rest. People whose main regular exercise is swimming may have a lower bone density than those who exercise by walking or running because of the much decreased load on the bones during swimming. Astronauts suffer from calcium loss during space flight either due to weightlessness or due to their relative immobility.

Ageing: Calcium absorption is decreased during old age. Associated with Vitamin D deficiency and hyper parathyridism may increase the risk of fractures.

Caffeine: High intakes of caffeine affect the bioavailability of calcium by increasing the loss of calcium in urine and stimulating the secretion of calcium into the gastrointestinal tract.

Drugs: Some medications including anticoagulants, cortisone and thyroxine, reduce calcium absorption as a side effect.

Cola beverages and bone fractures

Drinking cola beverages, which contain phosphoric acid and often caffeine may increase the fragility of bones in children and adolescents. Consumption of 0.7 or more cans or bottles of cola beverages per day can increase the incidence of bone fractures. Noncola carbonated soft drinks do not contain phosphoric acid and may not affect the bones.

Mayo Clinic Proceedings, 77, 2002

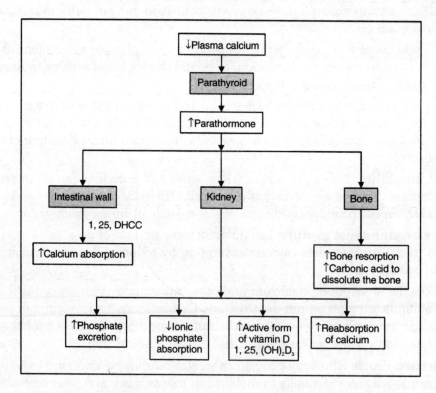

Figure 9d. Role of parathyroid hormone in maintaining calcium levels.

METABOLISM

Once calcium has been absorbed, it is transported in the blood and re-leased into the fluids bathing the tissues of the body. From these extracellular fluids the cells take up the amounts of calcium needed for their normal functioning and growth. As blood is filtered through the kidneys about 99 per cent (normally amounting 100-120 mg/ml) is excreted in urine. Some calcium is secreted within the digestive secretions of the stomach and intestine. Much of this calcium is reabsorbed. In faeces about 100 to150 mg calcium is lost per day regardless of dietary intake.

Most of the calcium absorbed by the body is used in the calcification of bones, a process that is facilitated by vitamin D. About one third of the calcium in bone acts as a reservoir of calcium that can be drawn on to maintain blood plasma calcium level, (9-11 mg/dl) when required.

Hormonal Control

The external balance of calcium, i.e., the difference between intake and output is determined by exchange between the skeleton, the intestine and the kidney. These fluxes are controlled by the action of the calciotrophic hormones, parathyroid hormones, 1,25, dihydoxy cholecalciferol and calcitonin. They are also influenced by a variety of locally acting hormones. Physiological changes in calcium balance occur during growth, pregnancy, lactation and with increasing years.

Calcium metabolism is regulated at three levels — absorption, renal reabsorption and bone resorption.

Parathyroid hormone: Decreased plasma free Ca^{2+} due to dietary deficiency or increased complex formation with phosphate triggers the secretion of parathyroid hormone. It helps in many ways in maintaining normal calcium levels.

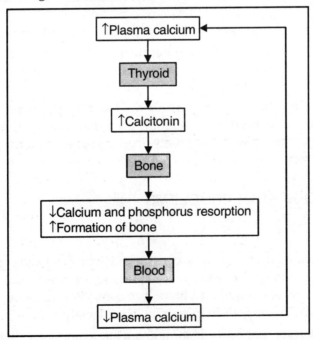

Figure 9e. Role of Calcitonin in maintaining plasma calcium level.

- Within minutes it increases reabsorption of calcium from the distal tubule of the kidney.

- Parathyroid hormone lowers serum phosphate concentration by enhancing phosphate excretion. PTH also inhibits the renal absorption of ionic phosphate at the proximate tubule of the nephron. Increase in serum phosphate concentration may cause fall in serum calcium concentration.

- Within hours of its release, the parathyroid hormone stimulates the release of bone calcium and phosphate into the blood. It achieves this effect on bone by stimulating the synthesis of carbonic acid by the enzyme carbonic anhydrase, generating the acid for the dissolution of bone.

- Parathyroid hormone also stimulates the absorption of calcium from the gastrointestinal tract. Parathyroid hormone activates the renal 1-α-hydroxylase which converts 25-hydroxy vitamin D_3 to 1,25 dihydroxy vitamin D_3 which brings about increase in the intestinal absorption of Ca^{2+} by probably increasing Ca^{2+} binding proteins.

In hyper parathyroidism the calcium level in serum may increase from the normal level of 9 to 11mg to 16 to 20mg. Rarefaction of the bones and spontaneous fracture may occur.

Calcitonin: Calcitonin is released from the thyroid gland when plasma calcium levels rise too high. Calcitonin lowers plasma levels of both calcium and phosphorus by inhibiting the release of these minerals into the blood from bone.

The combined efforts of parathyroid hormone and calcitonin maintain normal calcium levels of blood.

Vitamin D: In calcium deficiency, 1–25 $(OH)_2 D_3$, the most active form of vitamin D causes enhanced intestinal absorption and renal reabsorption of calcium and increased bone formation and resorption.

The bone undergoes metabolic turnover of decalcification and recalcification continuously. This process is controlled besides parathyroid hormone, by factors like vitamin D, vitamin C, vitamin A and anterior pituitary hormone. Nondiffusible plasma calcium is affected by increase or decrease in the albumin fraction.

Cytokines: Changes in calcium metabolism are also brought about by locally acting hormones. Immune cell products such as lymphotoxin, tumour necrosis factor TNF and the interleukins promote bone resorption and a variety of osteotrophic cytokines may have a central role in normal bone remodelling.

CALCIUM RELATED HEALTH PROBLEMS

Osteoporosis

It is a condition associated with a loss in bone density and bone mass and is primarily found in middle age and elderly women. Its major symptom is an increased vulnerability to bone fractures. The term is of Greek origin and literally means "Porous bone". Figure 9f shows osteoporotic bone density in comparison to normal bone density.

The bones of the skeleton are "remodelled" throughout life, a process involving the breakdown of existing bone and formation of new bone is a perpetual cycle that affects 10 per cent of the skeleton at any one time. When existing bone is being broken down, calcium is resorbed into the blood plasma. Plasma calcium must be deposited in the new bone during its phase of mineralisation. In young people in good health, the rate of calcium reabsorption equals that of bone formation. As people age, resorption begins to predominate over the bone formation, eventually resulting in osteoporosis. In osteoporosis the total amount of bone is reduced, but the remaining bone is of normal composition and quality.

Risk Factors

Although ageing is one universal and unavoidable factor that brings a risk of osteoporosis, a variety of other factors contribute to a person's over all risk.

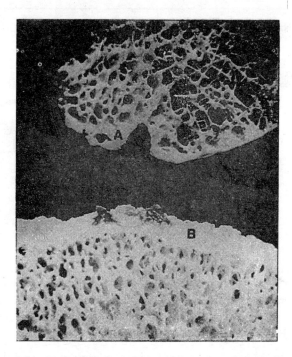

Figure 9f: Osteoporosis weakened bone (A) is much more fragile than normal bone (B).

Gender: Females are eight times more at risk of getting osteoporosis than are males. They have approximately 25 per cent less bone mass than do men and have an accelerated rate of bone loss after menopause because loss of hormones that act to maintain bone mass and density. Men tend to have higher levels of bone preserving hormones. Half of all postmenopausal women can expect to develop some degree of osteoporosis.

Race : People of white or Asian ancestry are more likely to develop osteoporosis than those with a black African ancestry. This presumably is related to the fact that black people have a 10-15 per cent greater bone density than do whites or Asians. Black women over 60 have only half as many hip fractures as do white women of the same age.

Body size : Small-boned people are at greater risk of osteoporosis than those who are large boned due to their lower body weight which puts less stress and makes bones less dense. There is reduced risk of osteoporosis in the presence of a significant amount of body fat. Fat also helps to produce the hormone estrogen, which has been proven to slow down the loss of bone.

Family history: A family history of osteoporosis puts a person at increased risk of developing osteoporosis.

Disease: Over activity of the thyroid gland, can over stimulate the cells that destroy bone during bone remodellings, malfunctions of the parathyroid gland can disturb the calcium balance of blood plasma; gastrointestinal tract disorders, may restrict the body's ability to absorb and use calcium and other nutrients needed for bone formation; liver disease, interferes with the absorption and use of minerals; and kidney disease leads to increased acidity of blood and increased phosphate levels in the blood with consequent damage to bones.

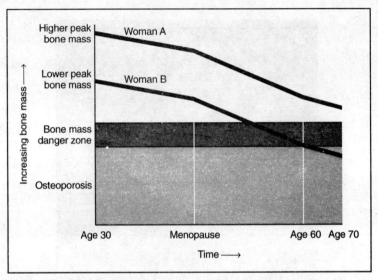

Figure 9g: Comparison of peak bone mass. Woman A entered adulthood with enough calcium. Woman B had less bone mass at the age of 30 years.

Source: Sizer Frances and Eleanor Whitney, 2000, Nutrition, concepts and controversies, University of Phoenix Wadsworth/Thomson learning, Belmont.

Drug therapy: Some drugs can accelerate the loss of bone mass and density. Some drugs can cause vitamin D deficiency and an associated impairment of calcium absorption. Anticonvulsants, thyroid hormones (given to counteract malfunction of the thyroid gland) and corticosteroids (used to treat rheumatoid arthritis and asthma) may have an effect on bone density.

Avoidable Risk Factors

Alcohol: Drinking an average of three or more alcoholic drinks per day is clearly associated with an increased risk of osteoporosis. It has been well established that even small doses of alcohol interface with the absorption and use of both calcium and vitamin D.

Caffeine: Daily consumption of the amount of caffeine in 3½ cups of coffee or seven cups of tea, has been shown to almost double the risk of developing osteoporosis. There is evidence to suggest that this is caused by caffeine's ability to interfere with the normal bone remodelling cycle, leading to increased loss of calcium in urine.

Salt intake: The daily addition of 3 g and 6 g of sodium chloride to the regular diet of healthy postmenopausal women would mobilise 7.5 and 10 per cent respectively, of skeletal calcium over a 10 year period, constituting a potential risk factor for osteoporosis.

Smoking: Greater incidence of osteoporosis was found among smokers than among nonsmokers. Smokers tend to have less body fat than do nonsmokers and low levels of body fat can increase the risk of osteoporosis because of decreased strain on the bones and reduced production of estrogen.

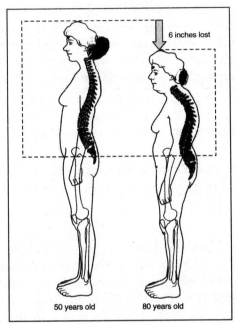

Figure 9h: Loss of height in a woman caused by osteoporosis. Her legs have not grown shorter; only her back has lost length, due to collapse of her spinal bones (vertebrae). When collapsed vertebrae cannot protect the spinal nerves, the pressure of bones pinching the nerves causes excruciating pain.

Source: Sizer Francis and Eleanor Whitney, 2000, Nutrition, concepts and controversies, Wadsworth, Thomson learning, Belmont.

Sedentary life-style: Bones subjected to the stresses and strains involved in exercise become more dense and therefore stronger than otherwise.

Emotional Stress: This increases the secretion of hormones, such as adrenaline, known to increase the breakdown of bone tissue during bone remodelling, without causing any balancing increase in bone formation. Stress is also known to interfere with the body's ability to absorb minerals, including calcium.

Reproductive status: Pregnancy and child birth are known to improve the general bone condition of mothers for two main reasons. During pregnancy a woman's body weight is significantly increased and she produces greater quantities of the hormone estrogen-both factors known to increase bone mass.

Inappropriate diet: Lack of sufficient calcium in the diet increases the chance of getting osteoporosis. Fibre can reduce the efficiency with which the calcium is absorbed. Some studies have also shown that excessive consumption of meat may be linked with an increased risk of osteoporosis. A meat based diet should probably contain not more than 180 g of meat per day. Two other dietary factors that can adversely affect calcium balance are the consumption of carbonated beverages and excess salt. Carbonated beverages contain phosphate ions and some caffeine which can bind to calcium in the gastrointestinal tract and so reduce its absorption.

Infusion of amino acids and glucose to patients receiving total parenteral nutrition results in urinary calcium loss and negative calcium balance, which can be ameliorated by the administration of additional phosphorus in the TPN solution.

A study to assess the incidence of osteoporotic fractures was conducted among women admitted to the hospital (NIN 98–99). It was observed that over 55 per cent of women above the age of 40 years had osteoporotic fractures, which confirms the problem of early onset of osteoporosis particularly among low socio-economic groups.

Fractures in osteoporosis are painful and atleast temporarily disabling, but many of them can be life threatening. Fractures of the hip are among the most serious and in many old people a hip fracture can cause a person to become bedridden and lead to complications that ultimately result in death.

Diagnosis of osteoporosis is based on the amount and quality of bone which is measured as bone mineral density. Duel Energy X-ray Absorptiometer (DEXA) measures bone density.

Treatment

Calcitonin and oestrogen are prescribed for osteoporosis. Calcitonin inhibits the reabsorption of bone calcium into the blood but has only a relatively short lived beneficial effect of 1 to 2 years. Oestrogen therapy in post menopausal women has been shown to slow the rate of bone loss although it does not stimulate new bone formation. It is much more effective as a preventive measure begun immediately after menopause than as a treatment of osteoporosis that has already developed. In the longer term, oestrogen treatment, results in increased parathyroid hormone and $1,25(OH)_2D$ synthesis, which may explain the observed improvement in the intestinal absorption and renal reabsorption of calcium.

An intake of 1000 to 1500 mg of calcium is prescribed for postmenopausal women.

Weight Bearing Exercise

Exercise combined with adequate calcium and vitamin D intake may have a modest effect on slowing the decrease in bone mineral density in postmenopausal women. Studies suggest that increased frequency duration and intensity may significantly affect the results of a weight bearing exercise programme on BMD. However, even moderate activity may be beneficial.

Resistance training represents a viable exercise alternative to combat bone loss in postmenopausal women who have preexisting fractures and are at an increased risk for falls, it is also an important adjunctive therapy for those at lower risk. In resistance training, muscles are strengthened making the muscle work against resistance in a controlled deliberate manner.

List of weight bearing exercises: Running, skiing, soccer, squash, stair climbing, table tennis, tennis, volley ball, walking, weight lifting, aerobics, archery, badminton, basket ball, dancing, gardening, golf and hiking.

List of non-weight bearing exercises: Chair exercises, cycling, swimming and yoga.

The most effective preventive measures are, ensuring calcium intake adequate amounts throughout life and adopting a life style that involves regular exercise and avoiding the avoidable risk factors.

Hypocalcaemia

Hypocalcaemia in clinical conditions is rarely caused by inadequate calcium ingestion. This may occur after operations on the thyroid gland, if too much parathyroid tissue is removed, or due to impaired alimentary absorption. It may also occur in patients with the malabsorption syndrome.

When plasma ionic calcium is reduced, nerve and muscle become more readily excitable. Sensation of tingling and numbness may be present and on the motor side twitching of muscles, known as tetany, which may be followed by spasm, involuntary muscle contraction. The face, hands and feet are mainly affected; characteristically the wrist and metacarpo phalangeal joints are flexed and the interphalangeal joints extended. The larynx may be affected and this causes a coarse stridor, harsh sound. Paresthesia of lips, tongue, fingers and feet may occur in hypocalcaemia. There is generalised muscle ache.

Pre-menstrual syndrome

Women who were on low calcium diets during pre-menstrual phases exhibited increased negative effect greater pain, more water retention and poorer concentration.

High Blood Pressure

Recent research has shown that low calcium intake (100 mg/day) is associated with increased blood pressure. Increasing the calcium intake in people with hypertension associated with low calcium intake has been found to lead to a marked decrease in blood pressure.

Colon Cancer

Calcium supplementation has been found to reduce the proliferation of colon epithelial cells associated with these cancers in people at risk for familial colon cancer. Increasing dietary calcium and vitamin D intakes reduces a person's risk of developing colon cancer.

Hypercalcaemia

This occurs in adults as a result of hyperparathyroidism or excessive doses of vitamin D. Hypercalcaemia can occur in infants as a result of high intakes of vitamin D. It is best corrected by reducing the vitamin D content of the diet, rather than by reducing the dietary calcium intake. It has also been reported in patients with peptic ulcer and impaired renal function treated with a milk diet and large doses of alkali. It may also occur in patients with cancer of the lung and at other sites due to "inappropriate" secretion of a parathyroid hormone-like substance by tumour cells.

In hypercalcaemia, gastrointestinal symptoms include anorexia, nausea, vomiting, constipation, abdominal pain. Renal stones and muscle weakness can also occur. Hypercalcaemia can be reduced by treatment with calcitonin.

RECOMMENDED DIETARY ALLOWANCES

Table 9.1 gives ICMR recommended dietary allowances.

Children up to ten years of age require 400 mg calcium per day to meet the increased rate of bone accumulation. The higher bone accretion rates during rapid skeletal growth in preadolescents and adolescents demand 400–600 mg per day of calcium in order to achieve the peak bone mass. Calcium is deposited in the foetus at a rate of about 330 mg per day during the last trimester of pregnancy.

Table 9.1: ICMR Recommended Dietary Allowances of calcium

Group	Calcium mg/day
Man	400
Woman	400
Pregnant woman	1000
Lactating woman	1000
Infants 0–12 months	500
Children 1–9 years	400
Boys and Girls 10–15 years	600
Boys and girls 16–18 years	500

During lactation, 200–300 mg per day of calcium is lost through breast milk. Hence an additional requirement of 600 mg per day of calcium is recommended for pregnant and lactating women.

During the entire lifetime of an adult, bone is continuously resorbed and new bone is formed as a result of which 400 mg of calcium leaves and enters the bone each day. Therefore 800 mg of calcium per day is advocated to maintain peak bone mass and the calcium balance after compensating for the obligatory calcium losses of 200–400 mg per day through urine, faeces and sweat. However, the body can reduce this loss on a low calcium intake through a process of adaptation involving reduced excertion. The capacity of the skin to synthesise vitamin D decreases with age which means that the dietary intake of vitamin D is more important among the elderly.

SOURCES

Calcium is present in both animal and plant foods. The richest source of calcium among animal foods is milk and among the vegetable sources it is green leafy vegetables. Among the leafy vegetables, amaranth, fenugreek and drumstick leaves are particularly rich in calcium. Most cereals and millets contain some amount. Ragi is a particularly rich source of calcium. Some of the pseudocereals like grain amaranth (Rajkeera) is a good source of calcium.

Calcium content of foods is given in Table 9.2.

Table 9.2: Calcium content of foods

Name of the foodstuff	Calcium mg/100g
Crab small	1606
Colacasia leaves	1546
Gingelly seeds	1450
Skimmed milk powder	1370
Agathi	1130
Whole milk powder	950
Cheese	790
Drum stick leaves	440
Milk, Buffalo	210
Aavin milk	120

PHOSPHORUS

Phosphorus constitutes approximately 1 per cent of the weight of the human body, largely in the form of phosphate (PO_4). Upto 90 per cent of phosphorus in the body is found within calcium phosphate (apatite) crystals in the bones and teeth.

FUNCTIONS

Mineralisation of Bones and Teeth

The mineral crystals laid down during bone calcification are actually composed of calcium phosphate, and a mixture of calcium phosphate and calcium hydroxide called hydroxyapatite. If phosphate levels are low, series of reactions are initiated that trigger vitamin D metabolism and ultimately raise the level of plasma phosphorus.

Facilitation of Energy Transactions

Energy released during the oxidation of carbohydrates, fats, proteins and alcohol is stored by cells within the structure of the phosphate - containing compound adenosine triphosphate (ATP). The presence of phosphorus in ATP and also adenosine diphosphate (ADP) and various coenzymes involved in energy transaction makes phosphorus essential for the capture and use of energy by all cells.

Absorption and Transport of Nutrients

Many nutrients must be combined with phosphate groups before they are able to be transported across cell membranes and hence absorbed into the body and distributed among its various cells and tissues. Thus the phosphorylation of nutrients and other biochemicals is essential for their proper distribution within the body.

Regulation of Protein Activity

Many proteins including many enzymes are turned 'on' or 'off' by phosphorylation reactions that attach phosphate groups to particular amino acids within the proteins concerned. These phosphorylation reactions are involved in controlling the activities of proteins that in turn control the rate of cell growth and cell division and the extent to which the specific genes within cell nuclei are active.

Component of Essential Body Compounds

ATP, ADP and various co-enzymes and regulated proteins require phosphorus as part of their chemical structure. Many other vital compounds like DNA of genes, RNA that carries the genetic message from the nucleus to the cytoplasm, the phospholipids of cell membranes and some vitamins contain phosphorus as a necessary part of their structure.

Regulation of Acid-Base Balance

Phosphate ions, hydrogen phosphate ions and dihydrogen phosphate ions are the major anions in blood plasma. These ions maintain acid base balance by combining with excess hydrogen ions when condition becomes too acidic and yet release hydrogen ions when conditions threatens to become too alkaline. The phosphate ions and phosphate containing compounds act as buffers against excessive variation in the pH level of fluids in the body.

ABSORPTION AND METABOLISM

Phosphorus can be released from phosphorus-containing compounds in food by the action of intestinal enzymes known as phosphatases and is then absorbed into the blood plasma with the help of vitamin D. The level of phosphorus in the blood is regulated by parathyroid gland, which interacts with vitamin D to control the amount of phosphorus absorbed, the amount retained by the kidneys and the amount either released from or deposited in bone.

In healthy people the rate at which phosphorus is absorbed from the gastrointestinal tract and excreted via the kidneys is equal, maintaining total body phosphorus at a steady level. Approximately 90 per cent of ingested phosphorus is excreted via the kidneys, with the remaining 10 per cent lost directly from the gastrointestinal tract without being absorbed. If plasma phosphorus levels decline, reabsorption of phosphorus by the kidneys increases to compensate and if plasma phosphorus levels rise too high, no phosphorus is reabsorbed in the kidneys.

If plasma phosphorus levels fall below 2.5 mg/100 ml hypophosphatemia results. This can result from either inadequate absorption of phosphorus from the gastrointestinal tract or increased excretion of phosphorus via the kidneys. Loss of phosphours occurs in diarrhoea, by use of laxatives and when there is loss of intestinal tissue for any reason. Conditions that increase phosphorus excretion are generally those that lead to increased secretion of parathyroid hormone such as hyperthyroidism, certain forms of kidney disease and certain cancers.

DEFICIENCY

Because of the widespread distribution of phosphorus in foods, deficiency is hardly found in humans. However, people who consume large amount of antacids (interfere with absorption) people who suffer excessive losses in urine (dialysis) and prematurely born infants may suffer from deficiency of phosphorus. Vitamin D deficiency and prolonged parenteral nutrition can cause phosphorus deficiency.

Deficiency of phosphate may produce osteomalacia, myopathy, growth failure and defects in leucocyte function.

RECOMMENDED DIETARY ALLOWANCES

The RDA for phosphorus for children and adults corresponds to an intake that is at least equal to the calcium allowance during the growth period but no more than twice that amount. During infancy the Ca:P ratio suggested is 1:1.5.

Table 9.3: ICMR Recommended dietary allowance of calcium and phosphorus mg/day

Group	Calcium	Phosphorus
Man	400	400
Woman	400	400
Pregnancy and lactation	1000	1000
Infants	500	750
Children		
1–9 Years	400	400
10–15 Years	600	600
16–18 years	500	500

Calcium: Phosphorus Ratio

During rapid growth and calcification the diet should have a calcium: phosphorus ratio 1:1. When calcium is required only for maintenance as in adults, the calcium requirement is lower both absolutely and relatively to the phosphorus requirement. Thus the Ca: P ratio is highest at the earliest age: (1:1), decreases with the attainment of adult status (1:2) and then in the case of the female increases again (1:1) in the latter part of pregnancy and during lactation. In the normal adult mammal the calcium: phosphorus ratio of the whole body is a little under 1:1 and that of the bone is a little over 2:1.

SOURCES

Practically all foods contain significant amounts of phosphorus, although it is particularly abundant in protein rich foods. Meat, fish, poultry, eggs, dairy products and cereal products like rice are the primary sources of phosphorus in the average diet.

SUMMARY OF SOME MACRO MINERALS

Magnesium, sodium, potassium, chlorine and sulphur are also macro minerals. Their metabolism, physiologic function, clinical application and food sources are briefly given in Table 9.4.

Table 9.4: Summary of some macro minerals

Mineral	Metabolism	Physiologic function	Clinical application	Food source
Magnesium	Absorption according to intake load, hindered by excess fat, phosphate, calcium, protein, excretion regulated by kidney	Constituent of bones and teeth, coenzyme in general metabolism, smooth muscle action, neuro muscular irritability, cation in intracellular fluid.	Low serum level following gastro intestinal losses, tremor, spasm in deficiency induced by malnutrition, alcoholism.	Milk, cheese, meat, seafood, whole grains, legumes, nuts.
Sodium	Readily absorbed, excretion chiefly by kidney, controlled by aldosterone	Major cation in extracellular fluid, water balance, acid base balance. Cell membrane permeability, absorption of glucose	Losses in gas tro-intestinal disorders, diarrhoea. Fluid electrolyte and acid base balance problems, muscle action Losses in tissue catabolism. Treatment of diabetic acidosis, rapid glycogen production reduces serum potassium level Losses wit Diuretic therapy.	NaCl – salt sodium compounds in baking and processing milk, cheese meat, egg, carrots, beats spinach, celery.
Potassium	Readily absorbed, secreted and reabsorbed in gastro-intestinal circulation, excertion chiefly by kidney, regulated by aldosterone	Major cation in intracellular fluid, water balance, acid-base balance normal muscle irritability glycogen formation, protein synthesis	Losses in gastro intestinal disorder, diarrhoea fluid electrolyte acid-base balance problems muscle action	Fruits vegetables, legumes, nuts, whole grains meat. Especially Heart action.
Chlorine	Readily absorbed excretion controlled by kidney	Major anion in extracellular fluid, water balance, acid-base balance, chloride-bicarbonate shift, gastric hydrochloride digestion	Losses in gstroitestinal disorder, vomiting diarrhoea, tube drainage Hypochloremic alkalosis	NaCl-Salt
Sulphur	Elemental form absorbed as such, split from amino acid sources (Methionine and cystine in digestion and absorbed into portal circulation. Excreted by kidney in relation to protein intake and tissue catabolism	Essential constituent of protein structure. Enzyme activity and energy metabolism through free sulphahydryl group (-SH) Detoxification reactions	Cystine renal calculi, Cystinuria	Meat, egg, milk, cheese, legumes, nuts.

Source: Williams Sue Rodwell, 1985, Nutrition and diet therapy, Times Mirror/Mosby College Publishing St. Louis.

QUESTIONS

1. Explain the functions of calcium.
2. Explain the role of calcium in blood clotting.
3. Discuss the causes and treatment of osteoporosis.
4. What are the factors affecting the absorption of calcium?
5. Why is milk considered the best source of calcium?
6. What is tetany? '
7. Explain the inter relationship of calcium, phosphorus and vitamin D.
8. Explain the impact of the following factors on calcium absorption.
   a. Oxalic acid
   b. Lack of exercise
   c. Lactose
   d. Protein
9. What is hydroxy apatite?
10. How do hormones help in maintaining normal calcium levels?
11. Explain briefly the importance of sodium and potassium in the diet.
12. How much calcium should be taken by post menopausal woman? Explain the ways of meeting this requirement.
13. What is the best strategy to reduce the risk of developing severe osteoporosis?
14. How can an individual with lactose intolerance obtain adequate calcium?
15. Give the importance of phosphorus in human nutrition.
16. Explain deficiency symptoms of calcium in women and children.

SUGGESTED READINGS

- Youclas Peter P. 2002. Osteoporsis: How much exercise is enough in bone health? Consultant, 42, 7.
- Pierre Colleeu, 1997, Calcium in your Life, The American Dietetic Association, Chronimed publishing, Minneapolis
- Information on osteoporosis : www.osteo.org

CHAPTER 10

MICRO MINERALS—IRON

The minerals present at levels less than 0.05 per cent in the human body are defined as micro-mineral. The micro minerals are also known as the trace elements. Some micro nutrient minerals are iron, iodine, zinc, copper, fluorine, selenium, chromium, manganese, cobalt and molybdenum.

Iron was first recognised as a constituent of the body by Lernery in 1713. In 1800, Lecanu identified iron in the metalloprotein haemoglobin. It is now known that virtually all the iron in the body exists in combination with protein molecules. Overall, the body contains 2.5 to 4.0g. The precise amount in any individual is dependent on gender, age, size, nutritional status, general health and level of iron stores.

DISTRIBUTION

Most of the iron in the body is found in the blood, but some is present in every cell, bound to iron containing enzymes. Over two-thirds of body iron is usually in the form of functional iron and most of this iron is bound within the structure of haemoglobin and a small portion in myoglobin.

Most of the nonfunctional iron of the body is held in iron storage compounds within the liver, spleen and bonemarrow. Some of the iron in these stores is held in large internal cavity within the protein ferritin. Ferritin is a soluble iron-storage compound, but other stores of iron are in the form of an insoluble iron-protein complex called haemosiderin which is up to one half iron. In men iron stored is 1000 mg and in women 400 mg.

Non-functional iron is the iron being transported within the blood, either bound to the protein transferrin or within molecules of ferritin. Transported iron is exchanged rapidly with the iron in both functional forms and non-functional storage forms. Table 10.1 gives percentage distribution of iron in the body.

Table 10.1: Percentage distribution of iron in the body

Type of Iron	Percentage
Functional	
Haemoglobin	60–70
Myoglobin	3–4
Tissue iron (enzyme)	5–15
Storage and Transport	
Storage iron (liver, spleen and bone marrow)	15–30
Transport iron (transferrin)	0.1
Serum ferritin	< 1

Source: Guthrie Helen A., Mary Frances Picciano, 1999, Human Nutrition, McGraw-Hill, Boston.

FUNCTIONS

Transport and Storage of Oxygen

Each gram of haemoglobin contains about 3.34 mg of iron. Iron within the metalloproteins haemoglobin and myoglobin can bind to oxygen molecules and transport them through the blood or store them within muscles. The iron in a haeme group itself is bound to the protein chain.

Myoglobin is found only in muscle, where it serves as a reservoir of oxygen. The oxygen is needed to combine with nutrient molecules to release the energy to power muscular contraction.

Co-factor of Enzymes and Other Proteins

The iron containing haeme group is also a part of several proteins involved in the release of energy during the oxidation of nutrients and the trapping of that energy within adenosine triphosphate (ATP). Also iron on its own is a co-factor bound to several nonhaeme enzymes required for the proper functioning of cells. Iron along with copper is a metal co-factor for cytochrome oxidase. Some of the other processes that depend on the activities of iron containing enzymes are the following:

- Conversion of β-carotene to the active form of vitamin A.
- Synthesis of purines, which form an integral part of deoxyribonucleic acid and ribonucleic acid.
- Synthesis of carnitine, a vitamin like substance needed for the transport of fatty acids.
- Synthesis of collagen, one of the proteins of the body.
- Detoxification of drugs and other toxic compounds in the liver and intestine.
- Synthesis of the neurotransmitter dopamine, serotonin and norepinephrine.
- Essential for catecholamine metabolism.

Formation of Red Blood Cells

Bone marrow produces immature cells known as erythroblasts. As erythroblasts mature in the bone marrow, many synthesise the iron containing haeme group in a process requiring the help of vitamin B_6 and copper. The haeme group becomes bound to globin molecules, also synthesised by the erythroblasts, to form completed haemoglobin molecules. The haemoglobin containing cells are known as reticulocytes and are released from the bone marrow into the blood. Within 24 to 36 hours after their release the nuclei of the reticulocytes disintegrate and the cells become mature erythrocytes ready to begin the transport of oxygen to the tissues and that of carbon dioxide away from the tissues.

Because a red blood cell has no nucleus, it cannot produce the enzyme and proteins necessary for long term survival. The life of RBC is 120 days. When red blood cells die, they are removed from the blood by cells of the liver, bone marrow and spleen which are part of the reticuloendothelial system. In the spleen, the iron and amino acids derived from haemoglobin are salvaged and recycled. The iron is stored as haemosiderin and ferritin in the liver and spleen or is returned to the bone marrow for incorporation into new haemoglobin molecules. In this way, iron is effectively conserved and reused. The amino acids are released to the blood, where they are available to all cells for the synthesis of new proteins or for the oxidative release of energy. The remaining portion of haemoglobin molecule, its haeme group are converted to bilirubin, which is transported to the liver and then excreted in bile.

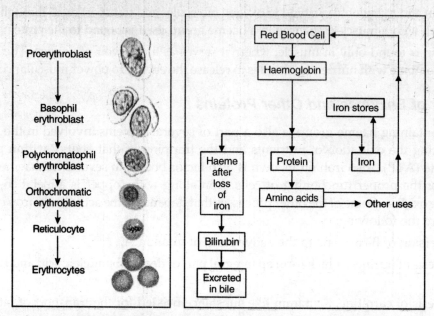

Figure 10a. Genesis and destruction of red blood cell.

ABSORPTION AND METABOLISM

Dietary iron exists in two chemical forms. Haeme iron is found in haemoglobin, myoglobin and some enzymes, and nonhaeme iron is found predominantly in plant foods but also in some animal foods, as in nonhaeme enzymes and ferritin.

Haeme iron is absorbed across the brush border of intestinal absorbing cells (enterocytes) after it is digested from animal sources. Once haeme enters the cytosol, the ferrous iron is enzymatically removed from the ferroporphyrin complex. The free iron ions combine immediately with apoferritin to form ferritin. Ferritin serves both as an intracellular store and as a ferry that carries bound iron from the brush border to the basolateral membrane of the absorbing cell.

The absorption of haeme iron is affected only minimally by the composition of meals and gastrointestinal secretions. Haeme iron is absorbed as high as 25 per cent.

Iron absorption is enhanced by the co-ingestion of vitamin C because ascorbic acid reduces ferric to ferrous iron and it also binds or chelates the ferrous form, which allows the two entities to be absorbed together at the brush border. Other food molecules such as sugars and sulphur-containing amino acids may also enhance iron entry by forming chelates with ionic iron. As chyme moves down the duodenum the addition of pancreatic and duodenal secretions increases the pH of the contents to 7, at which point, most ferric iron is precipitated unless it has been chelated. Ferrous iron, however is significantly more soluble at a pH 7 so these ions remain available for absorption in the remainder of the small intestine.

The efficiency of nonhaeme (but not heame) iron absorption appears to be controlled by intestinal mucosa which allows amounts of iron to enter the blood from the cytosolic ferritin pool according to the body's needs. The signal from the body to the absorbing cells may be transferrin saturation, that is, the percentage of iron bound to transferrin. Normally transferrin saturation is 30–35 per cent in healthy, iron consuming, individuals. The percentage can vary greatly, depending on both iron intake and bioavailability.

A low percentage, 15 per cent, of the total iron-binding capacity (TIBC) of transferrin would stimulate the absorbing cells to transport iron by the exit step at the basolateral membrane to the blood. In individuals with chronic low consumption of iron, the number of receptors may chronically be upregulated to maximise the efficiency of absorption of iron.

The metabolism of iron is given in Figure 10b. Most of the iron in the body is reutilized and about 1–3 mg of iron from the diet is absorbed.

Iron Balance

The body has three unique mechanisms for maintaining iron balance and attempting to prevent iron deficiency and iron overload.

- The continuous reutilisation of iron from catabolised red cells.
- The regulation of the absorption of iron from the intestines with increased iron absorption with decreasing iron stores and an almost complete cessation of iron absorption, when iron stores have reached a certain upper normal level.
- The access to the specific storage protein, ferritin, which can store and release iron to meet excessive iron demands, such as in the last trimester of pregnancy.

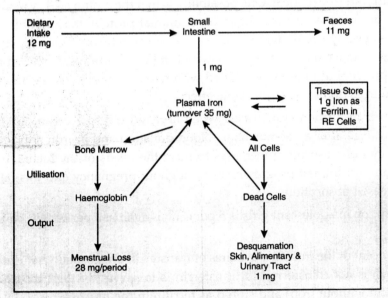

Figure 10b. Summary of daily iron metabolism in man.

Source: Passmore R., M.A. Eastwood 1986, Human Nutrition and Dietetics, ELBS, Churchill Livingstone.

Table 10.2: Iron absorption in different conditions and from different sources

Condition	% Absorption
General condition	3–8*
Anaemia	50
Deficient state of iron	20–30
Iron from plant source	2–10
Iron from animal source	10–30
Haeme iron	25

* Man – 3%; Woman – 7.5%; Pregnancy – 8%

FACTORS AFFECTING ABSORPTION OF NONHAEME IRON

Enhancing Factors

Increased acidity: Increased acidity can be either from food or through gastric secretions. This promotes iron absorption by maintaining more soluble ferrous form or by forming soluble and readily absorbable complexes of iron. Organic acids known as iron chelates — ascorbic acid, citric acid, lactic acid, malic acid, tartaric acid, hydrochloric acid, acidic amino acids enhance the solubility and absorbability of iron. In adults, the inclusion of 25 to 30 mg of ascorbic acid in a meal enhances iron absorption by 85 per cent by converting Fe^{3+} to F^{2+} by reducing action. Gastric secretion also appears to increase the absorption of haeme iron.

Animal tissue protein: Meat, poultry and fish also called MPF factor, increase the absorption of iron two to four fold from a meal. One possibility is that the amino acid cysteine or cysteine-containing peptides released during digestion of animal protein, may combine with iron to form soluble chelates, which allow the iron to be more effectively absorbed. It is found that 1 g of meat has the same enhancing effect as does 1 mg of ascorbic acid. The protein must not only be animal protein but must be contained within animal tissue. Hence animal protein in milk, cheese and eggs do not have the same effect.

Body Need: Iron absorption is increased when new red cells are being rapidly formed in the bone marrow, e.g., after a haemorrhage, blood donation and in iron deficiency anaemia. During pregnancy iron absorption increases to meet the needs of the foetus. Iron stores, as assessed by serum ferritin, fall progressively throughout pregnancy and this fall may be the stimulus to increased absorption.

The iron absorption in adolescent girls is 5 per cent as against 3 per cent in boys and girls of other ages.

Only 20–33 per cent of the iron binding sites of transferrin are normally saturated with iron. Excess iron which is not transferred to transferrin is taken up by the iron storage protein, apoferritin (ferritin without iron) and stored as ferritin in the mucosa.

There are specific transferrin receptors located at various sites in the body, particularly bone marrow which take up iron from blood borne transferrin for their metabolic functions.

Transferrin receptors present on cell surface interact with serum transferrin and sequester the iron for transport across plasma membrane. Depending on the number of receptors, the cell's need for iron is fulfilled. Proliferating tissues like placenta exhibit strong transferrin receptor expression which correlates with the higher number of receptors found in these tissues. Thus the greater need for iron in these cells is met by increasing the number of receptors, which regulate the inflow of iron into these cells.

Lactoferrin and lactalbumin: Although the iron content of human milk is very low, it is highly bioavailable because of the presence of milk lactoferrin, which enhances iron absorption. Infants retain more iron from human milk than from cow's milk or infant formulas because of the presence of lactoferrin in breast milk. When protein, lactalbumin, which constitutes a greater percentage of the total protein in human milk than in cow's milk may also improve iron absorption.

Calcium: An adequate amount of calcium helps bind and remove agents such as phosphate and phytate which if not removed would combine with iron and inhibit its absorption.

Inhibiting Factors

Low gastric acidity: Decreased secretion of hydrochloric acid in the stomach, over consumption of antacids or gastric surgery can lead to decreased absorption of nonhaeme iron. The secretion of hydrochloric acid into the stomach often decreases naturally with ageing.

Increased gastric motility: Dietary fibre like hemicellulose causes reduction in absorption. Cellulose has no such effect. Fibre reduces iron absorption by increasing peristaltic movements. Foods high in fibre are also high in phytate whose absorption strongly inhibit iron absorption. Malabsorption syndrome or any disturbance that causes diarrhoea or steatorrhoea hinders iron absorption.

Phytates and oxalates: These combine with iron ions and convert iron into an insoluble form which is unavailable to the body. Phytic acid is a phosphorus containing organic acid found in whole grains, bran and soya products. Ascorbic acid in sufficient amounts can partly counter act this inhibition. Fermentation degrade phytate and increase iron absorption. Oxalic acid is an organic acid found in spinach, rhubarb and chocolate form insoluble salts with iron.

Polyphenols: These are organic compounds present in coffee, tea, cocoa and some vegetables. They are able to reduce the absorption of iron from a meal by as much as 70 per cent by their ability to form insoluble complexes with iron. Phenolic compounds having mainly galloyl groups are responsible for the inhibition of iron absorption.

Minerals: Cobalt, zinc, cadmium, copper and molybdenum are competitive absorption inhibitors for iron. Manganese and iron appear to share same absorption pathway. One which is taken in high quantity can inhibit the other.

Infection: Severe infections hinder iron absorption.

Table 10.3 shows that rice based diets have better absorption of iron than wheat/millet based diet. Iron absorption is better during pregnancy, anaemia and in female adolescence.

Table 10.3: Dietary iron absorption from habitual Indian diets in different physiological groups

Groups	% Mean dietary Iron absorption		
	Rice based diet	Mixed cereal diet	Wheat/Millet diet
Adult males	5.0	3.0	2.0
Adult females	8.0	5.0	3.3
Children	5.0	3.0	2.0
Adolescent males	5.0	3.0	2.0
Adolescent females (10–18)	8.3	5.0	3.3
Post menopause females	5.0	3.0	2.0
Pregnancy	13.3	8.0	5.3
Anaemic males	10.0	6.0	4.0
Anaemic females	16.7	10.0	6.7

Source: Expert group of the Indian Council of Medical Research, 2000, Nutrient requirements and recommended dietary allowances for Indians, ICMR, National Institute of Nutrition, (Hyderabad) 500 007.

IRON OVERLOAD

Haemochromatosis: It is an inborn error of metabolism. There is a failure to control iron absorption from the small intestine. The excess iron is then deposited in the tissues. The characteristic features are an enlarged and cirrhotic liver, pancreatic diabetes, a slate-gray discolouration of the skin and hypogonadism probably secondary to iron deposition in the pituitary. The disease is fatal if the iron content in the body is not reduced.

Siderosis: In this condition, nutritional iron overload occurs due to high iron intake usually over 100 mg/day. Such intakes are usually due not to iron originally present in the food but to adventitious iron from iron vessels used in cooking and more frequently in the preparation of alcoholic beverages. The condition is common in Bantu population of Johannesburg who drink beer brewed from maize or sorghum in iron vessels. Siderosis is common among people who drink cheap wines made from iron vessels.

A minor degree of overload probably has no adverse effect on health, but it might be a contributing cause of liver cirrhosis.

REQUIREMENTS OF IRON

Iron requirements are determined by iron-balance studies as in the case of other nutrients. This method, however, yield abnormally high values due to cumulative errors. Iron requirement is established by determining body iron loss through long-term turnover studies in adult men using radio isotope of iron. Daily loss of body iron in well-nourished adult men has been estimated to be 12–15 µg/kg with an average of 14 µg/kg. This figure is also used for determining the basal loss of body iron in women and children. The total body iron requirement of different groups is computed factorially as follows.

Adult man: Basal loss of iron (through GI tract, urine and sweat) = 14 µg/kg.

Adult woman: Basal loss (14) + average loss of iron through menstrual loss of blood (16) = 30 µg/kg.

Children: Basal loss (14) + growth + expansion of blood volume (15) + improved iron stores = 29 µg/kg.

Pregnant woman: Basal loss (14) + foetal growth + expansion of blood volume (46) = 60 µg/kg

Lactating woman: Basal loss (14) + loss through breast milk (16) = 30 µg/kg

RECOMMENDED DIETARY ALLOWANCES

Iron requirements of different groups are derived by the factorial approach, in which the requirements for different physiological functions are added up. Basal loss, menstrual loss, expansion in blood volume, foetal growth and loss through milk are taken into consideration as the case may be to determine the RDA.

Table 10.4: ICMR recommended dietary allowances of iron

Group	Iron mg/day
Man	28
Woman	30
Pregnancy	38
Lactating	30
Children	
1–3 years	12
4–6 years	18
7–9 years	26
Boys	
10–2 years	34
13–15 years	41
16–8 years	50
Girls	
10–2 years	19
13–15 years	28
16–18 years	30

SOURCES

Rich sources of iron are cereals, millets, pulses and green leafy vegetables. Of the cereal grains and millets, bajra and ragi are very good source of iron. Iron from animal foods is better absorbed than from plant foods. Inclusion in our daily diet about 50 g of green leafy vegetables which are rich in iron can meet a fair proportion of iron needs.

Iron content of food can be increased by cooking in iron vessels. Studies have shown that iron pots released significantly more available iron into food than the other pots. Food in villages is likely to be contaminated with iron from water, soil residues or dust. Cooking in iron pots is less expensive compared to iron fortification and this should be one of the strategies to prevent anaemia.

Sources of iron are given in the Table 10.5.

Table 10.5: Iron content of plant and animal foods

Plant Foods	mg/100g	Animal Foods	mg/100g
Cauliflower green	40	Crab muscle	21
Manathakkali leaves	21	Ribbon fish fresh	14
Rice flakes	20	Herring, Indian	9
Beet greens	16	Liver sheep	6
Mint	16	Prawn	5
Paruppukeerai	15	Mackerel	5
Soyabean	10	Mutton muscle	3
Colocasia leaves	10	Sardine	3
Bengalgram roasted	10	Pomfrets black	2
Gingelly seeds	9	Pork muscle	2
Cow pea	9	Egg hen	2
Bajra	8	Shark	1
Onion stalks	7	Beef	1
Dates dried	7	Rohu	1
Rice puffed	7		

NUTRITIONAL ANAEMIA

Nutritional anaemia may be defined as the condition that results from the inability of the erythropoietic tissue to maintain a normal haemoglobin concentration on account of inadequate supply of one or more nutrients leading to reduction in the total circulating haemoglobin.

Nutritional anaemia is caused by the lack of any dietary essential that is involved in haemoglobin formation or by poor absorption of these dietary essentials. Some anaemias are caused by lack of either dietary iron or high quality protein, by lack of pyridoxine (vitamin B_6) which catalyses the synthesis of the heam portion of haemoglobin molecule, by a lack of vitamin C, which influences the rate of iron absorption into the tissues; or by a lack of vitamin E, which affects the stability of the red blood cell membrane. Copper is not part of the haemoglobin molecule but aids in its synthesis by influencing the absorption of iron, its release from the liver or its incorporation into haemoglobin molecule. Folic acid, Vitamin B_{12} and pantothenic acid also play a role in erythropoiesis. Ascorbic acid acts as hydrogen donor in conversion of folic acid into folinic acid and thus helps in DNA synthesis and haemopoiesis. Anaemia can be microcytic, normocytic or macrocytic.

PREVALENCE

Recent World Health Organisation (WHO) Statistics indicate a worldwide anaemia prevalence of about 30 per cent with higher rates in developing countries. Young children and pregnant women are the most affected group with an estimated global prevalence of about 40 per cent and 50 per cent respectively. Anaemia is also prevalent in non-pregnant women (35 per cent) and among adult males (18 per cent).

A prevalence rate of over 65 per cent in pre-school children has been reported in various studies undertaken in rural and urban India by Seshadri 1994 (Proc. of Nutr. Society of India, **41**, 1994).

Nearly 70 million of all children below 6 years suffer from varying degrees of anaemia in our country.

A recent report on prevalence of anaemia amongst adolescent girls (UNICEF Study, 1998) indicates that incidence of anaemia increases from 10 years onwards and continues to remain high till 18 years of age.

Table 10.6: Agewise percentage prevalence of anaemia

Age	Prevalence of anaemia
< 8	33.9
9 – 10	38.5
10 – 11	48.5
11 – 12	49.8
12 – 13	52.9
13 – 14	50.2
14 – 15	51.2
15 – 16	49.3
16 – 17	47.8
17 – 18	49.2
+ 18	37.0

UNICEF, 1998

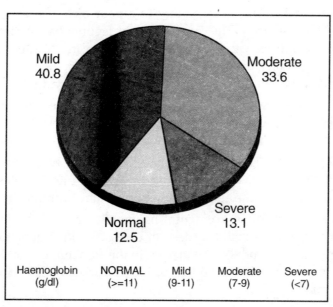

Figure 10c. Prevalence of Anaemia among pregnant women in India (Percentage).

Source: Reddy Vinodini, 1993, Nutrition trends in India, National Institute of Nutrition, ICMR, Hyderabad.

In Asia, 65 per cent of the pregnant women are anaemic compared to 14 per cent in Europe. In India its incidence varies from 20–70 per cent and it is an important public health problem affecting people from all walks of life. Anaemia is very widespread, more among females than males and higher among infants and children than adults. Severe anaemia (with haemoglobin levels < 8 g/dl) is more frequently seen in severely undernourished children who also exhibit signs associated with deficiencies of calories, proteins, vitamins and minerals.

According to National Institute of Nutrition (1991) anaemia is most common in all the groups of adolescent girls to the tune of 20–25 per cent irrespective of the social class.

Figure 10c shows that only 12.5 per cent per cent of pregnant women are normal and the rest of them suffer from different degress of anaemia.

IRON DEFICIENCY ANAEMIA

If there is an insufficiency of iron for the formation of haemoglobin, the red blood corpuscles are pale and small and the anaemia is said to be hypochromic and microcytic.

This is the most common form of anaemia throughout the world affecting mainly women in their reproductive years, infants and children. In both rural and urban areas in the tropics, this type of anaemia is extremely common. Iron deficiency is the case for 1/3 of patients suffering from anaemia.

Aetiology

Deficiency of iron may occur as a result of the following:

- **Inadequate iron intake:** This is secondary to a poor diet such as vegetarian life-style with insufficient haeme iron. The average cereal legume based diets as consumed in most developing countries would appear adequate in iron content (20–22 mg) for an adult. But the availability of iron from such diets is very poor. Only 3–5 per cent of dietary iron is absorbed in normal apparently healthy individual.

  Infants and children suffer from iron deficiency anaemia due to premature birth, iron deficiency in the mother and prolonged breast feeding. The elderly often have restricted diets hence may suffer from iron deficiency anaemia.

- **Inadequate utilisation:** This can take place secondary to chronic gastrointestinal disturbances, defective release of iron from iron stores into the plasma and defective iron utilisation owing to a chronic inflammation or other chronic disorder.

- **Blood losses:** It can occur in accidental haemorrhage, in chronic diseases such as tuberculosis, ulcers or intestinal disorders, or excessive blood donation or due to occult (blood or its breakdown products are present in the stool but cannot be seen) blood loss in hookworm infestation. Excessive loss of blood during menstruation and childbirth can cause anaemia.

  In rural areas post partum haemorrhage on account of poor obstetric care leads to iron depletion to a considerable extent. Repeated and closely spaced pregnancies and prolonged periods of lactation deplete iron stores with successive pregnancy and this is reflected in the high incidence of anaemia with higher parity. Resurgence of malaria is another important factor resulting in high incidence of anaemia. In women, using intrauterine contraceptive device, menorrhagia (increased blood loss) may result in further depletion of already poor stores of iron.

Histologic abnormalities of the mucosa of the G.I. tract, such as blunting of the villi are present in advanced iron deficiency anaemia and may cause leakage of blood and decreased absorption of iron, further compounding the problem. Chronic diarrhoea in early childhood be associated with considerable unrecognized blood loss.

Chronic intestinal blood loss can occur by exposure to a heat labile protein in whole cow's milk. Loss of blood in the stools can be prevented either by reducing the quality of whole cow's milk or by using heated or evaporated milk.

- **Increased demand:** Deficiency of iron in the diet during periods of accelerated demand like in infancy (rapidly expanding blood volume), adolescence (rapid growth and onset of menses in girls) and pregnancy and lactation can result in anaemia. Losses of iron may occur due to excessive sweating in tropical climate.

- **Inadequate absorption:** This can occur in diarrhoea (sprue and pellagra) or when there is lack of acid secretion by the stomach or in chronic renal diseases when antacid therapy is given. Gastrectomy impairs iron absorption by decreasing hydrochloric acid and transit time through the duodenum. Excessive amounts of phytates and phosphates in the diet and excess consumption of tea can decrease the absorption of iron.

- **Decreased iron stores:** Pre-term babies, small for dates and twins may have decreased iron stores and susceptible for anaemia.

Ascorbic acid intake of pre-school children is low in poor income group, hence absorption of iron may be affected.

Diagnosis

Progressive stages of iron deficiency can be evaluated by four different measurements.

1. The plasma ferritin level provides a measure of iron stores.

2. Transferrin saturation can be used as a gauge of iron supply to the tissues. It is calculated by dividing serum iron by Total Iron Binding Capacity. Levels less than 16 per cent are considered to be inadequate for erythropoiesis.

3. Both haemoglobin and hematocrit measurements can indicate anaemia. Most patients develop symptoms of anaemia when the haemoglobin level is approximately 8–11 g/dl.

4. The ratio of zinc protoporphyrin to haeme is a sensitive indicator of iron supply to the developing red blood cells.

When insufficient substrate iron is available to incorporate into porphyrin, zinc is then substituted. Although it can combine with globin and circulate, this zinc-containing molecule cannot bind oxygen.

The peak incidence of iron deficiency in children occurs 6 months to 3 years and 11 years to 17 years.

Anaemia in the newborn is defined as venous haemoglobin less than 13 g/dl in the first two weeks in a term baby and less than 12 g/dl in premature baby. According to National Insititute of Nutrition (2001–2002) serum transferrin receptor together with haemoglobin can be used for defining iron deficiency in population surveys.

Table 10.7: Causes of anaemia in different age groups

Age	Causes
Infancy	• Inadequate iron stores at birth due to low birth weight or due to preterm • Multiple births • Infant who is breast fed by a mother who is a strict vegetarian (vegan) • Infant who is on milk diet without proper weaning foods • Late weaning • Impaired absorption of folate • Regional enteritis, crohns disease, celiac disease
Childhood	• Dietary deficiency • Due to hook worm infestation—occult blood loss • Inflammatory bowel disease • Neglect of female child • Chronic diarrhoea may be associated with considerable unrecognized blood loss.
Adolescence	• Menarche • Growth spurt with a suboptimal haematopoitic contents • Gender discrimination • Intensive exercise conditioning as occurs in competitive athletics iron depletion in girls • Early marriage with pregnancy . • Excess blood loss during menstruation
Pregnancy	• Increased requirements • Increased parity • Hemodilution • Low maternal age • Cultural beliefs, taboos and inappropriate food practices • Infections which may interfere with intake, absorption and assimilation of nutrients • Pregnancy related complications
Old age	• Dietary deficiency • Atrophic gastritis • Gastro intestinal blood loss from malignant disease, like peptic ulcer • Use of nonsteroidal antiinflammatory drugs • Psychological problems • Poor absorption • Chronic inflammatory disease
Adults	• Chronic infection—tuberculosis, malignancy, chronic diarrhoea, malaria • GI surgery • Histologic abnormalities of the mucosa of the GI tract, such as blunting of the villi are present in advanced iron deficiency aneamia and may cause leakage of blood and decreased absorption of iron, further compounding the problem. • Infestation with tapeworm, diphyllobothrium latum infests the upper intestine.

Table 10.8: Haemoglobin and hematocrit cut offs used to define anaemia in people living at sea level

Age or Sex group	Haemoglobin below g/dl	Haematocrit below %
Children 6 months – 5 years	11.0	33
5 – 11 years	11.5	34
12 – 13 years	12.0	36
Non-pregnant women	12.0	36
Pregnant women	11.0	33
Men	13.0	39

Source: WHO/UNICEF/UNV,1998, Cyanmethaemoglobin (HiCN) is the preferred method for measuring Hb as per recommendations of International committees.

Table 10.9: Diagnosis of iron deficiency

Indicator	Interpretary guidelines
Peripheral smear	Microcytic hypochromic
MCHC pg*	<30
Serum Iron µg/dl	<60
Total Iron Binding capacity µg/dl	>300
Transferrin saturation %	<15
Erythrocyte protoporphyrin	>100
Protoporphyrin Heame ratio	>32
Serum ferritin mg/l	<12
Bone marrow iron (by perlstain)	0 or +

* Picogram – One trillionth of a gram.

Source: Raman Leela and K.V. Rameshwara Sarma. Nutrition and Anaemia. Textbook of Human nutrition, 1998, Edited by Bamji M.S.et al. Oxford and IBH Publishing Co. Pvt.

By itself haemoglobin concentration is unsuitable as a diagnostic tool in cases of suspected iron deficiency anaemia for three reasons:

- It is affected only late in the disease.
- It cannot distinguish iron deficiency from other anaemias.
- Haemoglobin values in normal individuals vary widely.

Three stages of iron deficiency have been described:

a. First stage is characterised by decreased storage of iron without any other detectable abnormalities.

b. An intermediate stage of latent iron deficiency, that is, iron stores are exhausted, but anaemia has not occurred as yet. Its recognition depends upon measurement of serum ferritin levels. The percentage saturation of transferrin falls from a normal value of 30 percent to less than 15 percent. This stage is the most widely prevalent stage in India.

c. The third stage is that of overt iron deficiency when there is a decrease in the concentration of circulating haemoglobin due to impaired haemoglobin synthesis.

In case of selecting indicators for detecting iron deficiency anaemia in the community, the filter paper method is found to be the most suitable to carry out haemoglobin estimation in field conditions.

Clinical Findings

The end result of iron deficiency is nutritional anaemia which is not a disease entity. It is rather a syndrome caused by malnutrition in its widest sense.

Besides anaemia the following clinical findings are observed:

Immunocompetence: A sign of early iron deficiency is reduced immunocompetence, particularly defects in cell-mediated immunity and the phagocytic activity of neutrophils, which may lead to an increased propensity for infection.

Diminished work performance: Inadequate muscle function is reflected in decreased work performance and exercise tolerance.

Cognitive development: In man, the iron content in the brain increases continuously during the development of the brain and through the teenage period. About 10 per cent of brain iron is present at birth; at the age of 10 the brain has only reached half its normal iron content and optimal amounts are first reached at the age of 20–30 years. Early iron deficiency may lead to irreparable damage. Iron deficient young adolescents have been shown to score relatively lower in tests of academic performance. Iron deficiency without significant anaemia affects attention span, alertness and learning in infants and children.

Behavioural implications: Anaemic children have been found to be more disruptive, irritable and restless in the classroom. Such changes may be related to functional changes in iron enzymes at cellular level. Iron deficiency is also sometimes associated with pica especially pagophagia (ice eating). Temper tantrum and breath holding spells are also observed in anaemic children. When the haemoglobin level falls below 5g/dl irritability and anorexia are prominent.

Structure and function of epithelial tissues: Mostly tongue, nails, mouth and stomach are affected. The skin may appear pale and the inside of the lower eyelid may be light pink instead of red. Finger nails can become thin and flat and eventually koilonychia (spoon shaped nails) develops as shown in figure 10e, Appendix 10. Mouth changes include atrophy of the lingual papillae, burning redness an in severe cases a completely smooth waxy and glistening appearance to the tongue (glossitis). Angular stomatitis and dysphagia may occur. Gastritis occurs frequently and may result in achloryhydria. Progressive, untreated anaemia results in cardiovascular and respiratory changes that can eventually lead to cardiac failure.

Chronic long term iron deficiency symptoms reflect a malfunction of a variety of body systems. The general symptoms are lassitude, fatigue, breathlessness on exertion, palpitations, dizziness, tinnitus, headache, dimness of vision, insomnia, paraesthesia in fingers and toes and angina. Growth abnormalities are also observed in anaemic children.

Treatment

Treatment should focus primarily on the underlying disease or situation leading to the anaemia Oral administration of inorganic iron in the ferrous form -ferrous sulphate 50–200 mg (60 mg elemental iron) 3 times daily for adults and 6 mg/kg for children. Other salts absorbed at about same degree are ferrous forms of lactate, fumarate, glycine, sulphate, glutamate and gluconate. Carbohydrate iron complexes were initially used only by parenteral route, but recent studies have shown that the therapeutic efficacy and absorption of these compounds are comparable to those of iron salts with lack of adverse effects.

Table 10.10: Response to iron therapy in iron deficiency anaemia

Time after iron administration	Response
* 12 – 24 hrs	Replacement of intracellular iron enzymes; subjective improvement, decreased irritability, increased appetite.
* 36 – 48 hrs	Initial bone marrow response, erythroid hyperplasia
* 48 – 75 hrs	Reticulocytosis, peaking at 5–7 days
* 4 – 30 days	Increase in haemoglobin level
* 1 – 3 months	Repletion of stores.

Source: Behrman R.E., et al. 2000, Nelson Text Book of Pediatrics, Asia PTE Ltd, Singapore – 238884.

Iron is best absorbed when the stomach is empty. However, under these conditions, it tends to cause gastric irritation. Gastrointestinal side effects of nausea, epigastric discomfort and distention, heart burn, diarrhoea or constipation can be minimised by increasing the dose slowly over a few days until the required dosage is reached and by giving the iron in divided doses atleast three times per day. Use of chelated form of iron (bound to amino acids) can result improved absorption and can reduce the likelihood of gastrointestinal distress. Ascorbic acid greatly increases iron absorption through its capacity to maintain iron in the reduced state.

Iron therapy should be continued for several months even after restoration of normal haemoglobin levels, to allow for repletion of body iron stores.

Some behavioural symptoms of iron deficiency seem to respond to iron therapy before the anaemia is cured, suggesting they may be the result of tissue depletion of iron-containing enzymes rather than of a decreased level of haemoglobin.

In iron deficiency anaemia when dietary folate is also low, treatment with iron alone precipitates folate deficiency because more is needed for production of erythrocytes and the supply of folate becomes insufficient.

An improvement in riboflavin status may stimulate iron absorption and turnover to effect an increase in iron store and help in the release of iron from ferritin.

PREVENTION

Policies for combating micronutrient malnutrition must be firmly rooted in food based rather than drug based approaches.

Dietary Improvement

Proper diet can definitely prevent anaemia though anaemia cannot be cured by diet alone.

 * The absorption of haeme iron which is derived from meat and flesh foods is better while that of non-haeme iron derived from cereals, pulses vegetables and fruits is low. Liver is an excellent source of iron. The absorption of non-haeme iron could however be enhanced by increasing the vitamin C content of the diet. The consumption of tea or coffee along with meals greatly reduces the absorption of non-haeme iron.

 * Regular consumption of iron rich foods (whole grain cereals and pulses, whole grains, nuts, dates, jaggery and foods of animal origin) and vitamin C rich foods (amla, all citrus fruits, guava, green leafy vegetables and salads and seasonal fruits) by all, with special emphasis during pregnancy, lactation, infancy, childhood and adolescence.

 * Consuming sprouted pulses regularly after giving some heat treatment as sprouting increases bio-availability of iron as well as increases the content of vitamin C and B-Complex vitamins in the grains and heating destroys the inhibiting factors.

 * Incorporating green leafy vegetables, (cauliflower greens and arakeerai) seasonal vegetables and fruits in the diet of infants and pre-school children once or twice daily.

Supplementation

Under Reproductive and Child Health Programme (1997) young children and adolescent girls are given iron and folic acid.

Children 6-24 months old are at the greatest risk of the irreversible long term consequences of iron deficiency namely impaired physical and mental development. They are given 20 mg elemental iron and 100 μg of folic acid in syrup form. Children below 5 years are given 20 mg of elemental iron and 100 μg of folic acid.

Adolescent girls on attaining menarche should consume weekly dosage of one IFA tablet containing 100 mg elemental iron and 500 μg of folic acid.

All pregnant mothers are given 60 mg of elemental iron and 500 μg of folic acid. Low birth weight infants need iron supplementation from the age of 2 months.

Fortification

Salt fortification with iron has been considered as one of the practical approaches for the prevention and control of iron deficiency anaemia.

Salt is considered as an eminently suitable vehicle for iron fortification in India as it satisfies all the criteria for an ideal vehicle. Salt is consumed in India by all segments of population, rich as well as poor perhaps more by the poor. Salt consumption lies within a narrow range of 12–20 g/day with an average intake of 15 g/day/person. Salt is fortified with ferrous sulphate and one gets 1 mg of iron per gram of fortified salt.

Fortification with iron has been successfully tried for wheat flour, rice, sugar, milk, fish sauce and curry powder.

Education

Nutrition education related to iron and anaemia should be given to the community.

- Promotion of consumption of pulses, green leafy vegetables, other vegetables (which are rich in iron and folic acid) and meat products rich in bioavailable iron, particularly by pregnant and lactating mothers.
- Creation of awareness in mothers attending antenatal clinics, immunisation sessions, anganwadi centres and creches about the prevalence of anaemia, ill effects of anaemia and its preventable nature.
- Addition of iron rich foods to the weaning foods of infants.
- Regular consumption of foods rich in vitamin C such as oranges, guava, amla etc. need to be encouraged to promote iron absorption.
- Promotion of home gardening to increase the availability of common iron rich foods such as green leafy vegetables.
- Discouraging the consumption of foods and beverages like tea and tamarind that inhibit iron absorption especially by the vulnerable groups like pregnant women and children.
- Control of parasitic worms and malaria.

Anaemia can be prevented by food based strategies and by supplementation, fortification and education.

QUESTIONS

1. Write the importance of the following:
   a. transferrin   *b.* ferritin   *c.* haeme iron
2. Discuss the factors that affect iron absorption.
3. Explain clinical findings of iron deficiency anaemia.
4. What is haemochromatosis? How is it different from siderosis?
5. Give the RDA of iron and iodine for different age groups.
6. Name 3 haeme iron sources and 3 non haeme iron sources.
7. Explain the cycle of haemoglobin.
8. The body recycles iron. Inspite of that, iron deficiency anaemia occurs. Why?
9. What is the role of hydrochloric acid in the absorption of iron?
10. Give the causes of anaemia in preschool children.
11. Define anaemia.
12. What measures are taken to prevent anaemia in India?
13. Explain prevalence of anaemia in India.
14. Explain the criterion used to diagnose iron deficiency anaemia.

SUGGESTED READINGS

- Nair Madhavan K, 2000, Recent advances in iron absorption and role of excess iron. Proceedings of the Nutrition Society of India, NIN, Hyderabad, **48.**
- Floreutino, RF, 2003, The Burden of iron deficiency and anaemia in Asia: Challenges in prevention and control. IX Asia Congress of Nutrition.
- Information on iron : www.healthfinder.gov/searchoptions/topicssaz/htm
- Information on iron overload : www.ironoverload.org

CHAPTER 11

MICRO MINERALS—IODINE

Iodine is one of the essential micronutrients required for normal growth and development of the human brain and body.

This trace mineral is present in a minute amount, accounting for approximately 0.00004 per cent of body weight. The body contains a total of 15 to 23 mg of iodine. Over 75 per cent of this is present in thyroid gland. The rest is distributed in salivary, mammary and gastric glands and the kidneys. Within the circulation, iodine occurs either in the form of free iodide ions (I) or as protein-bound iodine (PBI).

FUNCTIONS

Iodine plays an important role in the synthesis of triiodothyronine (T_3) and thyroxine (T_4). The thyroid hormones play a major role in regulating growth and development. They can stimulate the metabolic rate by as much as 30 per cent, resulting in an increased rate of oxygen use and increased generation of heat.

The activities of the thyroid hormones are critical for the normal development of the brain. They increase the proliferation of brain cells and regulate other processes involved in brain function. Thyroid hormones are important from the 4th month of intranterine life to the third year of postnatal life. Hypothyroidism (in which insufficient thyroid hormones are produced) is associated with defective and disorganised development of the brain, resulting in serious impairment of brain function.

Thyroid hormones regulate the conversion of carotene into active vitamin A, the synthesis of protein and the absorption of carbohydrate from the intestine. High cholesterol levels are associated with hypothyroidism, whereas hyperthyroidism leads to low levels of cholesterol.

Thyroxine is also known to be essential for reproduction.

ABSORPTION AND METABOLISM

Iodine occurs in food as iodide ions or as free inorganic iodine or in the form of iodine atoms covalently bonded within organic compounds from which they must be freed before absorption. Iodide ions are absorbed rapidly primarily in the small intestine and then become distributed throughout the extracellular fluid. Free iodine is reduced to iodide ions, and absorbed.

One-third of iodine absorbed is taken up by the thyroid gland. The remainder is removed as it passes through the kidneys to be excreted in urine. Iodine is also lost through perspiration and faeces. The excretion of iodide protects against the accumulation of toxic levels.

The iodide that enters the thyroid gland is oxidised back to iodine, which combines with residues of the amino acid tyrosine within the iodine-storage protein thyroglobulin. If the hypothalamus detects a fall in the blood thyroxin level, it releases a substance known as thyroxine releasing factor into the plasma. The TRF travels to the pituitary gland, where it stimulates, the release into plasma of a hormone called Thyroid Stimulating Hormone—TSH.

The TSH is transported to the thyroid gland, where it stimulates the production of an enzyme that acts on thyroglobulin to release the iodine-containing tyrosine residues from the protein. These residues are then converted into the two thyroid hormones T_3 and T_4 which are released into blood plasma in a ratio of four T_4 molecules for each T_3 molecule.

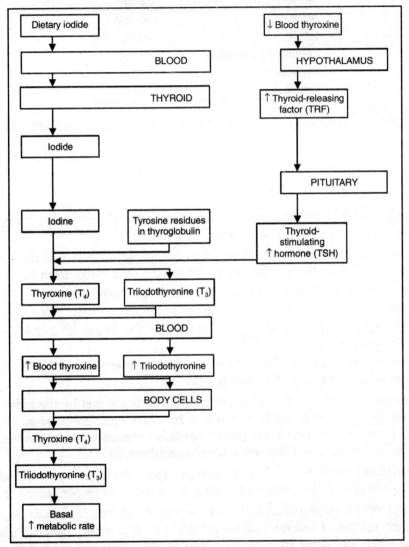

Figure 11a. Absorption and metabolism of iodine, including the synthesis of thyroxine and triiodothyronine.
Source: Guthrie Helen A. and Mary Frances Picciano, 1999, Human Nutrition, WCB McGraw-Hill Boston.

They travel to every cell in the body to regulate the processes of energy release, which determine the overall metabolic rate of the body. Figure 11a gives absorption and metabolism of iodine.

RECOMMENDED DIETARY ALLOWANCES

Table 11.1 gives ICMR Recommended Dietary Allowances of iodine.

Table 11.1: The ICMR Recommended Dietary Allowances of iodine

Group	µg/day
Adult	100–200
Infant	40–50
Children (1–10 years)	70–120
Pregnancy	+25
Lactation	+50

The joint expert committee of FAO/WHO set the maximum acceptable daily intake at 1000 µg/day.

SOURCES

The National Institute of Nutrition, Hyderabad has carried out a systematic study to establish a database on iodine content of Indian foods.

The iodine content of drinking water (as iodides) in goitrous areas is 3–16 µg/l as compared to 5–64 µg/l in non-goitrous areas. The values for bovine milk range from 11–13 µg/100 g.

The iodine content of fish ranges between 28 and 55 µg/100g. Only certain types of fish which are occasionally seen in the sea-coast (cod/heddock) contain more iodine (175 µg/100g) than fresh water fish. The iodine content of egg is about 50 µg/100g and is concentrated more in the white portion.

Based on dietary pattern and analysis of raw foods it is observed that the iodine content of various regional diets range from 170–300 µg/day.

In a non-endemic area 60–75 per cent of the iodine needs are met by the iodine present in diet and the rest through iodine content of water. In an endemic goitre area, there is iodine deficiency in the soil, water and locally grown foods. In non-goitre area diet provides daily nearly 200 µg iodine which meet the entire body's requirement.

Iodine content of the food is lowered by cooking processes. Frying reduces the iodine content by 20 per cent, grilling by 23 per cent and boiling by as much as 58 per cent.

The iodine content of food depends on iodine content of soil. Sea foods such as marine fish, shell fish are rich sources of iodine. Animal products such as milk, meat or eggs are much richer in iodine when they come from animals consuming iodine rich foods. Other sources of iodine are legumes and cereal grains.

Since a populations mean requirement amounts to 100–150 µg/day, it is clear that food sources rather than water intake are the important contributors to iodine intake.

Table 11.2: Iodine content of some common Indian foods µg/100g in goitrous and non-goitrous regions

Foods	Region	
	Goitrous	Non-goitrous
Cereals and millets		
Rice	10	40
Wheat	15	32
Maize	11	33
Bajra	26	42
Sorghum	21	73
Pulses		
Soyabean	4	49
Bengal gram	13	33
Black gram	17	48
Red gram	19	28
Horse gram	17	26
Lentil	4	13
Cowpea	22	39
Oil seeds		
Mustard	-	55
Groundnut	14	47
Sesame	29	43
Vegetables		
Amaranth leaves	8	15
Cucumber	5	11
Curry leaves	-	16
Spinach	-	4
Mint leaves	-	9
Tomato	-	2
Lady finger	-	5
Cabbage	-	3
Carrot	-	6
Brinjal	-	2
Cauliflower	-	1
Snake gourd	-	3
Fruits		
Apple	-	5
Orange	-	11
Custard apple	-	3
Banana	-	16
Grapes	-	11
Papaya	-	12

Source: Ranganathan, S. and Vinodini Reddy, 1995 Human requirements of iodine and safe use of iodised salt, Indian J Med Res 102

IODINE DEFICIENCY DISORDERS

Wide variety of physical and neurological disorders associated with iodine deficiency are called "Iodine Deficiency Disorders" IDD. Iodine deficiency is now recognised by WHO as the most preventable cause of brain damage in the world today.

IDD is a major global public health problem. Iodine deficiency disorders affect about 15 per cent of the world's population, 834 million having goitre and 16.5 million cretinism (WHO 1998). As per the estimates of WHO in 1999, 130 out of the 191 member states are affected by IDD. A total of 68 per cent of the households globally have an access to iodised salt, this achievement is a singular feat in itself. In the developed countries, the problem of IDD has been virtually eliminated through implementation of effective control measures such as iodine fortification of bread, salt etc. but it continues to be a major nutritional problem in Latin America, Africa and Asia.

Incidence of IDD

- North America and Australia — No IDD
- India, Asia and South America — IDD is decreasing with control programmes
- Africa — IDD likely to be persistent problem as there is no control programmes

In India, the endemic belt of goitre and cretinism mainly lies along the slopes, foothills and plains adjacent to Himalayas extending over 2400 km. Several pockets of endemic goitre are being identified in the Aravalli Hills in Rajasthan, Subvindhya hills of Madhya Pradesh, Narmada Valley in Gujarat, hilly areas of Orissa, Andhra Pradesh; tea estates of Karnataka and Kerala and the districts of Aurangabad, Pune in Maharashtra. Inhabitants of most coastal areas are relatively free of goitre.

The overall prevalence of total goitre among 6 to 11 years old children was about 4 precent which is below the cut off to indicate endemicity of IDD. The proportion is higher in Maharashtra (11.9 percent) and West Bengal (9 percent) (NIN – 2003 – 2004).

IDD affects the normal development of about 250 million people in India and accounts for an estimated 90,000 still births and neonatal deaths every year. It has led to 2.2 million Indian children being afflicted with cretinism and another 6.5 million becoming mildly retarded, (Ministry of Industry, 1994).

AETIOLOGY

The factors responsible for IDD are classified as environmental factors and intrinsic factors.

Environmental factors

Iodine deficiency is a disease of the soil where the environment deficiency results in the manifestation of iodine deficiency disorders in human beings and livestock population. Iodine deficiency is likely to occur in all elevated regions subject to higher rainfall with run-off into rivers. High rainfall, snow and flooding increase the loss of soil iodine which has often been already denuded by past glaciation. This causes the low iodine content of food for man and animals.

Iodine exists in nature in large quantities in seawater 50–60 µg/l. Sea water along with iodine evaporates to form clouds which condense, in the form of rain and enrich the top layers of soil with iodine. The food crops that are grown on this soil and the animals while grazing on the plants assimilate iodine. Water from deep wells can provide a major source of iodine.

In India, though classical endemic belt of IDD is known to exist in sub-Himalayan belt, several studies have shown that IDD endemic pockets do exists in peninsular India as well. The data compiled by the Director General of Health Services, Govt. of India from the sample surveys conducted between 1959 – 99 in 25 states and 4 union territories revealed that 239 districts out of 282 districts surveyed were endemic for IDD with the goitre prevalence ranging from 10 – 68 percent.

Table 11.3: Current Status of NIDDCP in States/UTs

State/UT	Total No. of Districts	Districts Surveyed	Districts Endemic	State/UT	Total No. of Districts	Districts Surveyed	Districts Endemic
ANDHRA PRADESH	23	12	11	NAGALAND	8	7	7
ARUNACHAL PRADESH	11	11	11	ORISSA	30	8	7
ASSAM	23	18	14	PUNJAB	17	3	3
BIHAR	37	14	14	RAJASTHAN	31	3	3
CHHATISGARH	16	2	2	SIKKIM	4	4	4
GOA	2	2	2	TAMILNADU	29	29	18
GUJARAT	25	16	8	TRIPURA	4	3	3
HARYANA	19	11	9	UTTAR PRADESH	71	28	22
HIMACHAL PRADESH	12	10	10	UTTARAKHAND	13	9	9
JAMMU & KASHMIR	15	14	14	WEST BENGAL	18	5	5
JHARKHAND	18	9	8	A & N ISLANDS	2	2	2
KARNATAKA	27	20	6	CHANDIGARH	1	1	1
KERALA	14	14	12	DAMAN & DIU	1	1	1
MADHYA PRADESH	45	14	14	D & N HAVELI	1	1	1
MAHARASHTRA	35	29	21	NCT DELHI	1	1	1
MANIPUR	9	8	8	LAKSHADWEEP	1	1	0
MEGHALAYA	7	4	4	PONDICHERRY	4	4	2
MIZORAM	8	3	3	TOTAL	582	321	260

Source: IDD and Nutrition Cell, Directorate General of Health Services, Ministry of Health and Family Welfare, Government of India, New Delhi.

Iodine deficient areas have water iodine levels below 2 µg/l in Nepal and in India (0.1–1.2 µg/l) compared with levels of 9.0 µg/l in the city of Delhi, which is not iodine deficient area.

Goitrogens

Goitrogens are substances that interfere with iodine metabolism. They can interfere at various stages of thyroid hormone homeostasis. The steps include uptake of iodine, its oxidation followed by thyroxine to triiodothyronine. The corresponding enzymes for these steps are NADPH-oxidase, thyroid peroxidase and 5'-deiodinase. Inhibition of any of the enzymes would disturb the hormonal balance leading to deficiency of iodine.

Depending on the level of interference, the goitrogens have been categorized into three classes:

Class I: Thiocyanate, isothiocyanate and cyanogenic glycosides which inhibit iodine uptake by the thyroid gland.

Class II: Thiourea, thionamides and flavanoides which affect the stages of organification and coupling in the process of thyroxine synthesis are grouped.

Class III: Excess iodine and lithium which interfere at the stage of proteolysis —a step necessary for utilisation of thyroxine.

Table 11.4: Goitrogens and their sources

Name of Substance	Chemical substance involved as goitrogen	Source
Thio-oxazolidone derivatives	1-5-vinyl-2 thio-oxazolidone	Brassicae family-cabbages, turnips and brussel sprouts
Thiocyanates and isothiocyanates	Thioglycosides thiocyanogens formed from cyanoglycosides	Rape seed, mustard
Indolyl acetonitrile	1,2, diethiacyclopentyl-4-ene-3-thione, Phenolic glycoside	Brassicae family, red skin of groundnut

Goitrogens are present in tapioca, sorghum, finger millets, okra, sweet potato, almonds, peaches, soyabeans, bamboo shoots, lima beans and cassava. Presence of goitrogens in cassava is particularly significant because it is a dietary staple in many tropical countries. Groundnuts contain arachidoside which interferes with iodine use.

There is a seasonal and regional variation in thiocyanate content. The action of goitrogens may become inactive after cooking.

The antibiotic sulphonamide reduces the conversion of iodine to iodide. The vitamin like substance, para amino benzoic acid has a similar potentially goitrogenic effect.

People who live in goitrous areas should avoid goitrogens. People who live in nongoitrous areas can include goitrogens in moderation. Goitrogen cannot be used as staple food.

Intrinsic Factors

Rare congenital defects can occur in the hormone synthesis and secretion and peripheral resistance to thyroid hormones can also result in goitre.

THE SPECTRUM OF IDD

IDD covers a myriad of consequences of iodine deficiency at all stages of human growth and development—from foetus, neonate, childhood, adolescence and adulthood. Depending on the stage of development, the iodine deficiency leads to a variety of disorders.

Foetus	: Abortions
	Still births
	Congenital anomalies
	Increased perinatal mortality
	Neurological cretinism
	Myxoedematous cretinism
	Psychomotor defects
Neonate	: Neonatal goitre
	Neonatal chemical hypothyroidism
Children and adolescents	: Goitre
	Juvenile hypothyroidism
	Impaired mental function
	Retarded physical development.
Adults	: Goitre with complications
	Hypothyroidism
	Impaired mental functions.

Goitre

Goitre is defined as non-neoplastic (tumour) non-inflammatory and non-toxic enlargement of thyroid gland. The enlargement is apparently a compensatory adaptation to lack of iodine required for the synthesis of thyroid hormones. The direct stimulus of the enlargement is an abnormally high level of TSH, itself brought about by low plasma levels of the thyroid hormones. The excessive TSH causes an increase in both the number and size of the cells of the thyroid gland.

Simple goitre is a painless condition but if uncorrected it can lead to pressure on the trachea, which may cause difficulty in breathing. Administration of appropriate doses of iodine results in a slow reduction in the size of the thyroid gland.

The prevalence of goitre is generally more among adolescents, young adults and schoolage children. More females are affected than males. Figure 11b shows a woman with goitre.

The goitre rate

A new classification of goitre severity has recently been adopted by the World Health Organisation.

Table 11.5: Proposed classification of goitre

Grade	Signs and symptoms
Grade 0	No palpable or visible goitre.
Grade 1	A mass in the neck that is consistent with an enlarged thyroid that is palpable but not visible when the neck is in normal position. It moves upward in the neck as the subject swallows. Nodular alternations can occur even when the thyroid is not enlarged.
Grade 3	A swelling in the neck, that is visible when the neck is in a normal position and is consistent with an enlarged thyroid when the neck is palpated.

Source: Joint WHO/UNICEF/ICC/DD Consultation (World Health Organization, 1994)

Cretinism

Endemic cretinism is associated with severe iodine deficiency, during intrauterine life. Mental deficiency, deaf-mutism and spastic paralysis of legs in varying degrees are associated with this condition. Clinically two types of cretinism are known.

Neurological cretinism: Mental retardation, deaf-mutism, squint, spastic diplegia - spastic rigidity affecting the lower limbs leading to characteristic gait and brisk reflexes are the manifestations of neurological cretinism. Stunting is not a regular feature.

The inner ear or cochlea and the brain develop during second trimester of pregnancy and iodine deficiency during this critical time is responsible for neurological cretinism.

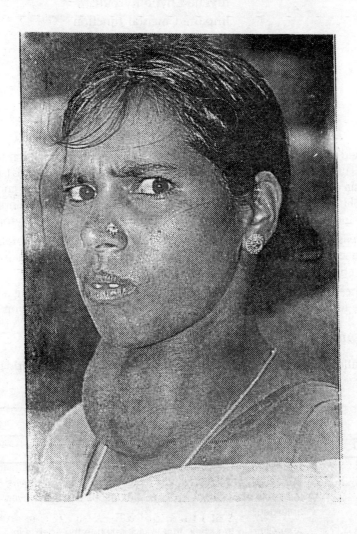

Figure 11b. A woman with goitre.

Myxoedematous cretinism: These cretins exhibit signs of hypothyroidism namely coarse and dry skin, swollen tongue, deep hoarse voice, apathy and mental deficiency. Associated skeletal growth retardation and weak abdominal muscles can be observed. They do not usually suffer from spasticity, goitre or deaf-mutism.

Neurological cretinism is seen in areas with evironmental iodine deficiency. Neurological cretinism appears in infants due to iodine deficiency in the mother during the first and second trimester of pregnancy.

Myxoedematous cretinism results from an iodine deficiency that develops later in pregnancy combined with continuing iodine deficiency during the infant's first few years of life. Myxoedematous cretinism is also seen predominantly in areas where goitrogens are consumed commonly. Tapioca eating population in Zaire (Africa) suffer from myxoedematous cretinism.

Hypothyroidism

This is characterised by coarse and dry skin, husky voice and delayed tendon reflexes. Low serum T_4 and normal T_3 and elevated TSH levels are found. This condition is common among adults. Recent studies show that iodine deficiency or mild maternal hypothyroidism can affect neuropsychological development in children.

Psychomotor Defects

Studies have shown that the child population from iodine deficient areas show poor scores on IQ tests and impaired school performance. They also exhibit poor motor coordination.

Impaired Mental Function

Communities residing in iodine deficient areas usually exhibit reduced mental function, low intelligence levels and high degree of apathy, reflected in lack of initiative and decision making capacity.

EPIDEMIOLOGICAL ASSESSMENT

This is necessary before initiating an iodisation programme and for surveillance of Iodine Deficiency Disorder Control Programmes. The following indicators are useful in this regard:

- Prevalence of goitre

  IDD is considered as public health problem if more than 5 per cent children aged 6–12 are found to be goitrous. (WHO 1994).

- Prevalence of cretinism

- Urinary iodine excretion

- Measurement of thyroid function

  Determination of serum levels of thyroxine T_4 and pituitary thyrotropic hormone TSH indicate the status of iodine. T_4 is more sensitive indicator of thyroid insufficiency than T_3. These can be estimated by Radio Immuno Assay. The normal levels of T_4 are 4–12 µg/dl. The normal levels of serum TSH are < 1 to 4 µU/ml. In case of hypothyroidism, the TSH is elevated.

- Prevalence of neonatal hypothyroidism is a sensitive indicator of environmental iodine deficiency.

  Cord blood of new born using filter-paper technique is used. A new born with T_4 level less than 3 µg/dl and TSH level 50 µU/ml is considered as having neonatal chemical hypothyroidism.

- Iodine content of water less than 2 µg/litre.

Grading of IDD

The different grades of IDD are given in Table 11.5

Table 11.6: **Parameters for Grades of IDD**

Parameter	Mild	Moderate	Severe
Urinary iodine µg/dl	5.0–9.99	2.0–4.99	< 2.0
Goitre prevalence per cent	10–30	20–50	30–100
Thyroid	Adequate	Impaired	risk of marked hypothyroidism
Mental and physical development	Normal	No overt cases of cretinism	Mental retardation, overt cretinism

Source: Brahmam G.N.V., 1998, Iodine deficiency disorders, Text book of Human Nutrition, Edited by Bamji *et al.*, Oxford & IBH Publishing Co. Pvt. Ltd, New Delhi.

PREVENTION

National IDD Control Programme

Since April 1992 this programme is being implemented by the Dept of Health, Govt. of India.

Salient Features

- Production of iodised salt is liberalised.
- To ensure the accessibility of iodised salt at a rate comparable to non-iodised salt. Manufacturers are being supplied potassium iodate free of cost or paid at subsidy.
- To arrange and supervise the transport of the salt by the Salt Commissioner in consultation with the Ministry of Railways.
- To ensure the use of iodised salt in goitre endemic areas simultaneously banning the sale of non-iodised salt under the provision of PFA act.
- To establish goitre control cells in all states and Union Territories for proper monitoring and implementation of NIDDCP.
- To impart training in undertaking simple surveys in States.

There are four essential components of National Iodine Deficiency Disorder Control Programme. These are iodine fortification, monitoring and surveillance, manpower training and mass communication.

Iodine Fortification

The only way to combat the problem of IDD is to provide iodine to the community. Fortification of food items such as wheat flour, bread, milk, sugar, drinking water and common salt are in practice in different parts of the world.

Criteria for selection and technical criteria for the food item to be chosen as a vehicle for fortification are given below:

Criteria for selection

- Should be consumed by high proportion of population
- Unrelated to socio economic status
- Low potential for excessive intake
- No change in consumers' acceptability

Technical Criteria

- Centrally processed
- Minimal segregation of fortificant and vehicle
- Minimal regional variation
- Good masking quality
- Simple, low cost technology
- Good shelf life
- High bioavailability

Iodised salt: Based on the above criteria, common salt has been selected as a suitable vehicle for fortification of iodine to control IDD. The technology involved in fortification of salt with iodine is simple. This involves either dry mixing or spray mixing of salt with iodine source. It is an economical, convenient and effective means of mass prophylaxis in endemic areas.

Salt is fortified with potassium iodate. National Institute of Nutrition developed double fortified salt with iron and iodine. In India the level of iodisation is fixed under the Prevention of Food Adulteration Act and is not less than 30 ppm at the production point and not less than 15 ppm of Iodine at the consumer level on dry weight basis. Goitre endemias of mild to moderate degree can be effectively controlled by using iodised salt.

National Iodine Deficiency Disorder Control Programme is being implemented in India by the Department of Health since 1992. 17 states and five union territories have completely banned the sale of non-iodised edible salt. Gujarat and Tamil Nadu produce 83 per cent of salt. A ban imposed will have a national impact.

Tamil Nadu has imposed a ban only in two districts—Tiruchi and Nilgiris. In Tamil Nadu the ban covers a population of 4.8 million, while nearly 50 million are yet to be covered. In places where the ban is enforced non-iodised salt must be sold with caption "not fit for human consumption" on the wrapper. Test kits are available to find iodine content of the salt. Only a total ban by all states can effectively help in liberating the country from iodine deficiency disorders.

The salt commissioner (based at Jaipur) is empowered to grant permission for establishing iodisation plants at any of the salt producing centres.

> With a decline in the iodine absorbed by food crops from the soil owing to geological and environmental factors, iodisation would be an effective programme even in non IDD - endemic areas. The iodisation of salt is an effective, low cost (about 30 paise per person a year), long term and sustainable solution. The Salt Corporation is involved in mass production of iodised salt and making it available to rural people at an affordable price through fair price shops.
>
> According to a 1994 UNICEF report on the state of the World's children, the results of such programmes are becoming apparent in Bhutan, Bolivia and Ecuador which are close to the point of preventing new cases of IDD.

The estimated iodine content of raw foods consumed in a day in nongoitrous areas is 170–300 µg of which 30–70 per cent is lost during cooking. Hence the daily iodine intake from diets is low (100–160 µg). The average salt intake among adults is about 10g/day and at the current level of fortification (15–30 ppm) the iodised salt provides an additional amount of about 100 µg. Thus, the total intake of iodine is much below the safe limit and therefore the iodised salt is unlikely to cause any harmful effects even in populations who are not iodine deficient.

CORRECT USE OF IODATED SALT	DON'TS
• Always use Iodated Salt and save yourself from goitre and other Iodine Deficiency Disorders	• Never store iodated salt near fire
• Whenever you buy salt, insist on iodated salt only	• Never use ordinary, unlined jute bags for transport of iodated salt
• Always store iodated salt in a container with a lid and keep it away from direct sunlight/heat and moisture	• Never store in the open or in a damp, poorly ventilated godown
	• Avoid transporting in open trucks or in open railway wagons
	• Never store iodated salt for more than six months

Iodised Oil: Oil fortified with iodine is available for oral or intramuscular injections. France is the only country in the world which is producing on a commercial scale, iodised oil from poppy seed oil for injection (Lipiodol) and oral (Oriodol) administration. An intramuscular injection of 1 ml of iodised oil containing 480 mg of iodine can maintain satisfactory iodine supply for 2–3 years, while the oral dose of 1 ml can give protection for one year.

In severe cases of cretinism and mental retardation supplementation of iodised oil should be given. Scientists at the National Institute of Nutrition, Hyderabad have now successfully developed a process to produce iodised oil with safflower oil.

The major problem of this programme when compared to salt is that direct contact must be made with each subject receiving the oil. It is very expensive and requires extensive manpower to carry out the programme.

The chief use of iodised oil is for areas where magnitude of the problem is large and severe and iodised salt is not available. This is the best method of preventing new cases of cretinism and mental retardation. Once the iodised salt distribution programme is well established, the iodised oil programme can be slowly phased out in these states.

Iodised Water: Iodine added directly to drinking water can correct iodine deficiency. Atleast 150 µg/l of iodine should be present in the drinking water. Iodisation is also achieved through a public water supply or through a common well. Iodiators consisting of canisters containing iodine crystals are connected to main water pipes and a fraction of the water diverted through them.

Iodine Monitoring

Countries implementing control programmes require a network of laboratories for iodine monitoring and surveillance. These laboratories are essential for

a. iodine excretion determination

b. determination of iodine in water, soil and food as part of epidemiological studies and

c. determination of iodine in salt for quality control. Neonatal hypothyroidism is a sensitive pointer to environmental iodine deficiency and can thus be an effective indicator for monitoring the impact of a programme.

Manpower Training

It is vital for the success of a control programme that health workers and others engaged in the programme be fully trained in all aspects of IDD control including legal enforcement and public education.

Mass Communication

Mass Communication is a powerful tool for nutrition education. It should be fully used in IDD control work. Creation of public awareness is a sign of successful public health programme.

The people in the endemic state at present do not perceive goitre as a health problem. They are the ones to be educated. People are still unaware that the swelling of the neck is the consequence of iodine deficiency. They are also unaware that pregnant goitrous mothers may give birth to children with mental handicap. They should know that cabbage, cauliflower, raddish, turnip, sweet potato and tapioca which are high in thiocyanate need to be avoided in endemic areas.

The need of the hour is planned education aimed at various levels- general public, health workers and all those concerned with the implementation of the programme.

IDD are declining rapidly possibly due to near—Universal Salt Iodisation (USI). The visible form of goitre is now (2003) seen in 2-3% and palpable goitre (invisible) above 10 per cent in the country. No cretins are born in recent years. Sustainable elimination is possible by 2010.

21st October is Global Iodine Deficiency Disorder Day.

The salt testing campaign is part of Global Iodine Deficiency Disorders Prevention Day. Children are required to bring from one tsp of salt to school and these samples are tested for enough content of iodine. The results are discussed and conveyed to block off.

QUESTIONS

1. Explain the incidence and aetiology of Iodine Deficiency Disorders.
2. What are goitrogens?
3. Discuss the spectrum of IDD.
4. What are the indicators used to initiate Iodine Deficiency Disorder Control Programme?
5. Explain grades of 1IDD.
6. What are the steps taken to prevent IDD?
7. What is the best vehicle to fortify iodine? Why?
8. Explain the following:

   Thiocyanate

   Myxoedematous cretinism

   Thyroid Stimulating Hormone (TSH).
9. Discuss absorption and metabolism of iodine.
10. Give five foods rich in iodine.
11. Give the RDA of iodine for different groups.
12. Explain functions of iodine.
13. Explain the role of hormones in preventing IDD.

SUGGESTED READINGS

- Hetzel Basil, S., 1989, *The story of Iodine deficiency*, Oxford University Press, Bombay.
- *Micro nutrient supplementation in health and disease*, 2002, Proceedings of symposium – organised by National Institute of Nutrition and center for Research on Nutrition Support systems, New Delhi.
- The micronutrient initiative : www.micronutrient.org

CHAPTER **12**

MICRO MINERALS—COPPER, FLUORINE, ZINC AND CHROMIUM

COPPER

Copper has been used therapeutically since at least 400 BC, when Hippocrates prescribed copper compounds for pulmonary and other diseases. Copper metabolism and Wilson's disease were linked as early as 1912, long before the condition was recognised as an in born error of metabolism in 1953.

The healthy human adult body contains about 100–150 mg of copper.

Functions

Copper is necessary for the maintenance of normal haemoglobin status and is also part of many enzyme systems. Many physiological functions in mammals such as erythropoiesis, skeletal mineralisation, connective tissue formation, myelin formation, melanin pigment synthesis, oxidative phosphorylation and others are dependent on the availability of copper. These functions are accomplished by enzymes that either have copper as prosthetic groups or require the participation of copper for their activity. A few of the copper metalloenzymcs and their respective physiological roles are as follows:

- tyrosinase—formation of melanin
- cytochrome oxidase—terminal step in the mitochondrial oxidative phosphorylation
- lysyl oxidase—cross linking of collagen and elastin in supportive connective tissue
- superoxide dismutase—quenching of free radicals.

Copper in blood exists in the form of copper protein complex—hemocuprin in red blood cells and ceruloplasmin in plasma. The role of copper in preventing anaemia may be due to an ability to assist the absorption of iron, stimulate the synthesis of the nonprotein haeme or globin parts of haemoglobin or to release stored iron from ferritin in the liver. As part of a multifunctional enzyme called ceruloplasmin copper is involved in the oxidation of ferrous ions to ferric ions.

Copper plays an important role in the metabolism of fatty acids and in the formation of ribonucleic acid. Copper in the body is capable of binding bacterial toxins and increase the activity of antibiotics.

Absorption and Metabolism

Typical diets provide about 1 mg of copper per day about 25–40 per cent of which is absorbed. Copper is absorbed from all parts of the gastrointestinal tract including the stomach and large intestine.

Once absorbed into the cells of the intestinal wall, most copper becomes bound to such proteins as metallothionein which slows absorption of copper. High intakes of either iron or vitamin C are found to decrease the absorption of copper.

Factors which increase the bioavailability are high levels of protein intake and low intake of dietary copper itself. It is found that the higher the Zn : Cu ratio in the diets, higher is the concentration of cholesterol in the plasma.

Copper is removed from plasma by the liver, from where it is either excreted into bile, or stored in a protein complex containing 2 per cent copper or used in the synthesis of the copper-containing enzyme ceruloplasmin, which is released back into the blood. Ceruloplasmin contains 90 per cent of plasma copper.

Some plasma copper enters the bone marrow, where it is used in the synthesis of the copper containing enzyme superoxide dismutase (SOD) found in red blood cells and it is responsible for protecting against the toxic effects of oxygen. SOD content of red blood cells can be used as an indicator of long standing copper status.

The total copper content of the body is estimated at 75 to 150 mg, 40 per cent of which is found in muscles. The liver with 15 per cent body copper is the major copper storage site. Normal serum copper level in the body is 0.64–1.56 µg/ml.

Deficiency

Copper deficiency is rare in humans. It occurs mainly in infants resulting in psychomotor retardation, hypotonia (low osmotic pressure of blood) hypopigmentation, pallor, anaemia, osteoporosis, low concentrations of plasma copper and ceruloplasmin.

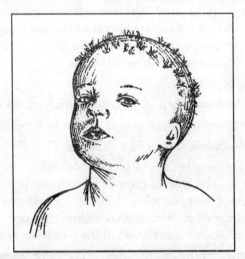

Figure 12a. Menke's kinky hair syndrome copper absorption disorder. *Note:* few clusters of hair that stand on end, turn white, and feel stiff.

Source: Williams Sue Rodwell, 1981, Nutrition and Diet Therapy, Times Mirror/Mosby college, Publishing St. Louis.

Low serum copper and ceruloplasmin levels are also found in an inheritd condition known as Menke's kinky hair syndrome as shown in figure 12a. This is characterised by slow growth, degeneration of brain tissue, hypothermia, seizures, defective arterial walls, depigmentation of skin and hair and peculiarly stubby white hair (Pili torti). The syndrome results from defective absorption of copper, abnormal transport of copper and increased excretion of copper through urine.

Toxicity

Copper poisoning occurs from contamination of food with copper from containers or ingestion of higher quantities of copper salt. Symptoms of acute copper poisoning include excessive salivation, epigastric pain, nausea, vomiting and diarrhoea. Consumption of milk based formula foods or weaning foods stored in brass containers may prove harmful. Liver failure is often associated with massive accumulation of liver copper.

Chronic copper toxicity is relatively rare but occurs in the hereditary condition called Wilson's disease. In this disease a failure to excrete copper in bile leads to accumulation of copper in the liver, brain, kidneys and cornea of the eyes, where it causes brown or green rings to appear. Pathway of copper metabolism leading to Wilson's disease is shown in figure 12b. Penicillamine, a penicillin derivative that forms a chelate with copper in a way that promotes its excretion, has been used to help reduce the copper levels of people with Wilson's disease.

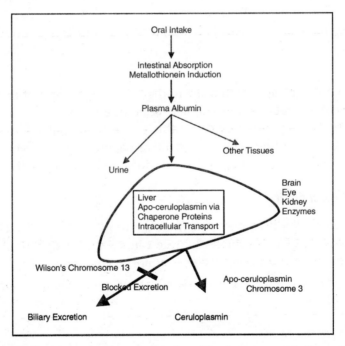

Figure12b. Pathway of copper metabolism. The bar represents the metabolic abnormality of Wilson disease. In the absence of normal ATP7B, intracellular trafficking of copper is inadequate, resulting in copper accumulation and increased degradation of the apoceruloplasmin form of the protein and subsequent low serum level. Excess copper eventually saturates the liver and other organs.

Source: Mayo clin proc., 2003, **78**.

Recommended dietary allowances

The desirable intake suggested by ICMR of copper for an adult man is 2.2 mg/day. Indian adults consuming rice and wheat based diets have been shown to ingest 4-6 mg of copper per day, which meets the requirement.

Sources

Some of the rich sources of copper are seafoods like oysters, crabs and lobster, meat sources followed by nuts and dried legumes like almonds, sesame, sunflower and soyabean contain 12–37 μg/g. Fruits and vegetables have only low content of copper about 0.3 μg/g. In seeds and other grains, most of the copper is present in the bran and germ. Refining of flour removes most of the copper.

FLUORINE

Fluorine occurs in the form of fluoride in nature. It is present in small but widely varying concentrations in practically all soils, water supplies, plants and animals and is a constituent of all diets.

It is an essential element and present in bones, teeth, thyroid gland and skin.

Functions

There is now, no doubt that traces of fluorine in the teeth help to protect them against decay. Fluoride imparts stability to bone and enamel tissue due to formation of highly insoluble fluoroapatite from hydroxyapatite. In view of this property, therapeutic use of fluoride has been recommended for preventing dental caries and osteoporotic fractures in elders. To prevent dental caries water should contain >1 ppm. The fluoride ions inhibit the activity of oral bacteria.

Absorption and excretion

Fluoride can be absorbed rapidly by passive diffusion through mouth, stomach, small intestine, lungs and skin. About 86-97% of soluble fluoride can be absorbed through gastrointestinal tract and the absorption from drinking water is almost complete.

Fluoride is excreted through urine faeces, sweat, saliva and milk, the main route being the urine.

Sources

The chief source is usually drinking water, which if it contains 1 part per million (ppm) of fluoride, supplies 1–2 mg/day. Soft water may contain no fluorine, whilst very hard water may contain over 10 ppm. Compared with this source, the fluoride in food stuff is of little importance. Sea fish contains large amounts of the order of 5 to 10 ppm. Another significant source is tea. Analysis done at NIN showed that the fluoride content of tea ranges between 110 μg/g to 140 μg/g of dry tea powder.

TOXICITY

Fluorosis occurs as an endemic disease in India in parts of Andhra Pradesh (Nalgonda, Prakasam and Guntur districts) and Punjab (Patiala district).

In India, an estimated 62 million people, including 6 million children in 17 states are affected with endemic fluorosis.

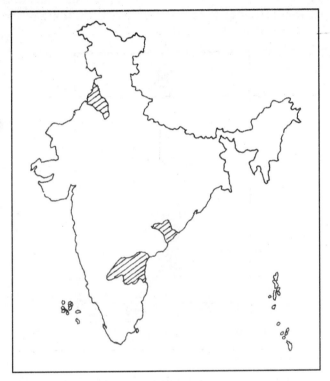

Figure 12c. India–Endemic areas of Fluorosis
Source: Murthy Ramadoss V, 'I am fluorine' Nutrition, **16**, 1982.

The heavy deposits of fluoride bearing minerals in the rock are mainly responsible for endemic fluorosis in India. The fluoride content of drinking water varies between 0.5 to 0.25 mg/litre in different parts of India.

Sorghum and Fluorosis

In communities where genuvalgum is prevalent, it is observed that their staple diet is generally sorghum and their calcium intake is low. Sorghum contains high levels of molybdenum as compared to other cereals. High molybdenum intake is known to increase copper excretion which is an essential element for bone development. It is observed that copper deficiency along with high fluoride intake is associated with high prevalence of genuvalgum. Substituting rice with sorghum may reduce the incidence of fluorosis.

Its presence in water > 2-3 ppm leads to fluorosis. Fluoride toxicity manifests in two major forms and skeletal fluorosis and dental fluorosis.

Skeletal fluorosis: The patients may develop stiffness, joint pain and deformities of the spine. The clinical manifestation of fluoride toxicity is called "genuvalgum" (knock knees), Young and adolescent people are affected with this syndrome with greater prevalence among boys. Studies conducted by NIN showed that genuvalgum results when fluoride intake was higher than 2 – 16 mg / litre. High levels of Mo and low levels of Cu might also contribute to genuvalgum. One important strategy to control fluorosis in these areas is to supply low fluoride water (figure 12d).

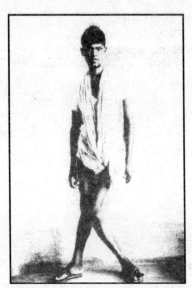

Figure 12d. Fluorine toxicity leads to genuvalgum.
Source: Murthy Ramadoss V, I am fluorine, Nutrition, **16**, 1982.

Dental fluorosis: Where the fluoride content of the water is high (> 3-5 ppm) mottling of permanent teeth is common as shown in Figure 12e. The enamel loses its luster and becomes rough. Bands of brown pigmentation separate patches as white as chalk. Small pits may be present on the surface. Incisors of the upper jaw are more affected. Dental fluorosis is not usually associated with any evidence of skeletal fluorosis or indeed with an impairment of health. Mottling is irreversible dental fluorosis occurs in children, who are exposed to high fluoride intake before completion of dental mineralisation both boys and girls are equally affected.

High fluoride intakes may also interfere with iodine metabolism, causing hypothyroidism. The hormones of bone metabolism like parathyroid hormone and growth hormone levels in serum are elevated in them compared to that in normals. High fluoride concentration in drinking water leads to vitamin D deficiency causing bone deformities in young children (NIN 2003 – 2004).

Supplementation of vitamin C is shown to alleviate the symptoms of endemic fluorosis. The National Environmental Engineering Research Institute (NEERI) developed a technique for defluoridation of water known as "Nalgonda Technique" using aluminium salts. Water should be consumed from alternative running water sources.

Apart from the naturally occurring minerals, fluoride gains access into the environment as particulate emission due to various industrial activities such as manufacture of fluoride containing fertilisers, aluminium smelting, nuclear power plants, electric power industry, petroleum refining industry in addition to automobile emission. Fluoride finds its way into sea water, surface water, under ground water and vegetation.

Household exposure to fluoride can occur with the use of fluoridated tooth paste, mouth wash and teflon coated pans. Use of fluoride based insecticide spray on horticulture may also contribute to the ingestion of large amounts of fluoride.

While high intake of fluoride is a health hazard, a minimum level of fluoride in water (< 1 ppm) is essential to protect against dental caries. To prevent fluorosis and dental caries fluorine levels of water should be >1 ppm but less than < 2 ppm.

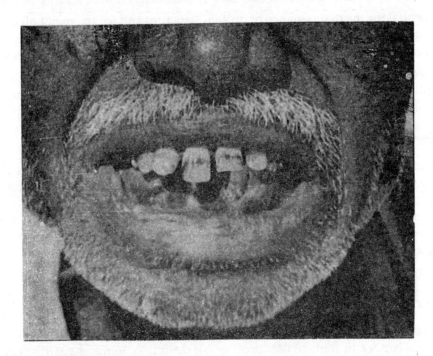

Figure 12e. Mottling of teeth due to fluorosis irreversible. Discolouration, pitting of teeth, the enamel loses its lustre and become rougher chalky white patches. Upper jaws are more affected.

Source: *Courtesy:* National Institute of Nutrition, Hyderabad-500 007.

ZINC

Adult contains between 1.5 and 2.5 g of zinc. Zinc is present in all cells, tissues, organs, fluids and secretions, although about 90 per cent of the body's zinc is in muscle and bone. Over 95 per cent of the body's zinc occurs bound within various metalloenzymes of cells and cell membranes. Blood plasma contains only 0.1 per cent of the body's zinc. Zinc plasma level is about 96 µg/100ml in adults and 8.9 µg/100ml in children.

Functions

Zinc performs many functions as a part of every cell in the body and so zinc is essential for normal growth, development, reproduction and immunity. Zinc is also involved in maintaining a healthy appetite, assisting in the perception of taste and maintaining capacity for night vision. Zinc is involved in these functions not just as a component of metalloenzymes, but also in specific interactions between zinc and various hormones. Zinc plasma level is about 96 μg/100ml in adults and 8.9 μg/100ml in children.

Human and animal tissues contain about 200 enzymes whose activity depends on the presence of zinc. Some of these enzymes are alcohol dehydrogenase, alkaline phosphatase, carbonic anhydrase, carboxypeptidase, deoxynucleotidyl transferase, DNA polymerase, glutamic acid dehydrogenase, superoxide dismutase etc. Zinc is considered as an antioxidant nutrient.

Zinc is essential for the maintenance of protein structure and for the metabolism of proteins and nucleic acids. The maintenance and replication of genetic material (DNA and RNA) and the use of genetic information to generate specific proteins are dependent on zinc.

Zinc is involved in cholesterol transport and in maintaining the stability of lipids within the cell membrane. Zinc-dependent enzymes are involved in the synthesis of long-chain fatty acids and various prostaglandins.

Absorption

Absorption may vary from 10 to 80 per cent depending on the chemical form in which zinc is present, constituents of the diet and the nutritional status of the subjects just before ingestion. Absorption of zinc is enhanced by low zinc status. The average absorption is 20 per cent unless the content of fibre and phytate are exceptionally high. Amino acids and peptides increase its absorption. Bioavailability of zinc from human milk is high. Elevated zinc concentrations of milk is found in early stages of lactation.

Normal zinc plasma level in an adult is 96 μg/100 ml and in a child 89 μg/100 ml.

Deficiency

Some of the predisposing factors of zinc deficiency are excessive phytates and phosphates in diet; excessive copper in diet; Malabsorption; sickle cell anaemia; hepatitis, chronic blood loss, chronic parenteral alimentation, rheumatoid arthritis, trauma surgery, burns and excessive sweating.

One form of severe zinc deficiency is Acrodermatitis Enteropathica, a rare genetic disease in which zinc absorption is significantly impaired. Severe dermatitis usually appear in the first few months of an infant's life, particularly when the infant is switched from its mother's milk to cow's milk. This can be successfully treated by giving 30 to 50 mg of zinc/day. Premature infants and PEM children are susceptible to zinc deficiency. Patients who are on parenteral nutrition may also suffer from zinc deficiency (Figure 12f – Appendix 10).

The manifestations of severe zinc deficiency in humans include bullous pustular dermatitis, alopecia, diarrhea, emotional disorder, weight loss, intercurrent infections due to cell mediated immune dysfunctions, hypogonadism in males, neuro-sensory disorders and problems with healing of ulcers. If this condition is unrecognised and not treated, it becomes fatal.

Moderate level of zinc deficiency can occur due to dietary factors, malabsorption syndrome, alcoholic liver disease, chronic renal disease, chronically debilitated conditions. The clinical manifestations of a moderate deficiency of zinc include growth retardation and male hypogonadism in the adolescents, rough skin, poor appetite, mental lethargy, delayed wound healing, cell mediated immune dysfunction and abnormal neuro sensory changes.

Hypogeusia and hyposmia, impaired taste and smell, appear in zinc deficiency that can be cured with zinc supplementation.

The clinical manifestations of a mild level of deficiency of zinc in humans include decreased serum testosterone level and oligospermia in males, decreased lean body mass, hyperammonemia and neuro sensory changes.

Zinc deficiency results in a variety of immunologic defects. Severe deficiency is accompanied by thymic atrophy. Even mild zinc deficiency can reduce immune function, producing impaired interleukin-2-production.

Zinc deficiency is associated with impaired glucose tolerance, implying a role for the mineral in carbohydrate metabolism. Zinc may interact with insulin and influences the uptake of glucose by the cells of adipose tissue. Zinc also interacts with growth hormone, various sex hormones, thyroid hormones, prolactin and corticosteroids.

Currently plasma zinc appears to be the most widely used parameter for assessment of human zinc status. Mild deficiency of zinc in humans is recognised by utilising assay of zinc in lymphocytes, granulocytes and platelets. Studies indicated that mild deficiency of zinc in humans affects clinical, biochemical and immunological functions adversely.

Zinc and vitamin A

Zinc and vitamin A appear to interact atleast at two levels. Retinal reductase that is alcohol dehydrogenase which converts retinol to its aldehyde analogue is a zinc metallo enzyme. Retinal oxidase which oxidises retinal to retinoic acid is a zinc modulated enzyme. In addition, the synthesis of plasma retinol binding protein (RBP) is significantly reduced in severe zinc deficiency and vitamin A release from the liver to the circulation is impaired.

Zinc is also essential for the conversion of β-carotene to vitamin A.

$$\text{Retinol} \xrightarrow[\substack{\text{alcohol dehydrogenase} \\ \textit{zinc metalloenzyme}}]{\text{retinal reductase}} \text{Retinal} \xrightarrow[\textit{zinc modulated enzyme}]{\text{retinal oxidase}} \text{Retinoic acid}$$

There is co-existence of vitamin A and zinc deficiency in PEM. In children with PEM, full restoration of dark adaptation may not occur until both the associated vitamin A and zinc depletion have been corrected. The assessment of dark adaptation could represent a promising new tool for the evaluation not only of vitamin A status but also of zinc status. Zinc is essential for the conversion of β-carotene to vitamin A.

Toxicity

Excessive intakes of zinc can cause toxicity. An acute toxicity with 1 to 2 g of zinc sulphate can produce metallic taste, nausea, vomiting, epigastric pain, abdominal cramps and bloody diarrhoea. Chronic ingestion of therapeutic doses as low as 18.5 mg daily can result in copper deficiency. This is due to the competition of these two minerals for intestinal absorption.

Recommended dietary allowances

ICMR has prescribed 15.5 mg/day as the RDA for an Indian adult man The body's need for zinc is greatest during periods of growth, infancy, adolescence, pregnancy and lactation.

Zinc status of pre-term infants and top fed babies is lower than the breastfed babies and additional zinc supplements are suggested for such babies to achieve better postnatal growth.

Sources

That there is no major body store for zinc, brings into focus the need for sustained dietary supply of this element.

Soil zinc status determines the concentration of zinc in foods. FAO rated India 'low' in rating soils for zinc concentration.

Zinc from animal products is more readily absorbed than zinc from plant products. Oysters contain 1 mg/g on a dry weight basis. Meats, poultry, eggs and dairy product are the best sources. Outer layer of grains also contribute to zinc. Nuts contain high amount of zinc. Fruit and most vegetables are fair sources. According to the studies conducted at NIN, Hyderabad, cereals, pulses and vegetables contain 2–4 mg/100 g. Analysis of a typical Indian vegetarian diet reveals an average zinc intake of 16 mg/day.

There is now sufficient information to indicate that programmes to enhance zinc status should be considered as a potential intervention to improve children's growth in those settings with high rates of stunting and/or low plasma zinc concentrations.

CHROMIUM

Chromium content of adult body is estimated to be 6 mg. It is present in all organic matter and appears to be an essential nutrient.

Functions

Chromium potentiates insulin action and as such, influences carbohydrate, lipid and protein metabolism. Although the chemical nature of the relationship between chromium and the activity of insulin has not been clearly identified chromium may have a beneficial effect on serum triglyceride levels in patients with non-insulin dependent diabetes mellitus.

The proposed role of chromium in a so-called glucose tolerance factor is controversial. Chromium may regulate synthesis of a molecule that potentiates insulin action. Another possible role for chromium, similar to that of zinc is in the regulation of gene expression.

Deficiency

Chromium deficiency results in insulin resistance and a few lipid abnormalities, which can be ameliorated by chromium supplementation. Chromium was not accepted as an essential nutrient until 1977 however, when patients received TPN exhibited abnormalities of glucose metabolism (impaired glucose tolerance or hyperglycaemia glycosuria) that were reversed by chromium supplementation.

Sources

Brewer's yeast, oysters, liver, and potatoes have high chromium concentrations; sea foods; whole grains and chicken are intermediate. Dairy products, fruits and vegetables are low in chromium.

Table 12.1 summarises the trace element deficiencies in humans.

Table 12.1: Effects of trace element deficiencies in humans

	Zn	Cu	Se	Cr	Mo	I
Growth retardation	+	+	±	±	−	−
Anaemia	±	+	+	−	?	?
Integumental(skin) lesions	+	+	±	−	?	+
Impaired immunity	+	+	+	−	?	+
Intestinal/pancreatic atrophy	+	+	+	−	?	?
Hepatic necrosis	−	±	?	−	−	−
Cardiac changes	−	+	+	−	−	+
Altered metabolism of carbohydrate/energy	+	+	−	+	−	+
Nitrogen and protein	+	−	−	+	+	+
Lipid	+	+	±	±	−	+

+ Prominent effect, ± marginal or needing confirmation, − Not reported.

Source: Iyengar Venkatesh, 1994 Dietary zinc in relation to human health, Proceedings of the NIN Platinum Jubilee, 41, National Institute of Nutrition, Hyderabad 500 007.

SUMMARY OF SOME TRACE ELEMENTS

Requirements of some trace elements is given in Table 12.2.

Table 12.2: Estimated requirements of trace elements other than iron (per day) (provisional)

Trace elements	Infants 6 m–1 yr	Children 1–5 yrs	Adolescents 12 + yrs	Adults
Zinc (mg)	5	10	14.5	15 (15.5)
Iodine (µg)	50	80	150	150
Copper (mg)	0.6	1.0	2.0	2.3 (2.2)
Manganese (mg)	0.6	1.5	3.5	3.5 (5.5)
Fluoride (mg)	0.5	1.5	2.0	2.5
Chromium (µg)	40	80	125	125
Molybdenum (µg)	30	50	150	150 (67)

Suggested for US population — Food and Nutrition Board, USA
Figures in parenthesis are the estimated requirement for Indian adults
Source: Narasinga Rao, B.S., Nutrient requirements (Edited) Bamji S.Mehtab, 2003, Textbook of Human Nutrition, Oxford & IBH Publishing Co.Pvt. Ltd. New Delhi.

The trace elements like manganese,' chromium, cobalt, selenium and molybdenum with their metabolism, physiological function, clinical application and sources are given in Table 12.9.

Table 12.3: Summary of some trace elements

Element	Metabolism	Physiologic Functions	Clinical Application	Sources
Manganese	Absorbed poorly Excretion mainly by intestine.	Enzyme component in general metabolism.	Low serum levels in diabetes, protein-energy malnutrition inhalation toxicity.	Cereals, whole grains, legumes, soya bean, leafy vegetables.
Chromium	Absorbed in association with zinc. Excretion mainly by kidney.	Associated with glucose metabolism, improves faulty glucose uptake by tissues, glucose tolerance factor.	Potentiates action of insulin in persons with diabetes. Lowers serum cholesterol LDL cholesterol.	Cereals, whole grains, animal proteins, Brewer's yeast.
Cobalt	Absorbed as component of food source, vitamin B_{12} Elemental form shares transport with iron, stored in liver.	Constituent of vitamin B_{12} functions with vitamin. Increases the biological effect of insulin.	Deficiency only associated with deficiency of B_{12}.	Vitamin B_{12} source.
Selenium*	Absorption depends on solubility of compound form Excreted mainly by kidney.	Constituent of enzyme glutathione peroxidase. Synergistic antioxidant with vitamin E, structural component of teeth.	Marginal deficiency when soil content is low. Deficiency secondary to parenteral nutrition (TPN) malnutrition.	Vary with soil, sea food legumes whole grains low-fat meat and dairy products, vegetable. Bioavailability is good from cereals and millets.
Molybdenum	Readily absorbed, Excreted rapidly by kidney, small amount excreted in bile.	Constituent of oxidase enzymes xanthine oxidase.	Deficiency unknown in humans.	Legumes, whole grains, milk, organ meats, leafy vegetables.

*Indian population is generally good in selenium nutritional status.

Source: Modified from Williams Sue Rodwell, 1985, Nutrition and diet therapy, Times Mirror/Mosby College Publishing St. Louis.

QUESTIONS

1. Explain the physiologic functions and deficiency of copper.
2. Discuss fluorine under sources, deficiency and excess.
3. Explain in short the following:
   (a) Menke's kinky hair
   (b) Wilson's disease

(c) Acrodermatitis Enteropathica

(d) Superoxide dismutase.

(e) Skeletal fluorosis.

4. Explain the interrelationships of

(a) Iron and Copper

(b) Zinc and vitamin A

5. Name five commonly eaten foods that contain zinc.

6. Bring out the relationship between glucose and chromium.

7. Discuss the role of trace elements in human nutrition.

SUGGESTED READINGS

• Effect of different cereals on fluoride deposition in bone, National Institute of Nutrition, Hyderabad, Annual Report 1999–2000.

• Bioavailability of selenium, National Institute of Nutrition, Hyderabad, Annual Report 2001–2002.

• Information on minerals from scientific and medical abstracts:

  http://www.ncbi.nlm.nih.gov/Pub Med/

• Khandare AL, Rao G.S. and Lakshmaiah, 2002, Effect of tamarind ingestion on fluoride excretion in humans. Europ J.Elin Nutr **58**

CHAPTER 13

FAT SOLUBLE VITAMIN—VITAMIN A

Vitamins are a group of unrelated organic substances occurring in many foods in small amounts and necessary in trace amounts for the normal metabolic functioning of the body. They may be water soluble or fat soluble.

Vitamin A was discovered in 1909, when McCollum and Davis observed that a fat soluble substance was necessary for the growth of animals. Although vitamin A was discovered as a vitamin in 1909, its chemical structure was not determined until 1931. Its chemical name is retinol and the structure of retinol is given in Figure 13a.

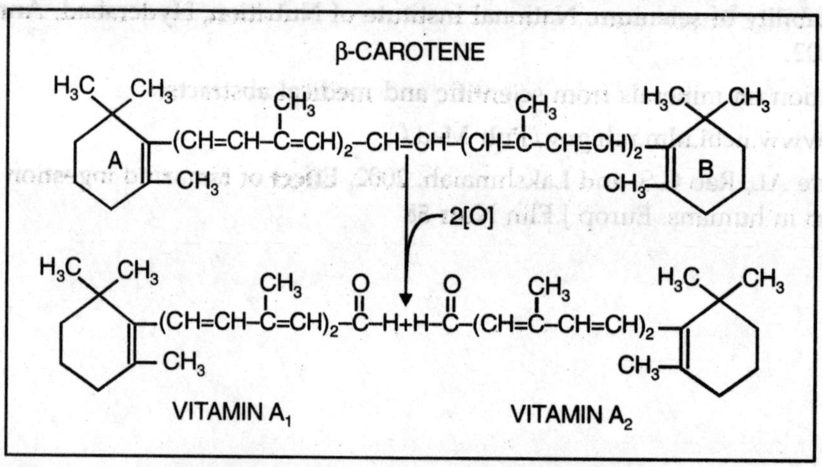

Figure 13a: Structure of Vitamin A and β-carotene.

It is an organic alcohol with the hydroxyl (OH) group characteristic of alcohols being attached to a polyunsaturated hydrocarbon chain that ends in a hydrocarbon ring. In the body, vitamin A can also function in the slightly different aldehyde (retinal) or acid (retinoic acid) forms. Retinol and retinal (retinaldehyde) can be readily inter converted but retinoic acid cannot be converted back into either retinol or retinal. The two other members of the vitamin A family of compounds are retinyl esters (produced when retinol combines with an organic acid, usually palmitic acid) and β-carotene. Retinol can be converted into all major members of the vitamin A family except β-carotene.

Carotenoids serve as precursors of vitamin A and these are structurally related to β-carotene.

Retinoids

The term retinoid is used to include retinol and its derivatives and analogues either naturally occurring or synthetic, with or without the biological activity of the vitamin. The main biologically active retinoids until the late 1990s, only retinol, retinoldehyde, all trans-retinoic acid and 9-cis-retinoic acid are known to be biologically active. However, a number of other retinoids are now also known or believed to have important functions, including 4-oxo-retinol, 4-oxo-retinoic acid and a variety of retroretinoids.

UNITS

Until 1967 the vitamin A activity of plant and animal tissue was measured in International Units. In 1967 FAO/WHO recommended that retinol equivalents (RE) be used.

1 µg of retinol	= 3.7. µg of β-carotene
	= 2.0 µg of carotenoids
	= 0.3 µg of Retinol Equivalents
1 Retinol Equivalent	= 3.3. IU. of vitamin A
	= 12 µg of carotenoids
	= 6 µg of all trans β-carotene
	= 1 µg of retinol
1 IU of vitamin A	= 3.6. µg of β-carotene
	= 1.12 µg of carotenoids
	= 0.30 µg of Retinol Equivalents
	= 0.162 µg of retinol
1 µg of β-carotene	= 1.6. IU of vitamin A
	= 2.0 µg of carotenoids
	= 0.16 µg of Retinol Equivalents
	= 0.25 mg of retinol

β-carotene forms a major source of dietary vitamin A in many developing countries including India. Although the enzymatic conversion of one molecule of β-carotene to retinol should theoretically result in two molecules of retinol, because of physiological inefficiency, the maximum conversion that has been shown in experimental animals is around 50 per cent Based upon available evidence the FAO/WHO expert group assumed that about one third of dietary β-carotene is absorbed. As a result, a factor of 0.16 was used to convert β-carotene to retinol. β-carotene from green leafy vegetables is absorbed upto 50–99 per cent β-carotene from carrots and-papayas are less well absorbed. Hence a factor 0.25 is used (50 per cent absorption and 50 per cent efficiency of conversion) to convert dietary β-carotene into retinol.

FUNCTIONS

Vision

Vitamin A plays a critical role in vision in dim light, in the retina of the eye. Retinol, supplied to the retina in blood is converted to retinal, which then combines with a protein called opsin to produce a purple pigment known as rhodopsin. Rhodopsin, also known as visual purple, is located in the light sensitive rod cells of the retina. When light strikes the retina, the rod cells are bleached as the rhodopsin splits to form retinal and opsin. As this occurs, a nerve stimulus is transmitted through the optic nerve fibres to the visual centre of the brain, where the sensation of vision is created.

Most of the retinal is rapidly converted to retinol. The retinol can then be converted to 11-cis-retinal that recombines with opsin to produce rhodopsin, ready to undergo the cycle again. At each "turn" of this cycle, however, a small amount of retinol is converted to retinoic acid or another inactive compound and is lost from the rod cells. This lost retinol must be continually replaced by fresh supplies of retinol brought by the blood. This means that the amount of retinol in the blood determines the rate at which rhodopsin is regenerated. If rhodopsin regeneration is slow, vision in dim light is poor. The speed with which the eye recovers it is full powers after exposure to bright light is directly related to the amount of vitamin A available to form rhodopsin . The recovery process is dark adaptation because it allows the eye to adapt to vision in dim light after exposure to bright light. The details of Rhodopsin-vitamin A, cycles are given in Figure 13b.

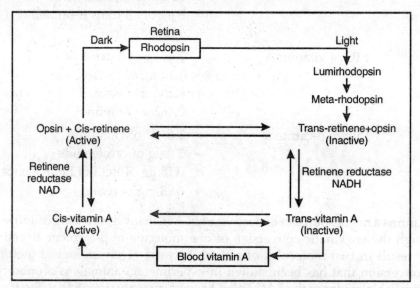

Figure 13b: Role of retinol in the visual cycle.

Source: Shaumugam Ambika, 1999, Fundamental Biochemistry for Medical students, **10**, 111-Cross Street, West C.I.T. Nagar, Chennai 600 035.

Retina of the eye also contains cone cells, which are involved in the perception of colour vision in good light. The light sensitive opsins of the cone cells also contain vitamin A as part of their structure. The functioning of the cone cells is not sensitive to variations in available vitamin A as is the case in the functioning of the rod cells.

The eye contains only 0.01 per cent of the total vitamin A in the body.

Growth

When animals are deprived of vitamin A, they stop growing once their reserves of the vitamin have been depleted. An early symptom of vitamin A deficiency is loss of appetite, followed by a cessation of growth (growth plateau) then rapid weight loss and ultimate death. It is well established that vitamin A is essential for the normal growth of bones. In vitamin A deficiency bones become weak, although thicker than normal. The cavities in the skull and spinal column do not enlarge to make room for the growing nervous system. Deficiency may involve failure of immature bone cells to mature into osteoclasts-responsible for the break down of bone during bone remodelling. As a result of vitamin A deficiency, bone remodelling does not occur properly Retinoic acid can support growth but will not maintain normal vision.

Cell differentiation and Gene expression

The likely involvement of vitamin A in the development or differentiation of immature bone cells into different types of mature cells is just one example of various forms of cell differentiation that depend on the vitamin.

Epithelial cells are found in many locations, including the skin, the eye and in the lining of the digestive system, genitourinary system and respiratory tract. Those within the body normally secrete mucus and are covered by hair like cilia. The cilia on the lining of the respiratory system prevent the accumulation of foreign material on the surface of the epithelial cells by their constant motion. The action of the cilia is involved in protecting the body against infection by sweeping the cell surfaces clear of invading microorganisms. In vitamin A deficient keratinised cells the cilia are lost. The keratinisation and the loss of cilia leave the body more vulnerable to infection. Hence, vitamin A is known as an "antiinfective" vitamin.

Epithelial cells are continually shed and replaced and because vitamin A is required for their formation, a constant supply of vitamin A is obligatory for normal health. The tissues that are most sensitive to vitamin A deficiency are the skin, trachea, salivary glands, cornea and testes.

The Regulatory Function of Retinoic Acid

Studies in the 1970s demonstrated that retinoic acid could induce the differentiation of embryonic stem cells, meaning their conversion from immature precursor cells into mature specialised cells such as muscle, skin and nerve cells. This process of differentiation is mediated by changes in gene activity. Retinoic acid is the active form of vitamin A involved in controlling cell development by influencing gene activity. This suggests a hormone like activity of retinoic acid. It is certainly one of the signals switching on the specific genes that allow immature skin cells (keratinocytes) to develop into mature skin cells. The results of some studies also suggest that retinoic acid or synthetic derivatives of retinoic acid can delay or prevent the progression of certain epithelial cancers.

In addition to its effects on cell differentiation, retinoic acid appears to regulate several aspects of vitamin A metabolism in general. For example, the rate at which vitamin A is degraded slows down as the body's reserves of the vitamin become depleted. Some kind of feedback mechanism allows retinoic acid to inhibit the degradation of retinol. The metabolism of vitamin A within the liver is also influenced by the availability of dietary vitamin A or retinoic acid.

Immunity

Several features of the immune systems are influenced by vitamin A. Vitamin A is required to maintain the normal health and function of epithelial layers, which provide a first line of defense against invading microorganisms. Humoral immune response (antibodies) and cellular immune response which involves the direct killing of infected cell are regulated by vitamin A or its metabolites. As an immune modulator vitamin A reduces the severity but not the incidence of certain type of infections like tuberculosis, diarrhoea and malaria. In children, there is evidence to indicate that vitamin A supplements are beneficial for reducing morbidity and mortality among HIV infected children.

Reproduction

The importance of vitamin A status during pregnancy on maternal and child health has been recognised only in the recent years. Serum retinol <20 µg/dl was found to be associated with pre-term deliveries, according to the studies conducted at NIN (2000–2001).

Neonatal complications of infants of mothers with and without night blindness is shown in Figure 13c.

Vitamin A is also known to be involved in the synthesis of glycoproteins. All-trans-retinyl-1 β-phospho-D-mannose which is formed from retinyl phosphate and UDP mannose is a good donor of mannose to certain glycoproteins. Retinoids are found to alter gene expression resulting in the prevention of some forms of neoplastic transformations.

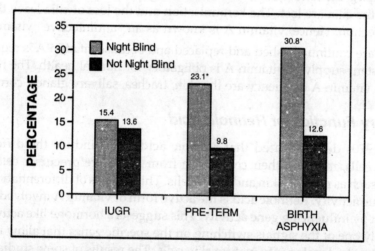

Figure 13c: Neonatal complications of infants of mothers with and without night blindness.

Sources: Annual report 2000-2001, National Institute of Nutrition, Hyderabad 500 007.

ABSORPTION, TRANSPORT AND METABOLISM

Retinol and retinyl esters account for virtually all of the preformed vitamin A available in the diet obtained exclusively from foods of animal origin.

β-carotene is widely available in fruits, vegetables and dairy fats and is converted to retinol in the body. Amount of protein and fat in the diet and variations in digestive function influence the bioavailability of β-carotene.

Retinol can be absorbed from food directly into the intestinal wall cells. Before retinyl esters can be absorbed, they must first be hydrolyzed to free retinol and an organic acid. This hydrolysis is catalysed by enzymes within pancreatic juice and the organic acid released is usually palmitic acid because retinyl palmitate is the predominant retinyl ester within food. Approximately 75 per cent of preformed dietary vitamin A (both retinol and the retinyl esters) is usually absorbed compared with between 5 per cent and 50 per cent of dietary β-carotene and other carotenoids. Reduced secretion of bile or obstruction in the bile duct leads to diminished absorption of vitamin A from the diet.

Only small amounts of retinoic acid are found in food. β-carotene is hydrolysed in the intestine to form retinol and about 10 per cent of the retinal is converted to retinoic acid.

Absorbed vitamin A in the form of retinol, retinyl esters, β-carotene or the retinal produced from β-carotene is transported from the intestine within chylomicrons. For this to happen, much of the retinol must be reesterified back into the form or retinyl esters. The chylomicrons are released into the lymphatic system, which transports them to the blood. Most of the retinol and retinyl esters are transported to the liver (with some uncleaved β-carotene) and some enter adipose tissue and other tissues.

When vitamin A is required by the rest of the body, it is released from the liver and transported to target tissues in the form of retinol bound to Retinol Binding Protein (RBP). The RBP within plasma itself, however, becomes bound to a protein called Transthyretin (TTR) or prealbumin (also produced by the liver). The proteins RBP and Transthyretin serve to make vitamin A more soluble in blood plasma. By incorporating the vitamin into a much larger structure, they protect it from being filtered from blood and excreted via the kidneys.

Once delivered into a cell, vitamin A is picked up by various binding proteins which are distinct from the proteins that serve to transport vitamin A within the blood.

The poor use of vitamin A in protein deficiency can be explained by the need for such a wide variety of proteins for the transport and metabolism of vitamin A. In addition to the wide range of binding proteins, many enzymes are required at various stages of vitamin A metabolism. In protein deficiency the synthesis of all these proteins is depressed. Low blood levels of vitamin A can be improved by administering protein alone for a PEM child.

Storage of Vitamin A

In the liver, vitamin A is stored in lipid droplets, mostly in the form of retinyl palmitate within special fat storing, stellate cells. Retinyl esters are also stored in other tissue including the adipose tissue, lungs, testes, bone marrow, eye and kidney.

The concentration of vitamin A in the liver (which holds 90 per cent of body stores) reflects long-term dietary intake of vitamin A. The amount of vitamin A in the liver ranges from 100–1000 IU/g of liver tissue. A healthy person stores an estimated 500,000 IU in the liver which is sufficient to meet the body's needs for several years.

Only 0.5 percent of the total body reserves are catabolised each day, which explains, why long periods on a vitamin A free diet are required to induce vitamin A deficiency in well nourished adults.

CAROTENE

Carotenes are important due to three attributes; their colour, their vitamin A activity and their potential as anticancer agent.

Only 50 of approximately 600 carotenoids found in nature are converted into vitamin A. Common provitamin A carotenoids in foods are β-carotene, α-carotene, γ-carotene and β-cryptoxanthin. The all trans isomer of each of these carotenoids is more active biologically than any of the cis isomers. Lycopone present in tomatoes has no vitamin A value.

β-carotene is the most important form and being the major dietary source of vitamin A it acquires nutritional significance.

That β-carotene can completely replace dietary vitamin A in rats was first shown by Moore, almost 50 years ago. The major site of conversion to vitamin A is the intestinal mucosa and the enzyme concerned is carotene dioxygenase. This enzyme resides within the mucosal cell. It needs molecular oxygen, bile salts and lecithin for its activity, is activated by thiol reagents and is strongly inhibited by sulphydryl inhibitors and iron chelating agents.

Experiments on human beings have revealed that β-carotene in food is better absorbed than are other carotenes; amounts of β-carotene absorbed varies from one food to another food. β-carotene in papaya is better absorbed than that in carrots. Absorption of β-carotene present in amaranth is less than that present either in papaya or carrots.

Table 13.1 Individual variability in absorption of β-carotene in man

Food source	% range
Amaranth	52-100
Papaya	73-99
Carrort	73-97
Leaf protein	58-90
Crystailline β-carotene	96-100

Source : Srikantia, S. G., The vitamin A equivalence of β-carotene, Pro. Nutr. Soci. India 35, 1989.

There is wide variation between individuals in the absorption of β-carotene from the same dietary source. Crystalline β-carotene is far more efficiently absorbed than β-carotene from any food source, including red palm oil.

Factors which influence conversion of β-carotene to vitamin A are given in Table 13.2.

Table 13.2: Regulation of conversion of β-carotene to vitamin A

Factors	Effects
Dioxygenase activity	Severe protein deficiency lowers activity (not mild deficiency) Starvation has no effect Vitamin A deficiency increases activity
Dietary protein	< 4–6% lowers conversion. Biological value influences conversion.
Amount of protein in intestinal lumen	X^2 at 40% vs 10% protein
Vitamin A status	Deficiency interferes
Zinc status	Deficiency interferes
Sex	On similar intakes, females have X^2 liver stores

Source: Srikantia, S.G., The vitamin A equivalence of β-carotene, Pro. Nutr. Soci. India **35**, 1989.

A single conversion factor is unlikely to be valid for all dietary situations.

After being released from plant cells during digestion, the carotene, precursors of vitaminA, are absorbed intact from the intestine in the presence of bile salts. Within the intestinal wall they are split to form retinol which then enters the general retinol pool. The conversion of carotene to retinol is subjected to regulation. Blood carotene levels reflect the dietary availability of carotene, rather than the body's overall vitamin A status.

Unconverted carotene, is stored in fat tissue and the adrenal glands, not in the liver. Because β-carotene can be converted directly into retinol, it can clearly serve as a direct precursor of both retinal and retinoic acid.

In addition, carotenoids may perform a function as antioxidants protecting the body from the potentially damaging effects of various oxidising agents.

Possible Health Benefits of β-carotene

Cancer: Many epidemiological studies have found that a high intake of foods rich in β-carotene is correlated with a reduced risk of certain cancers. The most definite correlation is with reduced risk of lung cancer. β-carotene has also been associated with reduced risk of cancer of the female reproductive system, gastrointestinal system and mouth, gums and trachea. These are all cancers of epithelial cells. The beneficial effects attributed to β-carotene may in some cases be due to other carotenoids or may be shared by all carotenoids.

In man the administration of β-carotene has been reported to reduce the number of micronucleated buccal mucosal cells in tobacco chewers as also lower the frequency of chromosomal breakages in betel nut eaters.

The mechanism by which β-carotene acts as an anticarcinogen is not established. It has been suggested that this effect may be mediated through its well known property of being an effective quencher of singlet oxygen or that it may deactivate certain reactive molecules, by altering hepatic levels of some drug metabolising enzymes, thus preventing cell damage. It has been suggested that β-carotene may act by enhancing the immune defense mechanism.

Cardiovascular disease: β-carotene may also be an important nutritional weapon in the fight against cardiovascular disease. Supplemental intake of β-carotene has been shown to reduce the incidence of angina in a small sample of men who had previously had heart attacks.

Cataracts: Cataracts are areas of opacity in the lens of the eye. Their formation has been linked to damage by oxidising agents and free radicals. People with low serum carotenoid levels had more than 5½times the risk of developing cataracts than those with high serum carotenoid levels. Although the lens of the eye contains little β-carotene, it has been suggested that β-carotene may protect against cataracts simply by decreasing the level of oxidative damage in the body as a whole.

Gastric inflammation: Carotenoids have inhibitory effect on gastric inflammation induced by *helico bacter pyroli* by inhibiting the activation of transcription factor.

RECOMMENDED DIETARY ALLOWANCES

Applying a factorial calculation and coefficient of variation of 20 per cent, the figure of 600 μg for a 65 kg man or 9.3 μg per kg body weight was derived by Expert Group.

The additional needs during lactation are calculated on the basis of vitamin A secreted in milk. The FAO/WHO Expert Group used an average milk secretion of 700 ml/day with a retinol content of 50 µg/dl and recommended adoption of an additional intake of 350 µg vitamin A per day during lactation. To have sufficient stores of vitamin A in the livers of newborn an additional intake of vitamin A (25 µg/day) is required throughout pregnancy. Since this constitutes a very small fraction of the recommended allowance for normal women, no additional dietary allowance during pregnancy is suggested.

On the basis of vitamin A ingested by breastfed infants in well nourished communities, the Expert Group has recommended a daily allowance of 350 µg retinol up to the age of 6 months. The same amount is also suggested for 6–12 months old children. Vitamin A requirements of the children of other ages have been computed from the requirement figures for infants (50 µg/kg) and adults (9.3 µg/kg) taking into account growth rates at different ages.

Table 13.3: ICMR Recommended Dietary allowance of retinol and β-carotene

Group	Retinol µg	β-carotene µg
Man	600	2400
Woman	600	2400
Pregnant woman	600	2400
Lactation	950	3800
Infants	350	1400
Children		
1-6 years	400	1600
7-9 years	600	2400
Boys and Girls		
10-18 years	600	2400

Sickness, particularly febrile conditions and lipid malabsorption, can markedly increase needs. Genetic defects in the handling of vitamin A can significantly affect requirements. Thus, the inability to convert β-carotene into vitamin A and genetic defects in the intestinal absorption and plasma transport of vitamin A, increase dietary needs.

SOURCES

In the animal foods, vitamin A is present in the form of retinol and its allied organic compounds, which are highly bioavailable. Though expensive, eggs are good sources of vitamin A and other nutrients and advocated as a measure to prevent vitamin A deficiency.

Over 80 per cent of the daily supply of vitamin A in the Indian diets is derived from its precursors, β-carotene, α-carotene, γ-carotene and β-cryptoxanthin which are present in many plant foods. Among these carotenoids, β-carotene has the highest vitamin A activity. Green leafy vegetables and yellow orange fruits and vegetables like mango, papaya and carrots are rich source of β-carotene.

Spirulina (fusiformis)

Blue green algae, spirulina is used as nutrient dense food. Spray dried spirulina is a rich source of β-carotene. About 70 per cent of β-carotene is absorbed. One gram spirulina contains carotenoids equivalent to 1 kg of vegetables and yellow fruits. 100 g of spirulina gives 3,20,000 μg of β-carotene.

Table 13.4: Total and β-carotene content of some food stuffs (μg/100g based on HPLC analysis)

Name of the foodstuff	Carotene	
	Total	Beta
Agathi	45,000	15,440
Amaranth Tender	20,160	8,340
Ambat chuka	9,400	2,800
Colocasia leaves	15,700	5,920
Coriander leaves	15,000	4,800
Spinach	9,440	2,740
Carrot	8,840	6,460
Pumpkin	2,100	1,160
Jack fruit	510	130
Mango ripe	2,210	1,990
Orange	2,240	190
Papaya	2,740	880
Tomato	3,010	590

Source: Gopalan, C.,B.V. Rama Sastri and S.C. Bala Subramanian, 2004. Nutritive value of Indian foods. National Institute of Nutrition, ICMR, Hyderabad 500 007.

Table 13.5: Vitamin A content of foods

Name of the foodstuff	Vitamin A μg/100g
Liver sheep	6690
Butter	960
Hydrogenated oil	750
Ghee (Cow)	600
Egg hen	420
Whole milk powder (Cow's milk)	420
Chesse	82
Buffalo's milk	53
Curds, cow's milk	31
Mutton	9

Effect of Processing, Cooking and Storage

Minimal losses in β-carotene occur when the vegetables are washed before cutting. Approximately, 30–40 per cent loss of β-carotene occur during cooking process. Steaming/ pressure cooking retains more β-carotene in foods than cooking without lid. The use of microwave oven for cooking is not superior to pressure cooking for retaining β-carotene in foods. Cooking greens along with tomato help in better retention of β-carotene because of the protection from lycopene. Cooking with lid is advisable for better retention of vitamin A activity in foods. Oils used for sauteing help in retaining β-carotene. Gogu (*Hibiscus*) one of the rich sources of β-carotene, is commonly used for preparing pickles in South India. Carrot pickles are also commonly prepared in North India. On storing for 60 days, these pickles retain only 10% of the actual β-carotene content. Preparation of dry curry leaf powder resulted in greater loss in carotene content 40–50 per cent which could be attributed to heat treatment.

Exposure of leaves to sun light destroys β-carotene. NIN studies revealed better retention of β-carotene with drying green leafy vegetables in shade or solar drying.

Table 13.6: Effect of processing on β-carotene content of a few common Indian recipes

Process	Recipe	β-Carotene mg/100g	% loss β-carotene
Cutting/	Amaranth dal	0.76	28.4
Sauteing	Palak dal	1.20	22.2
Grinding	Coriander Chutney	1.43	23.4
	Curry-leaf Chutney	1.57	23.1
	Curry-leaf powder	3.61	37.6
Grating/Heating	Pumpkin halwa	0.25	89.2
	Carrot Halwa	2.83	51.9

Sources: Bhaskarachary, K. 2000, Food-based strategy for combating vitamin A deficiency, Nutrition News National Institute of Nutrition, Hyderabad, 21, 2.

β-carotene Content of Leaf Curd

Preschool children cannot consume large quantities (106 g) of green leafy vegetables required to meet RDA. Hence NIN has made leaf concentrate. The leaf curds was prepared from green leafy vegetables by extracting the leaf juice and then curdling it through slight warming. The results showed that amaranth and spinach curds had 70–350 per cent more of β-carotene compared to the fresh leaves.

Addition of fat in the diets facilitates β-carotene absorption. Thus the food based approach can be adopted as an effective strategy in combating vitamin A deficiency in children.

TOXICITY

Symptoms of vitamin A toxicity have been reported after the consumption of polar bear liver (with 6000 RE/g of vitamin A). In adults the symptoms of vitamin A toxicity are headache, drowsiness, nausea, loss of hair, dry skin, diarrhoea, rapid resorption of bone and the cessation of menstruation in women. The symptoms in infants are scaly dermatitis, weight loss, anorexia, bulging of the head, hydrocephalus, hyper irritability and skeletal pain after dose of 8000 RE/day for as few as 30 days.

The most serious teratogenic effects of vitamin A includes fetal resorption, abortion, birth defects and permanent learning disabilities in the progeny. Generally 13-cis retinoic acid is implicated in producing human teratogenic effects.

Recovering from vitamin A toxicity proceeds rapidly after the vitamin is withdrawn in as few as 72 hours. It is rare for an episode of vitamin A toxicity to cause permanent damage. Problems of toxicity occur only from the use of preformed vitamin A not from the consumption of any vitamin A precursors, as intake of β-carotene increases, the percentage of absorption decreases.

Supplements are not needed by healthy persons ingesting a balanced diet.

QUESTIONS

1. What are the precursors of vitamin A?
2. Explain the relationship between carotenoids and vitamin A.
3. Explain the units and interconversions of vitamin A.
4. Discuss the functions of vitamin A.
5. Explain visual cycle.
6. Explain the effect of cooking and processing on carotenoids.
7. What is the importance of carotene to the body?
8. Name 5 best sources of vitamin A.
9. Give RDA of vitamin A during pregnancy and lactation.
10. Explain the regulatory function of retinoic acid.
11. Discuss toxicity of vitamin A.

SUGGESTED READINGS

- Sivakumar, B., 2000. Bioavailability of carotene and its conversion to vitaminA Proc. Nutr. Soc. India, **48**.
- Stephensen. CB., 2001. Vitamin A, infection and immune function–Annual Reviews of Nutrition, **21**.
- Vitamin update: bookman.com.au/vitamins.
- Fruits and vegetables to provide vitamins: www.dcpc.nci.nih.gov/5aday.

CHAPTER 14

VITAMIN A DEFICIENCY DISORDERS

The data collected by National Nutrition Monitoring Bureau (NNMB, 1999) indicate, that Indian preschool children continue to consume less than 50 per cent of RDI of Vitamin A despite considerable socio-economic development. The prevalence of Bitot spots (NNMB, 1999) is above the WHO cut-off level of 0.5 per cent to determine public health significance in all states except Kerala and Orissa (NIN 2003-2004).

Epidemiological evidence indicating that vitamin A deficiency, even at subclinical level is associated with increased risk of morbidity/mortality in children has shifted the focus from xerophthalmia to systemic effects. Vitamin A deficiency can limit growth, cause anaemia weaken host defenses, exacerbate infection and increase the risk of death. The term Vitamin A Deficiency Disorders – VADD – has been coined to cover the wide range of health effects. The over all prevalence of night blindness among preschool children is 0.3 percent and that of Bitot's spots is 0.8 percent.

EPIDEMIOLOGY

Age

Vitamin A deficiency is preponderant in children. While it is rare during infancy, preschool children are at a greater risk. The corneal lesions, however, are rarely seen in the children above the age of 6 years. A great majority of the cases of corneal xerophthalmia occur between 1 and 3 years, coinciding with the peak-prevalence of severe protein energy malnutrition.

Socio-economic Factors

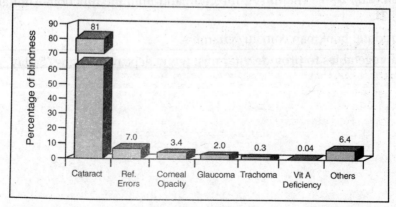

Figure 14a. Causes of blindness in India.
Source: NNMB Report of Repeat Surveys (1988-90).

Children from rural and tribal families belonging to low-income group are more vulnerable to vitamin A deficiency. Cases are common in remote villages. The mothers of vitamin A deficient children are generally illiterate and unaware of the importance of diet in disease. Because of food fads and false beliefs, foods like colostrum, green leafy vegetables and papaya which are rich in vitamin A are avoided. The poor families cannot afford animal foods which are rich in preformed vitamin A.

AETIOLOGY

Inadequate dietary intake: Vitamin A deficient diets are consumed by pregnant and lactating mothers, as a result, the off spring is born with poor liver stores of vitamin A.

Though during infancy mother's milk protects the child from vitamin A deficiency, the intake of vitamin A by the children either during the weaning period or at later ages is inadequate and provides only 25–30 per cent of recommended intake. Consequently the hepatic stores of vitamin in children are depleted gradually leading to hypovitaminosis A.

Animal foods like eggs, milk and liver provide preformed vitamin A. But these are expensive and the poor communities cannot afford these consequently they depend on plant foods which provide only provitamin A.

Inadequate intestinal absorption: The common childhood infections like measles, diarrhoea, respiratory tract infections and infestations like ascariasis and giardiasis interfere with the absorption of vitamin A.

Increased excretion: Vitamin A excretion is increased in cancer, urinary tract disease and chronic infectious disease.

Ignorance: Due to female illiteracy and consequent ignorance, supplementation with vitamin A rich foods is delayed and certain rich sources of β-carotene like green leafy vegetables and papaya are avoided with the belief that these are deleterious to the health of children.

Due to lack of awareness, the community does not make use of primary health services like diarrhoea control, immunisation, vitamin A supplementation and other basic health services.

Improper methods of cooking: Boiling or prolonged heating at high temperature has deleterious effects in the retention of carotenes. Cooking in the presence of oil helps in retaining β-carotene better. Vitamin A is lost by oxidation.

Levels of Vitamin A status

The **deficient state** is charaterised by the presence of clinical signs, which appear most strikingly in the conjunctiva and cornea of the eye. Bitot's spots in preschool age children are the most frequently used diagnostic indicator.

The **marginal state** also termed preclinical deficiency, is characterised by an inadequate concentration (< 0.07 μ mol/g wet weight) of vitamin A in the liver, and an increased susceptibility to severe infections. Clinical signs are not present. Marginal status can be measured by several relatively new procedures: the relative dose response test (RDR); the modified relative dose-response test (MRDR); frequency analysis of serum retinol concentrations before and after supplementation; conjunctival impression cytology; vision restoration time and the pupillary response test. The modified relative dose-response test is proving to be a highly reliable procedure.

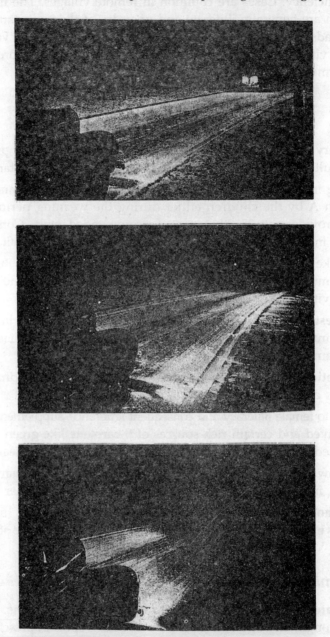

Figure 14b. Night blindness. (a) Safe driving at night depends, in part, on the ability of one's eyes to adjust to the glare of lights. (b) Properly focused headlights of an approaching automobile do not impede a good view of the road when the eye has an adequate supply of vitamin A. (c) The edge of the road and distances far ahead cannot be seen immediately after meeting an automobile when there is insufficient vitamin A available to the eye.

Source: Proudfit TF, Corinne H Robinson, 1957, Nutrition and diet therapy, The Macmillan Company, New York.

The Satisfactory state: This implies absence of clinical signs, full physiological functions that are dependent on vitamin A, and an adequate body reserve to meet stresses of various kinds and/or to provide adequate vitamin A during periods of low dietary intake. Mean total body contents of vitamin A that fulfil all functions of the vitamin and provide a 3-month reserve on a low vitamin A intake for a 76 kg male and 62 kg female are 0.18 and 0.14 µmol respectively. These values are derived from a satisfactory liver concentration of 0.07 µmol vitamin A per gram in both sexes.

CLINICAL FEATURES

Deficiency symptoms show up after liver reserves of the vitamin have been depleted. These symptoms can also be the result of a deficiency of protein or zinc, either of which reduce the amount of vitamin A released from liver stores. Symptoms may result from low dietary intakes, interference with absorption and storage or interference with the conversion of carotene to vitamin A.

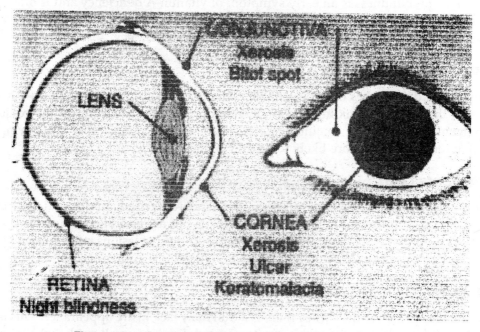

Figure 14c. Vitamin A deficiency in different parts of the eye.

Nutritional blindness due to xerophthalmia is an important public health problem among young children in India. The term xerophthalmia encompasses all ocular manifestations of vitamin A deficiency. It includes the structural changes affecting conjunctiva, cornea and occasionally retina and also the biophysical disorders of retinol rod and cone functions.

Night Blindness (XN)

The speed with which the eye recovers its full powers after exposure to bright light is directly related to the amount of vitamin A that is available to form rhodopsin. The recovery process is known as dark adaptation because it allows the eye to adapt to vision in dim light after exposure to bright light. The effects of vitamin A deficiency on the speed of dark adaptation is illustrated in Figure 14b.

Figure shows that a person with sufficient vitamin A and one with insufficient vitamin A see after exposure to a car's head lights on a dark road. The eyes of a person with sufficient vitamin A recover quickly after the car has passed, allowing him or her gain a virtually normal view quickly. The eyes of someone who is deficient in vitamin A takes much longer to recover because the reformation of the rhodopsin required for vision proceeds more slowly. As a result, vitamin A deficient persons can barely see any of the dim scene before than for a considerable time after the car has passed. This effect of vitamin A deficiency is known as night blindness.

People with vitamin A deficiency may find it difficult to see the way to their seats in a movie theatre, whereas those with sufficient vitamin A manage without difficulty. Those deficient in vitamin A usually cannot see in dim light, either at dusk or dawn.

When vitamin A is deficient, the formation of rhodopsin is impaired giving rise to night blindness. Night blindness is an early symptom of vitamin A deficiency and is often present without any signs of xerophthalmia. It responds well to treatment. It is a useful screening tool and correlates closely with other evidence of vitamin A deficiency.

Conjunctival Xerosis (XIA)

It manifests as dry patches of non-wettable conjunctiva. It may be associated with various degrees of thickening, wrinkling and pigmentation (muddy colouring) of the conjunctiva. The pigmentation gives the conjunctiva a peculiar "smoky" appearance. This symptom in children under 5 years is more likely to be due to dietary deficiency.

Bitot's Spots (XIB)

It is more an extension of the xerotic process. These spots are raised, muddy and dry triangular patches. Bitot's spots are not only easily diagnosable but are also of considerable diagnostic value in young children. In older children or young adults, the lesions may be due to physical factors like exposure to excess sunlight or dust (Figure 14d – Appendix 10).

Corneal Xerosis (X2)

When dryness spreads to the cornea there is a dull hazy lack lustre appearance. This is due to the keratinisation which is the result of vitamin A deficiency on all epithelial surfaces. The characteristic feature is a loss of substance (erosion) of a part or the whole of the corneal thickness. If there is secondary infection there is inflammation. The lesion only heals by scarring. If properly managed the corneal changes usually heal leaving useful vision. Corneal xerosis may progress suddenly and rapidly to keratomalacia.

Keratomalacia (X3B)

In this condition softening and dissolution of the cornea occurs. If the process is not stopped by treatment, perforation of the cornea leads to prolapse of the iris, extrusion of the lens and infection of the whole eyeball which almost invariably occurs. Healing results in scarring of the whole eye and frequently in total blindness (Figure 14d).

Increased Susceptibility to Infection

The action of the cilia of the epithelial cells is involved in protecting the body against infection by sweeping the cell surfaces clear of invading microorganisms. In vitamin A deficient keratinised cells, as shown in Figure 14e, the cilia are lost and the body is more vulnerable to infection.

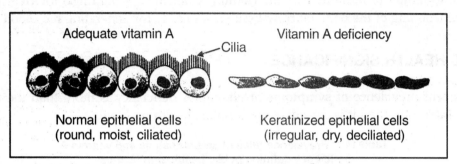

Figure 14e. Changes in epithelial cells in vitamin A deficiency.
Source: Guthrie Helen A and Mary Frances Picciano, 1999, Human Nutrition, WCB McGraw Hill, Boston.

In vitamin A deficiency, both specific and non specific protective mechanisms are impaired. The humoral response to bacterial, parasitic and viral infections; cell mediated immunity; mucosal immunity; natural killer cell activity and phagocytosis are impaired. The immune response to certain antigens in vitamin A depleted children are enhanced by vitamin A supplementation.

The primary immune response to protein antigens is markedly reduced in vitamin A deficiency. The T–helper cell is a major site of vitamin A action in the immune response. Retinol, probably via 14–hydroxy–retroretinol is also involved in proliferation of normal B cells and T cells.

Mortality and morbidity in PEM is four fold higher when they have xeropthalmia as well. This is due to the irreversible damage caused by vitamin A deficiency to the epithelial cells of the natural barriers lining the respiratory, genitourinary, GI tract which may lead to infection.

Vitamin A is known to be required for the proper activity of the immune system, which defends against infection. Once an infection has taken hold, it can aggravate a preexisting vitamin A deficiency, placing the individual at even greater risk of further infections and perhaps eventual death. Carotenoids, which do not act as a source of vitamin A also stimulate immune response. This may be due to their role as antioxidants.

Children with mild xerophthalmia are known to be at increased risk of respiratory infections and diarrhoea. Supplementation of vitamin A has been shown to reduce the prevalence of the infections and diarrhoea and lead to increased growth rates. It is also known that vitamin A deficiency is a significant factor in the course and severity of measles in developing countries. The presence of measles virus infection probably causes a depletion of the body's stores of vitamin A by increasing the use of vitamin A and so compounding the problems caused by decreased dietary intake and absorption of the vitamin.

The WHO and UNICEF have jointly recommended that high oral doses of vitamin A should be given to all children suffering from measles in communities that are known to be at risk of vitamin A deficiency.

Administering vitamin A to individuals with a vitamin A deficiency is followed by a rise in serum iron levels, increased saturation of transferrin and increased haemoglobin levels. Vitamin A deficiency may be associated with a failure to mobilise stored iron properly or could directly prevent normal differentiation of red blood cells. Infections brought on by the impaired immunity of individuals with vitamin A deficiency could also interfere with the normal functioning of the bone marrow tissue responsible for generating red blood cells.

PUBLIC HEALTH SIGNIFICANCE

If the percent prevalence of symptoms of vitamin A deficiency is more than the value as given in Table 14.1, then it is considered as a public health problem.

Table14.1: Prevalence rates of xerophthalmia and vitamin-A deficiency defining public health significance.

Sign/symptoms/Biochemical indicators	% prevalence
Night blindness (XN)	>1.0
Bitot s spots (X1B)	>0.5
Corneal xerosis (X2, X3A & X3B)	>0.01
Corneal scar related to xerophthalmia (XS)	>0.05
Serum retinol level less than 10 µg/dl	>5.0

Source: Bhaskaram, P. 1999, Programmes for preventing vitamin A deficiency – Indian status. Heinz Nutrition foundation of India, In Touch, 1,2

EVALUATION OF VITAMIN A STATUS

Liver vitamin A concentration: Liver vitamin A concentration in excess of 20 µg/g of wet liver are considered to indicate a sufficiency of vitamin A in the body as a whole. Concentrations lower than 5 µg/g of wet liver indicate that a person is at high risk of vitamin A deficiency.

Serum vitamin A : It is a less sensitive test than the liver vitamin A concentration. A serum vitamin A concentration below 10 µ/dl strongly suggests a state of vitamin A deficiency.

The relative dose response test: In this test, a small amount of vitamin A is given by mouth or intravenously after a period of fasting and the change in serum vitamin A concentration that occurs in response to this dose is monitored over several hours before serum vitamin A returns to initial low levels. In people with poor vitamin A status, the increase in serum vitamin A concentration is significantly greater and a longer time elapses before the concentration returns to the initial low levels.

While plasma vitamin A levels represent the liver stores over a wide range, they are not always reliable when the body stores are moderately depleted or when a superimposing depletion of other nutrients or acute infection exists.

Conjunctival impression cytology: A piece of filter paper is brought briefly into contact with the conjunctiva of the eye and then removed. The cells which adhere to the paper are examined under the microscope after suitable fixing and staining. In this way, the cell changes characteristic of xerosis conjunctiva can be identified before this symptom of vitamin A deficiency becomes apparent during a normal eye examination. It is difficult to obtain a suitable sample of cells from children younger than 3 years of age, which group are at high risk of vitamin A deficiency.

Dark adaptation test : The dark adaptation test, which measures the speed of recovery of vision in dim light, is accurate and sensitive measure of vitamin A status. It is a relatively complex and expensive test and is not very useful with children because it requires the subjects to describe accurately what they see.

Metabolic indicator: Circulating level of retinyl β-glucuronide has been proposed as a metabolic indicator of vitamin A status.

Functional tests: Two biochemical functional tests based on increased erythrocyte oxidative stress and Ammonia Nitrogen (Am N) excretion have been developed at National Institute of Nutrition. Am N/creatinine found very useful in both children and pregnant woman to show the functional inadequacy of vitamin A status.

Breast milk retinol : There is no single effective indicator in determining vitamin A deficiency in the community. In the case of children and pregnant women, a record of dietary intake and history of night blindness are found to be the most effective while in case of lactating women, dietary information and breast milk retinol are found to be the effective combination of indicators (WHO 1996). The ratio of vitamin A to fat in breast milk is a better indicator of maternal vitamin A status than vitamin A concentration alone which can vary greatly during the day.

Tear fluid retinol: Night blindness in young children as assessed by interview of the mother, tear fluid vitamin A concentration and other indicators have been used.

Table 14.2: Biochemical indices of Vitamin A Status

Liver Retinyl Ester	mg/kg
Adequate	>20
Deficient	<5
Plasma Retinol	µg/l
Normal	200–500
Unsatisfactory	100–200
Plasma Retinol Binding Protein	µg/l
Adults	40–90
Preschool children	25–35
Relative Dose Response	
Normal	<20%
Marginal deficiency	>20%

TREATMENT

Immediately on diagnosis, an oral dose of 200,000 IU of oil miscible vitamin A should be given to children in the age group of 1-6 years. In the case of those with persistent vomiting and diarrhoea an intramuscularly injection of 1,00,000 IU of water miscible vitamin A can be substituted for the oral dose.

This is followed by another dose of 2,00,000 IU one to four weeks later. In the case of infants and children weighing less than 8 kg, the same schedule may be followed using half the dose of vitamin A. Acute corneal lesions should be considered as medical emergency and should be referred to the nearest hospital for treatment of the general condition in addition to the treatment of the eye disease.

Table 14.3 gives treatment schedule.

Table 14.3: Treatment Schedules for Xerophthalmia — Oil Miscible oral Vitamin A

	< 1 year of age	> 1 year of age
Immediately	100,000 IU	200,000 IU
Next Day	100,000 IU	200,000 IU
2-4 weeks later	100,000 IU	200,000 IU
Severe Protein Energy Malnutrition (PEM)		
Additional monthly dose until PEM resolves	100,000 IU	200,000 IU

Source: WHO/ UNICEF/IVACG Task Force, 1988.

Xerophthalmic children with severe protein energy malnutrition should be closely monitored. They may require additional doses of vitamin A.

Even in the case of older children and adolescents the same schedule can be adopted. In the case of women in the reproductive age with either night blindness and/or Bitot's spot a daily oral dose of 10,000 IU of vitamin A in oil is recommended for 2 weeks. Pregnant women, unless absolutely essential, should not be given large doses of vitamin A because of teratogenic risk to the foetus.

PREVENTION

A comprehensive strategy simultaneously addressing the following issues is crucial to achieve the goals of elimination of vitamin A deficiency.

Nutrition Education

The Education of the people to promote dietary intake of vitamin A and β-carotene rich foods is the foremost requirement for alleviating the problem of vitamin A deficiency in all age groups. The strategy though it sounds simple is a complex one needing inputs from various sectors of the Government, Research Institutions, Home Science Colleges, NGOs and the private sector.

National programmes like Integrated Child Development Services (ICDS) and Child Survival and Safe Motherhood (CSSM) need to promote the following activities:

- Ensuring adequate intake of vitamin A and carotene rich foods by pregnant mothers for building up vitamin A stores in mothers and the foetus.
- Early initiation of breast feeding (within one hour of delivery) to establish good lactation.
- Feeding of colostrum to build up vitamin A stores in infants.
- Exclusive breast feeding for first 4-6 months.
- Ensuring adequate intake of vitamin A and carotene rich foods by pregnant mothers.
- Supplements of vitamin A and β-carotene rich foods like carrots, pumpkin, spinach and other dark green leafy vegetables to be given in puree form (boiled and mashed) with addition of a little ghee or oil and fruits like papaya, mango are to be given to the infants from 4-6 months onwards atleast once daily.
- Red palm oil is rich in β-carotene. Incorporation of RPO into national feeding programmes and supplementary feeding programmes has been shown to be feasible.
- Ensuring regular intake of vitamin A and β-carotene rich food by preschool children.
- School children to be used as "change agents" for communicating the information on vitamin A to their families and the community. For this purpose, adequate information on various aspects of vitamin A deficiency and its prevention and control is to be incorporated in their existing curriculum.
- Nutrition information on vitamin A is to be communicated extensively to all sections of population by all concerned sectors, NGOs, extension agencies and the food industry.

Horticultural Interventions Including Home Gardening

Ensuring an adequate supply of β-carotene rich foods for the population is one of the most important pre-requisites for promoting the dietary intake of vitamin A.

- Production of golden rice biofortified with provitamin A need to be encouraged.
- Specifying annual requirements of b-carotene rich plant foods at production level for the country.
- Department of Horticulture and social forestry should encourage production of green leafy vegetables, fruits and vegetables which are rich in micronutrients like vitamin A, iron and vitamin C.
- Development of village level community nurseries.
- Distribution of seeds, saplings and plant materials of species known to be rich in β-carotene.
- Identifying less familiar local fruits and vegetables with high b-carotene content and promoting them.
- Promoting production and consumption of non-conventional foods like red palm oil for combating vitamin A deficiency.
- Krishi Vigyan Kendras to emphasise on the production and consumption of fruits and vegetables, through demonstration, vocational training, in-service training and on-farm research.
- School gardens and kitchen gardens to be encouraged.
- Strengthening linkages between the infrastructures of Agriculture (Horticulture), Nutrition (ICDS, FNB) and Maternal Child Health (MCH) with a view to ensure nutrition oriented horticultural activities at the village level.

Nutrient Supplementation

"The National Prophylaxis Programme Against Nutritional Blindness" is being implemented in the country since 1970 through Health and family infrastructure. This involves oral administration of a massive dose of 2,00,000 IU of vitamin A in oil every six months to preschool children (Figure 15g).

Since, vitamin A can be stored in the liver for a prolonged period, it is possible to build up adequate stores of vitamin A through periodic administration of massive doses of vitamin A. This approach has been found to be feasible in extensive field studies carried out at the National Institute of Nutrition. Studies in pre-school children have shown that following a massive dose of 2,00,000 IU of vitamin A, there is a significant reduction in the prevalence of ocular signs of vitamin A deficiency.

Since 1992, the programme is included in the, Package of services, provided to children under the Child Survival and Safe Motherhood (CSSM)programme and it addresses children in the age group of 9 months to 3 years only. The first dose of 1,00,000 IU of vitamin A is administered at nine months of age along with measles vaccine. The subsequent doses of 2,00,000 IU are given at 18 months along with DPT Booster dose, at 24,30 and 36 months. It would be better if children in the age group of 3-6 years are also covered under the vitamin A deficiency control programme.

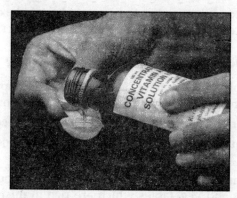

Figure14f. The National Prophylaxis Programme Against Nutritional Blindness.
An oral dose of a single spoon (2ml) gives 200,000 IU of vitamin A.

Prevention of Infection

Vitamin A deficiency is often precipitated by a range of infections including measles, diarrhoea and acute respiratory infection. Studies have documented corneal xerophthalmia, following episodes of these common infections of childhood. Frequent infections in children lead to greater requirement for vitamin A. These infections need to be prevented through immunisation and intensification of programmes on supply of safe drinking water and improved sanitation.

Fortification

The first food fortified with vitamin A in India was vanaspati. All hydrogenated fats, by legistatition are expected to be fortified with vitamins A and D. The general fortification of common foods with ligh levels of vitamin A is not recommended in view of the risk of toxicity caused by excess of vitamin A. Selective fortification of food with vitamin A is recommended.

- Foods meant for identified high risk areas of vitamin A deficiency such as tribal areas should be fortified with vitamin A.
- Low cost processed foods for supplementary feeding of infants, preschool children and school children (1CDS and Mid Day Meal Programme) to be fortified with vitamin A.
- All special foods meant for children to be fortified with vitamin A.
- All toned and double toned milk to be fortified with vitamin A so as to replace the amount of vitamin A lost during the process of toning. Aavix milk produced by Government of Tamilnadu is fortified with 1000 IU for 500 ml of milk.
- The legislation of fortification of vanaspati with vitamin A to be extended to include all vegetable oils in view of the greater consumption of vegetable oils than the hydrogenated fat in recent years.
- The scope of fortifying sugar and wheat flour with vitamin A needs to be explored.

The strategy to prevent vitamin A deficiency should be a combination of long-term programme of nutrition education and improvement in household food security and a short term periodic massive dose of vitamin A. There is also a need for intensification of research and development activities to identify technologies to increase the production and consumption of less familiar β-carotene rich foods such as red palm oil and spirulina, a blue-green algae. Involvement, motivation and mobilisation of community are essential for achieving the goal of prevention of vitamin A deficiency.

19th November is world sight day.

QUESTIONS

1. Which age group is susceptible to vitamin A deficiency? Why?
2. Discuss the aetiology of vitamin A deficiency.
3. Give the WHO classification of xerophthalmia.
4. Why does night blindness occur in vitamin A deficiency?
5. Give the clinical symptoms of vitamin A deficiency.
6. Give the prevalence rates of xerophthalmia and vitamin A deficiency of public health significance.
7. What methods are used to evaluate the vitamin A status?
8. Give the treatment schedules for xerophthalmia.
9. Discuss in detail methods to prevent vitamin A deficiency.
10. Give the role of ICDS in preventing vitamin A deficiency.
11. Explain "The National prophylaxis programme against Nutritional Blindness".
12. Explain the role of vitamin A in the prevention of infections.

SUGGESTED READINGS

- Effect of vitamin A deficiency during pregnancy on maternal and child health, National Institute of Nutrition, Annual Report 2000-2001.
- Scientific and medical abstracts : http://www.ncbi.nlm.nih.gov/PubMcd/
- Toteja G.S et al. 2002, Vitamin A deficiency disorders in 16 districts of India. Indian J. Pediatr **69**

CHAPTER 15

FAT SOLUBLE VITAMINS—VITAMIN D, E AND K

VITAMIN D

From ancient times, in folk medicine, sunlight is used in the treatment of rickets, a bone disease of infancy and childhood. In 1918, Sir Edward Mellanby presented evidence of a fat soluble substance with antirachitic properties. Shortly afterward, the antirachitic properties of cod liver oil which had been used as a folk remedy since the early 19th century were properly recognised. Mellanby's fat soluble substance and the active principle within cod liver oil were the same compound which was soon designated as vitamin D by McCollum and associates at John Hopkins University.

Later it has been demonstrated that ultra violet light promotes conversion of sterol to vitamin D and thus prevents and cures rickets.

Vitamin D exists in two forms, vitamin D_3 (cholecalciferol) of the animal origin and vitamin D_2 (ergocalciferol) of the plant origin. The precursors of vitamin D, 7-dehydro-cholesterol in animals and ergosterol in plants were discovered in 1922. Vitamin D was isolated in crystalline form in 1932 and its chemical structure had been determined by 1936. The structures of vitamin D_2 and D_3 are given in Figure 15a.

Units

1 IU of vitamin D = 25 Nanograms (25 NG) of vitamin D.

1 IU of vitamin D = 5 NG of 25-hydroxy vitamin D.

1 IU of vitamin D = 5 NG of 24, 25-dihydroxy vitamin D.

1 IU of vitamin D = 1 NG of 1,25-dihydroxy vitamin D.

1 µg of vitamin D = 40 IU of vitamin D.

1 µg of 25-hydroxyvitamin D = 200 IU of vitamin D.

1 µg of 24,25-dihydroxy vitamin D = 200 IU of vitamin D.

1 µg of 1,25-dihydroxy vitamin D = 1000 IU of vitamin D.

SYNTHESIS

In humans, the ultraviolet rays of sunlight, with a wave length of 290–315 nm, initiate the photo conversion of provitamin D_3, 7-dehydrocholesterol to previtamin D_3 in the skin. A heat induced isomerisation then converts previtamin D_3 to vitamin D_3 over a period of 2 to 3 days. Less vitamin

D is synthesised in dark-skinned people exposed to the same amount of sunshine as fair-skinned people because the pigments within dark skin restrict the access of ultraviolet radiation.

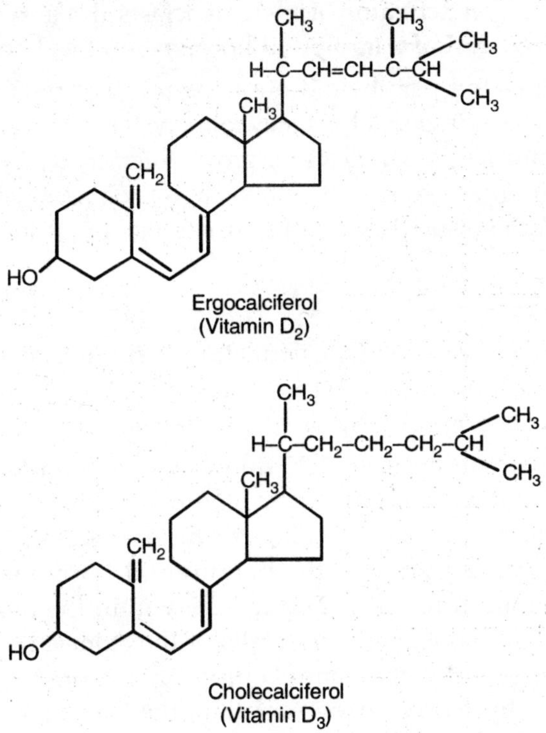

Figure 15a. Structures of Vitamin D_2 and D_3.

Functions

The metabolite of vitamin D that is believed to be directly responsible for bringing about the vitamin's physiological effects on target tissues is 1,25 dihydroxy vitamin D. This is the specific metabolite that is often considered to be a hormone, rather than a vitamin. Indeed, the regulation of calcium homeostasis involving the interaction between 1,25-dihydroxy vitamin D and parathyroid hormone is known as the vitamin D endocrine system.

Calcium Homeostasis and Bone Formation and Maintenance

In the small intestine, 1,25-dihydroxy vitamin D facilitates the absorption of dietary calcium and phosphorus. This is due to its ability to stimulate an increase in the level of calcium binding protein in the intestinal wall. In the bone, 1,25-dihydroxy vitamin D acts together with parathyroid hormone to stimulate the mobilisation of calcium and phosphorus. In the distal tubules of the kidney, 1,25-dihydroxy vitamin D and parathyroid hormone again work together to increase the reabsorption of calcium.

One major effect of 1,25-dihydroxy vitamin D in the body is to stimulate the mineralisation of bone, probably mainly because of the stimulation of the absorption of dietary calcium and phosphorus. 1,25-dihydroxy vitamin D is not itself directly involved in bone mineralisation but it does have significant effect on osteoblasts (the bone forming cells) which play an important role in bone formation. 1,25-dihydroxy vitamin D stimulates the osteoblasts in the production of non-bone matrix proteins. It is involved in bone remodelling (essential for healthy bone condition) as an activator of the osteoclasts (bone-reabsorbing cells) and in facilitating the stimulating effect of parathyroid hormone on this bone reabsorption process.

1,25-dihydroxy vitamin D and parathyroid hormone together regulate the concentration of calcium in blood plasma. This is important not only for bone formation and maintenance, but also for maintaining blood calcium levels to facilitate the proper interaction between nerves and muscles. One of the most serious disorders associated with vitamin D deficiency is the convulsive state of hypocalcaemia tetany, which is caused by insufficient supplies of calcium to nerves and muscles.

Other Functions

1,25-dihydroxy vitamin D is involved in the regulation of specific genes. To perform this role, 1,25-dihydroxy vitamin D binds to a receptor protein in the cell nucleus, stimulating the protein to bind to specific regions of DNA involved in controlling gene activity.

The discovery of receptor proteins for 1,25-dihydroxy vitamin D within cell nuclei was followed by various studies demonstrating direct binding of 1,25, dihydroxy vitamin D within the nuclei of cells of the intestine, bone, and kidney. Nuclear reception for vitamin D has been found in the islet cells of the pancreas, the parathyroid hormone secreting cells of the parathyroid glands, bone marrow cells, specific cells within the ovaries, some brain cells, epithelial cells within breast tissue, endocrine cells of the stomach and the keratinocytes of the skin. It is becoming apparent that vitamin D probably performs some functions required for insulin secretion, parathyroid hormone secretion, the operation of the immune system and the development of the female reproductive system and the skin.

Absorption, transport and metabolism

Dietary vitamin D_3 is absorbed from jejunum with the aid of bile salts and is incorporated within chylomicrons, which take it through the lymph and then into the blood. An average of 80 per cent of dietary vitamin D is absorbed by both infants and adults.

On release from lymph into the blood the vitamin D is removed from the chylomicrons and becomes bound to a specific vitamin D-binding protein (DBP), called alpha globulin and gets transported to the liver. The concentration of vitamin D in blood plasma varies in response to recent dietary intake of vitamin D and any recent synthesis of vitamin D in the skin. This makes the plasma vitamin D level a poor indicator of over all vitamin D status. The half-life of vitamin D in the blood plasma is only about 24 hours.

Vitamin D_3, derived either exogenously from the diet or endogenously from photobiogenesis in the skin is converted into biologically active metabolite 1,25-$(OH)_2$ D_3 by two steps.

The first metabolic step occurs in liver, where vitamin D_3 is hydroxylated to form 25-hydroxy vitamin D_3 (25-OH-D_3). The circulating levels of 25-OH-D_3 reflect the vitamin D nutritional status. It is further hydroxylated in the kidney to form 1,25-dihydroxy vitamin D_3 (l-25-$(OH)_2D_3$. It is the physiologically active hormonal form of vitamin D_3.

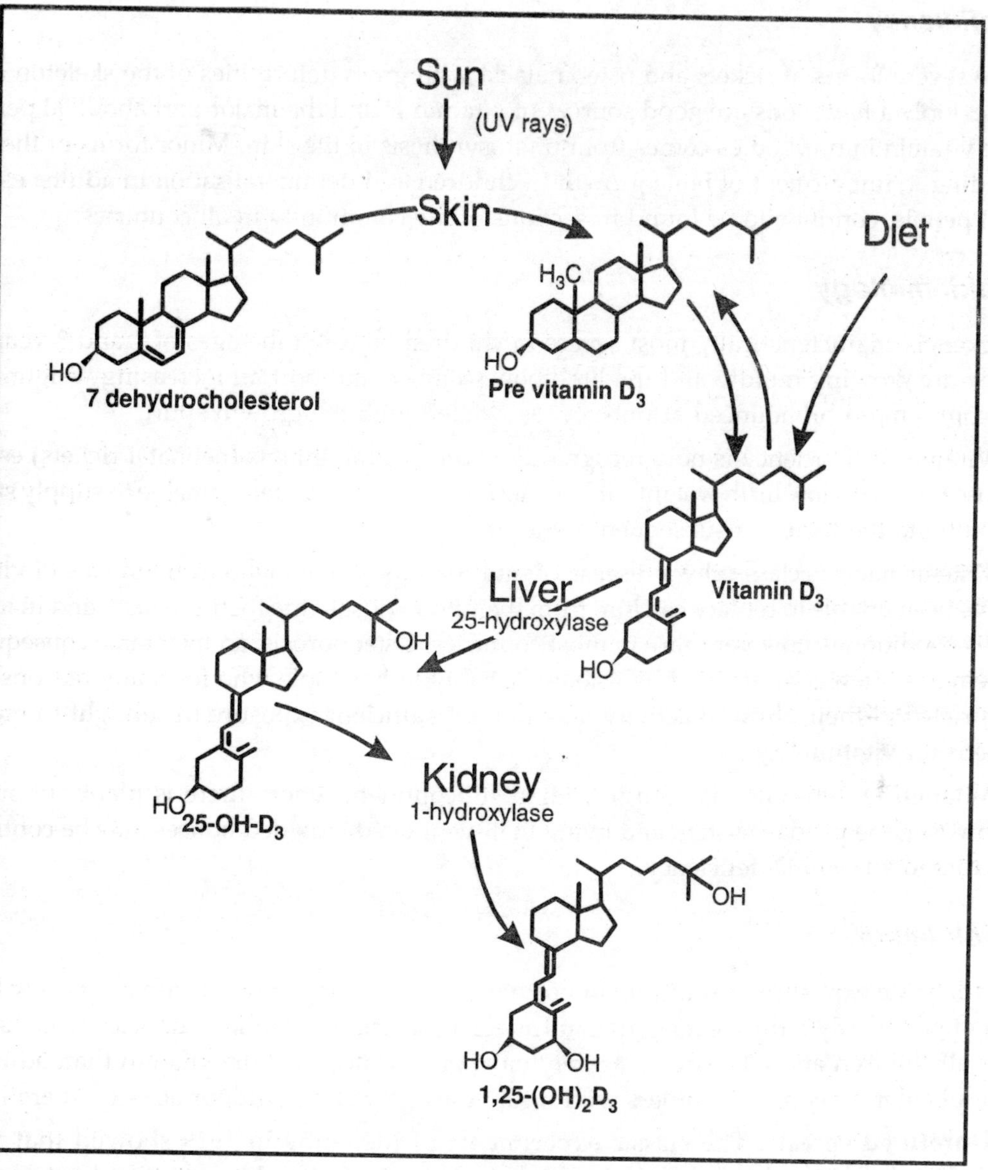

Figure 15b. Metabolism of vitamin D_3 in liver and kidney.

Source: Raghuramulu, N., Vitamin D_3 activity in some plants, Nutrition News. National Institute of Nutrition, Hyderabad, 21, **3**,2000.

Figure 15 b shows the metabolism of vitamin D_3. The production of 1,25 $(OH)_2 D_3$ is regulated by control of the vitamin D-1-hydroxylase enzyme of the kidney. The chief regulatory factors affecting the enzymes are 1,25-dihydroxy vitamin D itself, parathyroid hormone and the serum concentration of calcium and phosphorus.

Deficiency

The severe forms of rickets and osteomalacia with gross deformities of the skeleton are now rare. Only a few foods are good sources of vitamin D and the major part about 90 per cent of the vitamin in our bodies comes from photosynthesis in the skin. Minor forms of the disease leading to impairment of bone growth in children and demineralisation in adults, especially old people, continue to be found in sections of the community in all countries.

Epidemiology

Rickets is characteristically most severe in children between the ages of 1 and 3 years when they are growing rapidly and the limb bones have to support an increasing weight. It often becomes more pronounced at puberty, associated with the growth spurt.

Vitamin D deficiency is now recognised in very young infants (neonatal rickets) especially those born with low birth weights; it is attributable to a mother being unable to supply sufficient vitamin to the foetus or subsequent in her milk.

Osteomalacia is classically a disease of multiparous women who through lack of vitamin D have been unable to replace calcium from their bones lost to the foetus *in utero* and in lactation. This condition is now very rare in most countries. Osteoporosis, an inevitable consequence of ageing, is often accompanied by osteomalacia. Elderly people who for many reasons may be restricted in their physical activity may not get sufficient exposure to sunlight to meet their needs for vitamin D.

Vitamin D deficiency is seen in Indian subcontinent where there is plenty of sunshine. However, the purdah system and living in ill-ventilated crowded houses may be contributory factors to vitamin D deficiency.

Risk factors

Inadequate exposure to sunlight: In northern latitudes long winters with only a few hours of day light greatly reduce exposure to ultraviolet radiation. Vitamin D deficiency is then a risk for all children and adolescents as they have greater need for the vitamin than adults. Also for all elderly people and others with disabilities restricting outdoor activity, there is a risk.

Unrefined cereals: The classic experiments of Mellanby in 1919 showed that puppies developed rickets when white bread in their diet was replaced by unrefined oatmeal. Asian communities whose staple food is chapathis made from high extraction wheat flour appear to be at increased risk of both rickets and osteomalacia.

Vegetarianism: Strict Hindus and others who eat no animal food exhibit an increased proportion of cases of osteomalacia. This complete exclusion of vitamin D from the diet does not normally lead to rickets or osteomalacia but increases the risk.

Prolonged breast feeding: When an infant is fed exclusively on milk from a vitamin D deficient mother for more than three months, the risk of infantile rickets rises.

Skin pigmentation : Heavy pigmentation reduces synthesis of vitamin D in the skin. This can only be a minor risk factor.

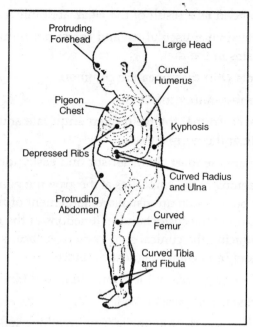

Figure 15c. Symptoms of rickets.

Source: Proudfit, TF., Corinne H. RRobinson, 1957, Nutrition and diet therapy, The Macmillan company, New York.

Secondary osteomalacia and rickets

Gastrointestinal disease: Osteomalacia may arise in patients with the malabsorption syndrome after many months. This is due to impaired calcium absorption.

Renal disease: Osteomalacia and other bone disorders arise in patients with chronic renal failure. Impaired formation of $1,25(OH)_2D_3$ in the kidney may be responsible.

Liver disease: Osteomalacia is sometimes found in patients with cirrhosis of liver due to failure to form $25(OH)D_3$.

Burnt Patient: A diminished capacity to make vitamin D is a characteristic of children with severe burns and such children should receive vitamin D supplements to stop their bones from weakening. Even skin that is not burned cannot make enough vitamin D, in burned children. Children with burns over more than 40 percent of their bodies do not make enough vitamin D. Incidence of bone fractures are high in burn patients later in life. Vitamin D supplements should become part of the burned children's therapy during their treatment and after they are discharged from hospital.

Clinical features

In children, vitamin D deficiency causes the following sign and symptoms:

* The child is restless, fretful and pale with flabby and toneless muscles which allow the limbs to assume unnatural postures.
* Excessive sweating on the head is common.

✳ The abdomen is distended as a result of the weak abdominal muscles.

✳ The atony of the intestinal musculature and intestinal fermentation may arise from excessive carbohydrates in the diet.

✳ Gastrointestinal upsets with diarrhoea are common.

✳ The child is prone to respiratory infections.

✳ Development is delayed so that the teeth often erupt late and there is failure to sit up, stand crawl and walk at the normal ages.

✳ The changes in bone are the most characteristic and easily identifiable signs of rickets.

- Extension and widening of the epiphyses at the growing points where cartilage meets bone. The earliest bony lesion are usually enlargement of the epiphyses at the lower end of the radius and at the costochondral junctions of the ribs (costo–rib, chondral – cartilaginous) producing the clinical sign known as "beading" of the ribs or "rickety rosary" an early and important diagnostic feature.

- Enlargement of the lower ends of the femur, tibia and fibula.

- 'Bossing' of the frontal and parietal bones.

- Delayed closure of the anterior fontanelle. This breathing space in a baby's skull usually closes by 2 years.

- Deformities of the chest such as undue prominence of the sternum (pigeon chest) and a transverse depression.

- Harrison's sulcus (groove) this is apparently caused by the sucking in of the softened ribs on inspiration during whooping cough or other respiratory infections to which rachitic children are prone.

- Craniotabes, that is, thinning and wasting of the cranial bones occur in infancy.

- If rickets continues into the second and third years of life, the signs may persist or be magnified. Deformities such as kyphosis (hunch back) of the spine develop as a result of the new gravitational and muscular strains caused by sitting up and crawling.

- When the rachitic child begins to walk, deformities of the shafts of the leg bones develop, 'knock knees' genu valgum or 'bow legs" genu varum occurs.

- Anteriolateral bowing of the tibiae at the junction of the middle and lower end is frequently noted in young children.

- The spinal kyphosis is often replaced by lordosis.

- Pelvic deformities may follow and later serious difficulties at child birth may take place.

Osteomalacia

In adults, vitamin D deficiency results in osteomalacia which is characterised by a wide scam of unmineralised matrix (osteoid) living the bone surfaces. Vitamin resistant rickets is an inherited disorder which is apparently caused by defective receptors for 1, 25 $(OH)_2D_3$

The common presenting features are pain and muscular weakness. Pain ranges from a dull ache to severe pain. Sites frequently affected are ribs, sacrum, lower lumbar vertebrae, pelvis and legs. Bone tenderness on pressure is common. Muscular weakness is often present and the patient may find difficulty in climbing stairs or getting out of a chair. A waddling gait is not unusual.

There is rarefaction of bone and commonly translucent bands (pseudo fractures, Looser's zones) often symmetrical at points submitted to compression stress. Common sites are the ribs, the axillary borders of the scapula, the pubic rami and the medial cortex of the upper femur. Looser's zones are diagnostic of osteomalacia.

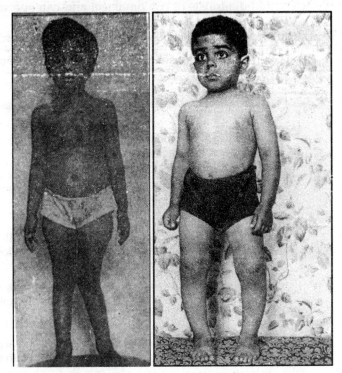

Figure15d. Rachitic children with knock knees and bow legs.

Source: Muratee Shobana, 1994, Vitamin D related bone disorders, Nutrition 28, 1, Muratee Passmore and M.A. Eastwood, 1990, Davidson and Passmore's Human Nutrition and Dietetics, ELBS, Churchill, Livingstone.

Diagnosis

Radiograph of the wrist may show characteristic changes at the epiphyses. The outline of the joint is blurred and hazy and the epiphyseal line becomes broadened. Later in older children, as a result of decalcification of the metaphysis and the effects of movements and stresses the classical concave 'saucer' deformity is clearly shown radiographically. The diagnosis is supported by a raised plasma alkaline phosphatase and confirmed if plasma 25(OH)D is low.

Treatment

A daily oral dose of 25–125 µg (1000-500 IU) of vitamin D cures rickets and osteomalacia. Because of the risk of toxicity this should be reduced to 10 µg, the prophylactic dose, when plasma alkaline phosphatase has returned to normal and radiographs show that healing is established. Children can be given 1 ml of halibut oil.

Advice on diet and general hygiene is needed. An adequate intake of calcium is essential. The best source is milk and at least 500 ml should be taken daily. An egg daily and butter or fortified margarine to increase the dietary intake of vitamin D are recommended. Children should enjoy playing in the sun.

Table 15.1 shows the differential diagnosis of osteomalacia and osteoporosis.

Table 15.1: The differential diagnosis of osteomalacia and osteoporosis

Features	Osteomalacia	Osteoporosis
General		
Type	It is a deficiency disease.	It is not a primary deficiency disease.
Age at which it occurs	It occurs in the reproductive stage due to repeated pregnancies.	It occurs in the post menopausal stage.
Composition of bone	Composition of bone changes. Amount of calcium and phosphorous is low and bone become translucent.	Composition of bone remains the same. Decrease in quantity of the bone.
Deficiency	Less accretion of calcium and phosphorous in the bone due to the deficiency of vitamin D.	Resorption of the bone is more due to the deficiency of estrogen.
Sex	It occurs mostly in women.	It occurs mostly in women but men can also get it.
Clinical features		
Skeletal pain	A major complaint usually persistent.	Episodic and usually associated with a fracture
Muscle weakness	Usually present and producing disability and when severe, a characteristic gait.	Absent
Fractures	Relatively uncommon; healing delayed.	The usual presenting feature; heals normally.
Skeletal deformity	Common, especially kyphosis.	Only occurs where there is a fracture.
Radiographic features		
Loss of density of bone	Widespread	Irregular and often most marked in the spine.
Looser's Zones (Rarefaction of bone and Translucent bands)	Diagnostic	Absent

Contd....

Features	Osteomalacia	Osteoporosis
Biopsy		
Histological changes	Excess osteoid tissue with bone present in normal quantity.	Bone reduced in quantity but fully mineralized.
Biochemical changes		
Plasma Ca and P	Often low	Normal
Plasma alkaline phosphatase	Often high	Normal
Urinary calcium	Often low	Normal or high
Response to treatment		
Vitamin D	Dramatic	None

Source: (Modified) Passmore, R. and M.A. Eastwood, 1990, Davidson and Passmore, Human nutrition and Dietetics, Modified ELBS, Churchill Livingstone.

Evaluation of vitamin D status

The half-life of 25-hydroxy vitamin D in plasma in 3 to 7 weeks, and the plasma concentration of this metabolite of vitamin D appears to be a reliable indicator of the amount of vitamin D stored in the liver. Thus, the plasma 25-hydroxy vitamin D concentration is a good indicator of overall vitamin D status.

Normal levels of 25-hydroxy vitamin D for infants is 10–40 ng/ml. In infant with rickets the level is less than 9 ng/ml.

Recommended dietary allowances

Vitamin D is now considered more as a prohormone than a vitamin. It can be synthesised in the body in adequate amounts by simple exposure to sunlight even for 5 mts per day. Indian diets do not supply even one tenth of the present recommendation for vitamin D which is made by the Committee. Only in those cases where vitamin D requirement is not met through adequate exposure to sunlight or due to metabolic or genetic reasons, therapeutic supplementation of vitamin D may be necessary.

In prescribing medicinal vitamin D under certain situations where there is minimal exposure to sunlight, a specific recommendation of a daily supplement of 400 µg is made by ICMR.

Sources

Most foods have negligible amounts of vitamin D. Certain marine fishes are known to be good sources of vitamin D. Egg yolk, butter and milk have some vitamin D and can be considered as poor sources. Recent work indicated that even the fresh water fishes have moderate amounts of vitamin D_3 in liver.

Table 15.2: Vitamin D content of foods

Name of the foodstuff	Vitamin D IU/100g
Cod liver oil	10,0000
Shrimp	150
Liver (Lamb)	120
Mackerel	120
Cod	85
Butter	35
Egg yolk	25
Beef steak	13
Cheese	12
Corn oil	9
Milk (cow)	03–4.0
Beet greens	0.2
Spinach	0.2
Cabbage	0.2

Source: Guthrie Helen, A. and Mary Frances Picciano, 1999, Human Nutrition, WCB McGraw Hill, Boston.

Studies carried out at NIN, Hyderabad identified to have vitamin D like activity in plants belonging to the family *solanaceae*. The vegetable plants belonging to *solanaceae* family like tomato plant leaves have vitamin D like activity. The chloroform extract of the leaves has free vitamin D_3, 25-OH-D_3 and 1,25-$(OH)_2D_3$. The concentration of free vitamin D_3 was the highest of the three vitamin D_3 metabolites in tomato plant leaves.

In addition the studies also provided the proof of presence of free vitamin D_3, 25-OH-D_3 and 1,25 $(OH)_2D_3$ in *c.diurnum* leaves, which suggests that 1,25-$(OH)_2 D_3$ is the active principle in the plant. With several potential uses in both human and animal health, these easily available plant materials could serve as an inexpensive source of vitamin D_3.

Even the best food sources of vitamin D are somewhat unreliable sources, because their vitamin D content varies with the diets and breeds of the animals concerned.

Toxicity

There is no extra benefit from intakes in excess of 200–400 IU/day, the currently recommended intake for infants, children, adolescents and young adults. Intake of 100 µg of vitamin D can cause hypercalcaemia in infants. Hypercalcaemia can cause irreversible damage by calcification of various soft tissues of the body, including the heart, lungs and kidneys.

Most cases of hypercalcaemia in adults have been caused by vitamin D intakes of 25,000 to 60,000 IU/day continued over a period of 1–4 months. The first symptoms include loss of appetite, nausea, weight loss and failure to thrive. The early symptoms all disappear quickly as soon as all sources of vitamin D are withdrawn from the diet. If the state of hypercalcaemia is allowed to persist for a long period, however, the calcification of soft tissues can eventually cause death.

There is no evidence that excessive vitamin D production ever becomes a problem simply as a result of over exposure to sunlight.

VITAMIN E

Vitamin E was first recognised in 1922 by Evans and Bishop as a dietary factor obtained from plant based foods that was essential for normal reproduction in rats. In 1933 it was identified as essential for humans and found to comprise a range of substances known as tocopherols and tocotrienols. Vitamin E is a generic term that includes all compounds that exhibit the biological activity of α-tocopherol. Eight compounds with vitamin E activity (including α-tocopherol) are found in nature; four are tocopherols and the other four are tocotrienols.

The various forms of vitamin E differ only slightly from one another. These slight chemical differences make differences in biological activity. α-tocopherol is the most active form. Much of the vitamin E used in supplements is naturally occurring a-tocopherol concentrated from vegetable oils. Most of the vitamin E activity in such supplements is due to the derivatives of vitamin E succinate and vitamin E acetate.

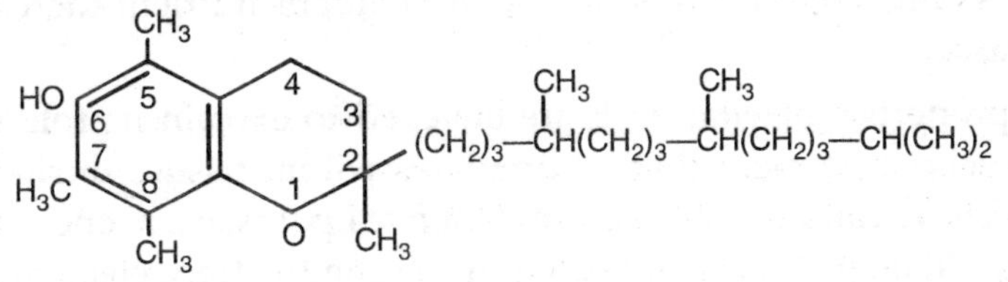

Figure 15e. Structure of α-tocopherol.

Tocopherols are yellow, oily liquids, freely soluble in fat solvents, stable to heat even above 100°C.

Units

The amount of vitamin E present in any sample of food or tissue is quoted in tocopherol equivalents (TEs)

$$1mg \ TE = 1 \ mg \ of \ \alpha\text{-tocopherol}$$
$$= 1 \ IU \ of \ tocopherol$$

Functions

It is generally agreed that the main function of vitamin E within the body is to act as an antioxidant. Antioxidants are substances that protect other chemicals of the body from damaging oxidation reactions by reacting with oxidising agents within the body.

Because vitamin E is a fat soluble vitamin, it is able to mix with and protect lipid molecules from oxidation. It is considered to be the body's first line of defense against a specific form of lipid oxidation known as lipid peroxidation, which involves formation of peroxide derivatives of lipids. In this role, vitamin E protects cell membranes against oxidising free radicals.

Free radicals are produced during the normal oxidation of energy yielding nutrients in the cell. Free radicals can also be produced by the presence in the body of various environmental pollutants (such as cigarette smoke, smog and pesticides) and many drugs. When free radicals attack the lipids of cell membranes they can initiate a highly damaging chain reaction, leading to widespread damage to the structure and therefore function of the membranes. Vitamin E is the main "chain-blocking" antioxidant in the body that is able to prevent these chain reactions from the starting. Polyunsaturated lipids are the ones most prone to oxidation. Vitamin E prevents the oxidation of β-carotene and vitamin A in the intestine.

The damage suffered by cells during vitamin E, deficiency has been linked to the onset of several types of cancer, the early stages of atherosclerosis, premature ageing the formation of cataracts and arthritis. Recent research also suggests that vitamin E may be required for the normal functioning of the immune system and by regulating the production of prostaglandins may control the aggregation of blood platelets during the formation of blood clots. Other suggested roles for vitamin E include some involvement in the metabolism of nucleic acids and proteins, the functioning of mitochondria and the regulation of the production of various hormones.

A WHO study found that improved vitamin E status was strongly correlated with reduced death rates from coronary vascular diseases. A 'synergy' with the other antioxidants, vitamin C and the carotenoids was also found, meaning that each antioxidant enhances the others' effects. In general, as nutritional status for the antioxidant nutrient increases, death rates are found to decrease.

The antioxidant properties of vitamin E are believed to explain its role in inhibiting the formation of lipofuscin, a pigment that accumulates within tissues during ageing. Brown spots in a variety of tissues caused by the accumulation of lipofuscin are one of the characteristic indicators of ageing. Vitamin E is also involved in sparing the trace element selenium within the body and in protecting vitamin A against oxidative damage.

Vitamin E protects the organism against the damage likely to be caused by nitrosamines which are strong tumour promoters.

Absorption and Metabolism

Absorption of vitamin E is similar to that of the other fat soluble vitamins. Absorption is facilitated by bile salts. Midgut is the site of maximal absorption. About 20–40% of vitamin E is absorbed.

Tocopherol predominantly enters blood via lymph, in which it is associated with chylomicrons and very low density lipoproteins. When vitamin E reaches the blood plasma, it becomes associated with lipoproteins, primarily LDL. It is exchanged rapidly between the LDL particles and lipid membranes, especially the membranes of red blood cells. Although most tissues store vitamin E, adipose tissue is the site of maximal vitamin E storage.

Plasma tocopherol concentrations are normally between 0.6 and 1.6 mg/100 ml. Most people have relatively abundant stores of vitamin E, sufficient to last for several months if no vitamin E is available from the diet.

Deficiency

Vitamin E deficiency occurs only in premature infants and adults who have some defect in fat absorption. In addition to a drop in blood tocopherol levels, the most common symptom observed in these cases is an increase in haemolysis of the red blood cells, which shows up also as vitamin E induced anaemia. These symptoms are also seen when the relative need for vitamin E increases resulting from increased intake of PUFA.

In infants, the anaemia that results from the break down of the red blood cells is exaggerated when large amounts of iron are given. Because premature infants have difficulty in absorbing lipid, it may be necessary to give them vitamin E by injection or by mouth in water miscible form, which is a form of the vitamin that is more readily absorbed. Vitamin E deficient infants are particularly sensitive to oxygen therapy, which is often used to help them through early critical periods; one unwanted result of oxygen therapy is damage to the retina of the eye, which can cause permanent blindness. Vitamin E in doses up to 100 mg/day protects against the severity of a condition known as retrolental fibroplasia, which is fairly common in newborns.

A lack of vitamin E in animals shows up in a variety of seemingly unrelated ways, with symptoms involving the muscles, nervous systems, reproductive organs, vascular system and glandular system.

Neurological Disorders: In animal studies vitamin E deficient diets have been found to produce uncoordinated movement (ataxia), weakness and sensory disturbances.

A 'pure' form of vitamin E deficiency in humans is caused by an inborn error of metabolism known as isolated vitamin E deficiency. This produces neurological disorders similar to those found in people with vitamin E deficiency for other reasons, such as impaired absorption of fat. At least some of the neurological disorders associated with vitamin E deficiency are believed to be caused by the peroxidation of membrane lipids. This can be corrected by vitamin E.

Haemolytic Anaemia: In vitamin E deficiency the body is depleted in its major fat soluble antioxidant defense against free radicals. The two types of cells that are most susceptible to damaging oxidation are red blood cells and the cells of the lungs. Oxidative damage to red blood cell membranes may cause the membranes to break, letting the cell contents escape in a process known as haemolysis.

In 1960s and 70s infant formula fed premature infants developed haemolytic anaemia. The vitamin E to PUFA ratio of the formula was low and the infants were often given high doses of iron, which acts as an oxidant in the body. As a result of having been fed a formula with a low vitamin E /PUFA ratio in the presence of a powerful oxidant, some of the infants developed haemolytic anaemia. The administration of vitamin E corrected the problem. This led to a modification of the formulas fed to premature infants, which now contain more vitamin E and less PUFA.

Retinopathy: Defective functioning of the retina of the eye (retinopathy), which can often cause permanent blindness is a danger in premature infants. Large doses (30 mg) of vitamin E have been found to offer some protection against this risk.

Platelet and Lymphocyte Malfunction: Vitamin E deficiency in children with severe liver disease or cystic fibrosis of the pancreas has been associated with increased aggregation of platelets in the blood. Studies in experimental animals have confirmed this effect. In several species of animals vitamin E deficiency has also been associated with a decreased ability of T and B lymphocytes to proliferate as part of body's immune defences.

Evaluation of Vitamin E Status

Serum Vitamin E: Serum levels below 0.6 mg/dl suggest a state of vitamin E deficiency whereas levels above 3.5 mg/dl may be associated with symptoms of vitamin E toxicity.

Erythrocyte Haemolysis Test: Vitamin E offers protection against the peroxide induced erythrocyte membrane damage responsible for haemolysis. Hence the resistance of erythrocytes to haemolysis provides an indirect but useful indication of vitamin E status.

Vitamin E and Selenium

There exists nutritional and biochemical relationship between selenium and vitamin E. Both are antioxidants These micronutrients may be inversely related to carcinogenesis due to their antioxidant properties. These two nutrients are interchangeable for the prevention of certain conditions but each one is by itself essential to cure particular disease states. In chickens both vitamin E and selenium can prevent exudative diathesis (to ooze out the fluid). Vitamin E is necessary to prevent muscular dystrophy and selenium is needed to prevent pancreatic fibrosis. Peroxide damage is found in tissues when either vitamin E or selenium is absent from the diet but their mode of action is unrelated. Selenium along with vitamin E is required for maintaining liver integrity.

Vitamin E is thought to help bind the fatty acyl chains of polyunsaturated phospholipids and hence prevent peroxidation. Selenium is part of the enzyme glutathione peroxidase, which while combining two glutathione molecules, changes lipid peroxides to alcohols and water. In some situations selenium and vitamin E can be partly replaced by sulphur amino acids because these allow greater synthesis of glutathione. It has been suggested that in tissues that normally contain little glutathione peroxidase, vitamin E is essential to prevent peroxidation. In other tissues, selenium may be essential to remove hydrogen peroxide because there is little catalase present in the tissues.

Vitamin E and Rheumatoid Arthritis

Studies on mice have indicated that fish oil and vitamin E are promising potential therapies for those suffering from rheumatoid arthritis. It probably can't prevent development but it may delay symptoms and allow a reduction in other medication. It reduces the levels of inflammation inducing cytokines, the proteins that cause the joint swelling, pain and tenderness, characteristics of the disease.

Clinical trials in humans have shown that dietary supplementation with ω-3 fatty acids found in fish oil provide significant benefits. Fish oil and vitamin E are beneficial in modulating levels of specific cytokines and thereby they may affect the immune system and the onset of autoimmunity.

Therapeutic potential of tocotrienols: Tocotrienols inhibit platelet aggregation and therefore prevent thrombus formation in arteries. They also possess a cholesterol lowering action. They are much powerful antioxidants than α-tocopherol. They protect the skin against harmful effects of ultraviolet radiation. They curb the initiation and spread of human cancer cells.

Recommended Dietary Allowances

Limited information suggests that Indians have blood levels of 0.5 mg/kg/ml, which is regarded as satisfactory. Vitamin E requirement is linked to that of PUFA. The requirements of vitamin E suggested by ICMR is 0.8 mg/g of essential fatty acids.

Sources

Vegetable oils, nuts and whole grams are the richest natural sources of vitamin E (wheat germ oil contains 120 mg/100 g oil) Rice bran oil contains a high amount of unsaponifiable compounds such as tocotrienols and oryzanol which have antioxidant activity. It is present in small quantities in lettuce, grasses and embryos of many seeds. In general plant foods are richer sources of vitamin E than animal foods.

Vitamin E content of vegetable oils is found to be higher than many other foodstuffs. Prior heating of the oil is a common method used for many of our food preparations. It is seen from Table 15.4 that oils when heated to their smoking points lost appreciable amounts of tocopherols; this loss correspondingly increased with the length of duration heating. When the oils are oxidised in the presence of air, peroxides are formed and tocopherols are destroyed.

Table 15.3: Vitamin E content of foods

Name of the foodstuff	Vitamin E mg%
Wheat flour	6.5
Bajra flour	8.8
Jowar flour	2.2
Maize flour	6.2
Rice flakes	3.4
Rice	3.7
Red gram dal	10.2
Green gram whole	12.4
Moth beans	10.0
Onion	1.1
Yam	3.2
Cluster beans	11.6
French beans	8.3
Cauliflower	6.8
Butter	5.1
Ghee	2.8
Vanaspati	6.7
Mustard oil	86.2
Groundnut oil	35.9
Sesame oil	53.1

Source: Gupta Soame and B.D. Punekar, 1978. Studies on vitamin E content of commonly consumed food stuffs and influence of heating vegetable oils. S.N.D.T. University, Bombay.

Table 15.4: Effect of heating vegetable oils on vitamin E content

Temperature and time of heating	Smoking Temperature °C	Vitamin E mg%	Percent loss
Groundnut oil			
Raw	165	35.9	–
At ST for 10 mts		23.1	35.3
At ST for 20 mts		12.8	64.4
Sesame oil			
Raw	175	53.1	–
At ST for 10 mts		36.5	30.9
At ST for 20 mts		31.7	39.9

ST = smoking temperature.
Source: Gupta Soame and B.D. Punekar, 1978. Studies on vitamin E content of commonly consumed food stuffs and influence of heating vegetable oils. S.N.D.T. University, Bombay.

In general, length and conditions of storage affect the vitamin E content of a foodstuff to a great extent.

Toxicity

In infants, there is stronger evidence linking large oral or intravenous doses of vitamin E with possible toxicity. The intravenous administration of 15 to 30 mg of DL α-tocopherol acetate to premature infants has been associated with liver and kidney failure, accumulation of fluid in the peritoneal cavity (ascites) decreased blood platelet numbers and eventual death.

VITAMIN K

Vitamin K was first discovered in 1934 by a Danish scientist named Dam. He found that bleeding in chickens can be prevented by giving lucerne and decayed fish meal. The active principle in these materials could be extracted with ether and thus a new fat soluble vitamin was discovered. Dam named it vitamin K (Koagulation vitamin) and isolated it in 1939 along with Swiss chemist Karrer and his colleagues.

Chemistry

The vitamin, a naphthoquinone exists in nature in two forms. Vitamin K_1 originally isolated form lucerne, occurs in plants as phylloquinone or phytylmenaquinone. Vitamin K_2 originally isolated from putrid fish meal is one of a family of homologous produced by bacteria, with 4 to 13 isoprenyl units in the side chain. They are called menaquinone-4-to menaquinone-13 according to the number of isoprenyl units. Menadione is synthetic vitamin K_3.

Figure 15f gives the structures of vitamin K_1, K_2 and K_3.

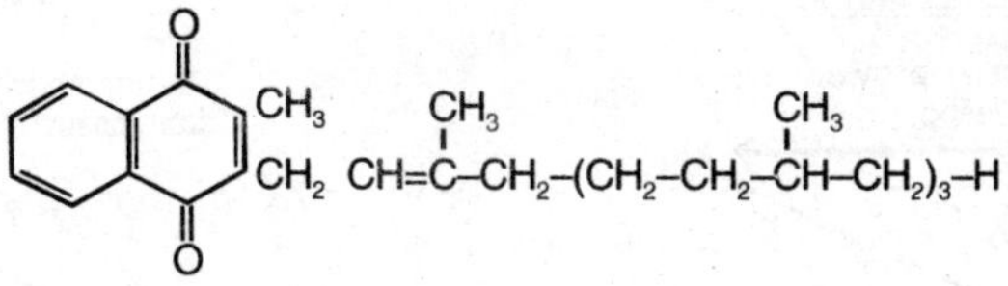

Vitamin K_1

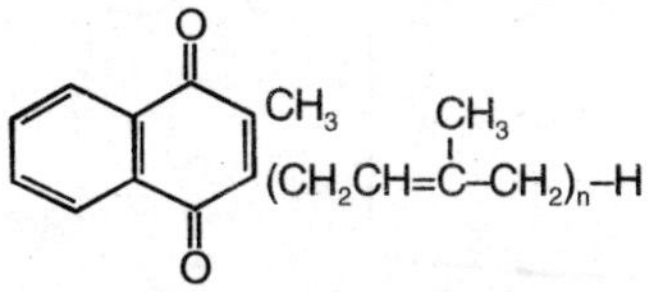

Vitamin K_2 (Menaquinone)
(n=6, 7 or 9)

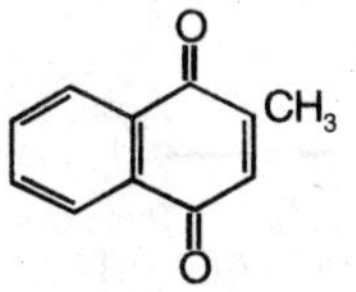

Vitamin K_3 (Menadione)

Figure 15f. Structures of vitamin K_1, K_2 and K_3.

FUNCTIONS

The only known function of vitamin K is its use by the liver in the synthesis of various substances needed for blood clotting. Among these substances are prothrombin factor II, proconvertin factor III, plasma thromboplastin component factor IX and stuart factor, factor X. Vitamin K appears to be necessary to catalyse the conversion of the precursor of prothrombin to prothrombin in the liver; it does this by helping to convert the glutamic acid of the protein to a new amino acid, gamma-carboxyglutamate acid. In turn, prothrombin in the blood catalyses the conversion of fibrinogen, another factor involved in blood coagulation, into fibrin. Prothrombin levels in the blood determine the rate at which the blood will clot.

For blood to clot, fibrinogen, a soluble protein must be converted into fibrin. Thrombin catalyses the proteolysis of fibrinogen to yield fibrin.

Two pathways, extrinsic and intrinsic can be used to generate prothrombin and thus thrombin for blood clotting. In the intrinsic pathway, the coagulation process is initiated by the adsorption of factor XII into a substance such as collagen. Once factor XII is activated XII_a, it proceeds to cleave factor XI to generate an active compound XI_a, which in turn cleaves IX. Factor IX is vitamin K-dependent. Thus once carbooxylated it binds calcium and with phospholipids made from aggregated platelets, converts X to X_a which is also vitamin K-dependent. X_2 in turn can hydrolyse prothrombin (factor II) into thrombin (II_a) which completes the conversion of fibrinogen to fibrin for clot formation.

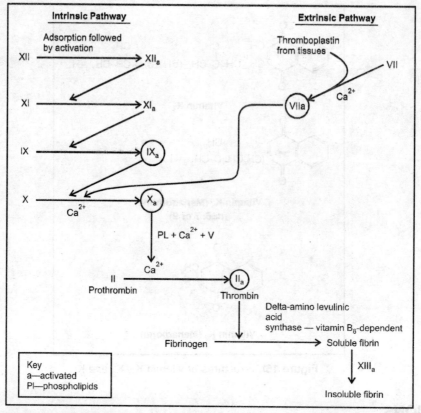

Figure 15g. The activation of prothrombin and the roles of vitamin K-dependent clotting factors. Circled letters require vitamin K for their formation.

Source: Groff James L. and Sareen S. Gropper, 2000, Advanced Nutrition and Human Metabolism, Wadsworth/Thomson Learning, Belmont.

In the extrinsic pathway (in tissue injury) compounds such as tissue thromboplastin activate VII. VII_a is vitamin K-dependent. Through a similar cascade of reactions as described for the intrinsic pathway results in the synthesis of thrombin from prothrombin.

An anticoagulant called dicoumarol which is chemically similar to vitamin K stimulates the formation of vitamin K oxide in the liver. This substance then interferes with the role of vitamin K in stimulating the conversion of the prothrombin precursor to prothrombin. The widespread use of anticoagulant drugs in treating phlebitis and thrombosin has made the use of vitamin K therapy important in counteracting undesirable side effects such as haemorrhaging. The function of osteocalcin, a vitamin K-dependent protein is not known its calcium binding properties and abundance in bone suggest that it may be involved in calcium metabolism, transport and deposition.

ABSORPTION

The absorption of vitamin K is affected by the same factors as those that affect fat absorption. Absorption from the intestine into the lymphatic system requires bile and pancreatic secretions. The absorption efficiency of vitamin K ranges from 40 per cent to 70 per cent. An obstruction of the bile duct, which limits the secretion of fat emulsifying bile salts, reduces absorption of vitamin K.

Fat soluble forms of vitamin K are excreted in both the bile and urine, whereas water soluble forms are excreted rapidly, primarily in the urine.

DEFICIENCY

Primary deficiency may arise in infants called neonatal haemorrhage. It is rare in adults. Newborn babies have a sterile intestinal tract and are fed on foods relatively free from bacterial contamination. The synthetic form of vitamin K, menadione about 5 mg is given either to the mother just before birth or to the infant in the first few days of life. Cow's milk contains small amounts of vitamin K but breast milk is a very poor source. Infants in the first week of life have less prothrombin in their blood than normal adults and sometimes have a prolonged prothrombin time. There is spontaneous improvement within a few days.

As vitamin K is fat soluble, it is not surprising that any defect in absorption of fats may result in vitamin K deficiency. Vitamin K, normally comes into the body from the diet. Vitamin K_2 is synthesized by bacteria in the lumen of the large intestine. Probably about half of our vitamin normally comes from gut bacteria and vitamin K deficiency may occur in patients given antibiotics or salicylic acid that reduce the intestinal bacterial flora.

The only known symptoms of vitamin K deficiency are a prolonged blood coaguation time and a consequent susceptibility to haemorrhage. Clotting time is relatively insensitive method. The level of prothrombin in plasma can be reduced by 50 percent because of vitamin K deficiency without producing any detectable prolongation of clotting time.

Individuals who are deficient in vitamin K possess an abnormal form of prothrombin known as PIVKA (for Protein Induced by Vitamin K Absence or Antagonism) or PIVKA-II, to specify that it is an abnormal form of factor II.

RECOMMENDED DIETARY ALLOWANCES

The ICMR committee considered that no recommendation need be made for this vitamin, since deficiency in India is seen only occasionally in premature newborn infants. A dose of 0.5–1.0 mg of vitamin K administered by the intramuscular route to deficient infants is suggested. Because much of the synthesis of vitamin K occurs in the lower intestine, only a small portion of the vitamin produced may actually be absorbed.

The committee on Medical aspects of food policy of the United Kingdom concluded that 1 µg/Kg/day of vitamin K is both safe and adequate for adults.

SOURCES

The concentration of vitamin K in foods is highest in dark green leafy vegetables but is also found in fruits, tubers, seeds and dairy and meat products. Vitamin K usually occurs in association with chlorophyll in the chloroplasts of plants. Alfalfa is a specially rich source. The average diet provides enough vitamin K hence there is no need for a supplement.

QUESTIONS

1. Why are Vitamins D and K of special concern in infant nutrition?
2. Explain the role of vitamin K in blood clotting.
3. Bring out the relationship between the following :
    (a) PUFA and vitamin E
    (b) Vitamin E and Selenium
    (c) Skin and Vitamin D
    (d) Large intestine and vitamin K
    (e) Osteomalacia and Osteoporosis.
4. Explain deficiency of vitamin D in children and adults.
5. How do we meet our requirement of vitamin D ?
6. Discuss the metabolism of vitamin D.
7. Explain Vitamin E as antioxidant.
8. The deficiency of vitamins E, K and D are not common. Give reasons.
9. Give the importance of Vitamin K.
10. How do we meet our requirement to Vitamins E, K and D?
11. Explain the interrelationship of calcium, phosphorus and vitamin D.
12. Give important sources of vitamin E and vitamin K.

SUGGESTED READINGS

- Mc Caffree Jim, 2001, Rickets on the rise, J.Amer. Diet Assoc. *101*.
- Vitamin update : bookman.com.au/vitamins.

CHAPTER 16

WATER SOLUBLE VITAMINS— THIAMIN, RIBOFLAVIN, NIACIN

THIAMIN

Thiamin also known as B_1, is widely known for its role in preventing the deficiency disease beriberi. The Philippino word *beriberi* means "I can't, I can't" and probably refers to the lack of neuromotor coordination in persons with the disease. The countries most affected by the disease were those in which cereals, such as rice, provided as much as 80 per cent of energy in the diet.

The discoveries of the water-soluble vitamins began at the turn of the last century with the recognition by Christian Eijkman, a Dutch physician in Java. He observed neurological abnormalities in chickens which were fed on a highly polished rice diet which disappeared on feeding bran. That discovery revolutionised the physiology of the day-giving birth to the field of nutrition.

In 1855, Takaki had cured beriberi in the Japanese navy by using meat and milk to supplement the men's regular diet. Physicians in Philippines and Indonesia recognised that consuming the rice bran extract brought about full recovery. It became obvious that a deficiency of some substance within rice bran which was removed during milling, was the cause of beri beri.

In 1936 the chemical structure of thiamin was fully established and chemists learned how to synthesise it.

The chemical structure of thiamin is shown in Figure 16a.

Functions

Thiamin is converted into the coenzyme thiamin pyrophosphate (TPP) when two phosphate molecules are added to the basic thiamin structure. The active coenzyme form of the vitamin has also been known as thiamin diphosphate and cocarboxylase.

$$\text{Thiamin} + \text{ATP} \xrightarrow[\text{Mg}^{++}]{\text{Pyrophosphorylase}} \text{TPP} + \text{AMP}.$$

TPP is needed for the decarboxylation of pyruvate (pyruvic acid) to form the acetyl Coenzyme A that enters the Kreb's TCA cycle and for the decarboxylation of a α-ketoglutarate to succinyl-CoA within the Kreb's TCA cycle. Pyruvic acid and α-ketoglutarate accumulate in those with thiamin deficiency.

A third vital role of TPP is as a coenzyme of the enzyme transketolase which is required for the metabolism of glucose via the hexose monophosphate shunt or pentose pathway. In the liver and the adrenal gland as much as 60 per cent of glucose can be used via the hexose monophosphate shunt. It is the only way in which the body can produce the ribose and deoxyribose sugars needed for the synthesis of ribonucleic acid, deoxyribonucleic acid.

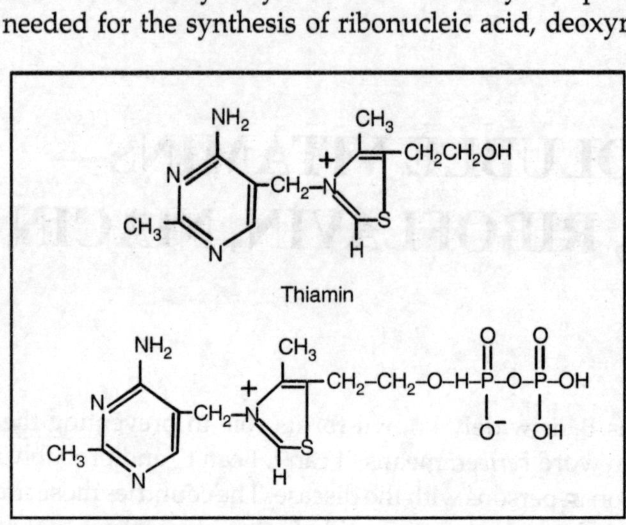

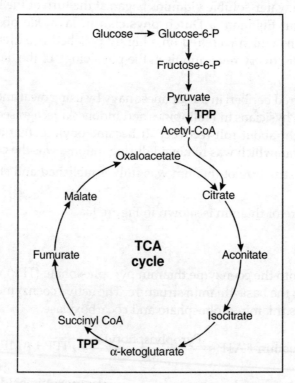

Figure 16a. Structure of thiamin and thiamin pyrophosphate.

Figure 16b. Role of thiamin in TCA cycle. In thiamin deficiency pyruvic acid and α-ketoglutarate are accumulated.

Thiamin is involved in the transmission of high-frequency impulses across nerve synapses, the junctions between neighbouring nerve cells, across which signals are carried by chemical neuro transmitters. Thiamin appears to be involved either in the production and release of the neurotransmitter acetylcholine or as the thymidine triphosphate (TTP) in the transport of sodium across neural membranes that are essential for the transmission of nerve impulses.

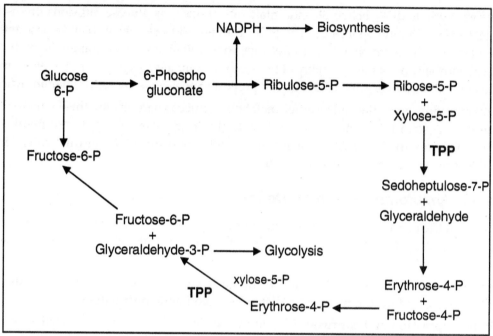

Figure 16c. Role of thiamin as transketolase enzyme which is required for the metabolism of glucose via the hexose monophosphate shunt or pentose path way.

Thiamin is also known to be involved in the conversion of the amino acid tryptophan to the vitamin niacin and the metabolism of the branched-chain amino acids leucine, isoleucine and valine.

Absorption and metabolism

Most absorption of thiamin occurs in the jejunum and ileum of the small intestine. If only small amounts of thiamin are consumed, the vitamin is absorbed by a sodium dependent active transport mechanism. If large amounts are consumed, passive diffusion can account for a substantial proportion of the absorption.

The coenzyme TPP cannot cross cell membranes apart from the membranes of red blood cells. TPP within food must be dephosphorylated to thiamin before it can be absorbed by humans. TPP is then reformed from thiamin and phosphate within cells whenever required.

The adult body contains 30 to 70 mg of thiamin, about 80 per cent of which is in the form of TPP. Half of the body's thiamin is within muscle tissue. The body contains no specific storage site for thiamin, but the normal levels in the muscles, brain, liver and kidneys can be doubled by thiamin therapy. Thiamin is excreted from the body as thiamin-acetic acid and as various other metabolites produced by its degradation.

DEFICIENCY

Causes

High carbohydrate diets, heavy alcohol intake or intravenous glucose infusions predispose to and aggravate thiamine deficiency. The body contains only 30 mg of thiamin and deficiency starts after about a month on a thiamin-free diet, sooner than any other vitamin. Poor absorption due to abnormality of GI tract, inability of tissues to accumulate adequate supplies of thiamin and failure of the tissues to use available thiamin properly are also the causes of thiamin deficiency.

In thiamin deficiency the cells cannot metabolise glucose aerobically; this is likely to affect the nervous system first, since it depends entirely on glucose for its energy requirements. There is accumulation of pyruvic acid and a lactic acid derived from it, which produce vasodilatation and increase cardiac output.

Specific Symptoms of Thiamin Deficiency

Loss of appetite or anorexia: This is accompanied by vomiting and it is the first sign of thiamin deficiency. Increased intake of thiamin restores the appetite but it does not stimulate appetite beyond a normal level.

Decreased muscle tone: In the wall of the gastrointestinal tract, decreased muscle tone results in decreased gastric motility, a distended colon and constipation.

Mental depression and confusion: Thiamin is called "morale vitamin". Deficiency causes mood changes, vague feelings of uneasiness, fear, disorderly thinking and other signs of mental depression, instability, fatigue and headache. The affected individuals voluntarily restrict their social-engagements. Thiamin excreted in urine drops dramatically. The most acute symptom of thiamin deficiency is the mental confusion that precedes coma.

Neurological changes: Thiamin levels in the brain can be reduced by 50 per cent without any noticeable symptoms. Further reduction to 30 per cent of normal levels leads to development of a slow and unsteady gait. At 20 per cent of normal levels, severe disturbance of posture and equilibrium occur, and neuro muscular coordination in general becomes impaired leading to deterioration in speed of movements and hand eye coordination.

Infantile Beri-beri

It occurs in infants between 2 and 5 months of age. The condition develops frighteningly quickly and if not treated can lead to death. The affected baby develops cyanosis, in which the lack of oxygen or accumulation of carbondioxide in the blood causes the skin to turn blue, tachycardia and a loud, piercing cry that changes to a thin, weak and almost inaudible one. The symptoms are sometimes accompanied by vomiting and convulsions. Beri-beri occurs more often in breast fed than in bottle fed infants because a lactating mother's intake of thiamin may be too low to allow a sufficient amount to enter her milk. The situation is complicated by the transfer into the milk of pyruvic aldehyde, a toxic product of carbohydrate metabolism that accumulates in thiamin deficiency.

Wet Beri Beri

Oriental beriberi is usually caused by eating diets in which most of the calories are derived from polished, highly milled rice. The disorder is often precipitated by infections, hard physical labour or pregnancy and lactation. In Britain and North America, beriberi heart disease is seen in alcoholics.

Owing to a lack of thiamin, glucose is incompletely metabolised and pyruvic and lactic acids accumulate in the tissues and body fluids. Also there is inability to use glucose efficiently. These metabolites cause dilatation of peripheral blood vessels as in normal exercise. In beriberi this vasodilatation may be extreme so that fluid leaks out through the capillaries, producing oedema. At the same time the blood flows rapidly through the dilated peripheral circulation. There is a high cardiac output and as the disease progresses the heart dilates because the myocardium is over worked. Serious cases can progress to low output cardiac failure — "shoshin" beri beri.

Soshin or pernicious beriberi is the sudden onset of cardiac pain, restlessness, cyanosis and peripheral circulatory failure. Patients with such an attack seldom survive.

Oedema is the most notable feature and may develop rapidly to involve not only the legs but also the face, trunk and serous cavities. Palpitations are marked and there may be pain in the legs after walking, probably due to the accumulation of lactic acid. There is usually tachycardia and an increase in pulse pressure. The heart is enlarged and the jugular venous pressure rises. Person finds it difficult to walk.

The best laboratory test is measurement of transketolase activity in red cells with and without added thiamin pyrophosphate *in vitro*. A TPP effect above 30 per cent is to be expected in beriberi or Wernicke's encephalopathy.

Dry Beriberi

This is essentially a peripheral neuropathy, formerly common in South East Asia. The nutritional background is similar to that of wet beriberi. In long standing cases there is degeneration and demyelination of both sensory and motor nerves, resulting in severe wasting of muscles. The vagus and other autonomic nerves can also be affected.

In both forms, the symptoms include numbness in the legs, irritability, vague uneasiness, disorderly thinking and nausea.

Wernicke's Encephalopathy

This cerebral form of thiamin deficiency occurs in Europe, North America and Australia. It often presents acutely usually in an alcoholic. But it is sometimes seen in people with persistent vomiting. It occurred in prisoners of war on small rations of polished rice.

In Wernicke's encephalopathy the patient is quite confused and the most valuable clinical sign is some form of bilateral, symmetrical opthalmoplegia-paralysis of eye muscles, nystagmus involuntary and jerky repetition movement of eye balls, may be present.

If Wernicke's encephalopathy is not treated, it can lead to death. If transketolase test is positive thiamin should be given. If Wernicke's encephalopathy is treated late, Korsakoff's psychosis may become permanent. The patient is fully conscious but has a profound impairment of memory recall and new learning ability. Amnesia also occurs. In South East Asia, cerebral forms are uncommon. Beriberi cardiomyopathy is seldom seen with Wernicke/Korsakoff disease.

Thiamin deficiency can produce high output cardiac failure and/or peripheral neuropathy and/or encephalopathy. These occur in various combinations in wet and dry beriberi, infantile beriberi and Wernicke's encephalopathy.

Table 16.1: Manifestation of Thiamin deficiency

	Infantile Beriberi	Wet Beriberi	Dry Beriberi	Wernicke's Encephalopathy
Cause	Lack of thiamin in mothers milk, presence of pyruvic aldehyde.	Intake of polished rice, physical Exertion, high carbohydrate diet.	Intake of polished rice.	Alcoholism, Persistant vomiting.
Symptom	Cyanosis, Aphoniainaudible cry, convulsion, coma.	Oedema, pain in the leg, tachycardia, dyspnoea, cold extremities cyanosis, shoshin beriberi, death.	Numbness in the leg, irritability, disorderly thinking, nausea degeneration, and demyelination of motor and sensory nerves wasting of muscle, calf muscle tenderness, burning, sensation of pins and needles in the extremities, muscle cramps, foot and wrist drop.	Opthalmaplegia, nystagmus, amnesia, korosakoffs psychosis, confused, impairment of memory, recall and new leaning ability.
Organ Affected	Heart	Heart in people doing heavy work.	Nerves and muscles	Brain, eyes
Treatment	2–5 mg	50 mg thiamin intramuscularly 3 days, 10 mg 3 times a day orally for a month.	5–10 mg orally for long time.	10–20 mg parenterally twice or thrice a day.

It is not very well understood as to why the brain is affected in one person, the heart in another and the peripheral nerves in a third. Possibly the cardiomyopathy occurs in people who use their muscles for heavy work and so accumulate large amounts of pyruvate, producing intense vasodilatation and increasing cardiac work while encephalopathy is the first manifestation in less active, people.

Treatment

Treatment of thiamin deficiency is simple and the response is dramatic. Severe manifestations such as cardiac beriberi and Wernicke's syndrome can be treated by 10–20 mg of thiamin given parenterally twice or thrice a day. Infantile beriberi may respond to 2–5 mg of thiamin within a few hours. Chronic beriberi requires prolonged therapy. Small doses of 5–10 mg of oral route given over long durations is better than large doses of thiamin by parenteral route as it is rapidly eliminated by the kidney.

The response of a patient with beriberi to thiamin is one of the most dramatic therapeutic events. Within a few hours the breathing is easier, the pulse rate slower, the extremities cooler and a rapid diuresis begins to dispose of the oedema. In a few days the size of the heart is restored to normal.

Prevention

As per the Indian Government regulations the extent of rice polishing should not exceed 5 per cent. If rice is milled beyond 10 per cent then most of the thiamin is lost. Avoiding excessive milling and polishing of cereal grains can increase the thiamin intakes from cereal diets.

Traditional family cooking practices need to be encouraged. Consumption of refined and processed foods and alcoholic drinks should be discouraged.

Thiamin deficiency can be prevented by supplementing vitamins in alcholic's diet. Bread and other staple cereal foods can be fortified with the vitamin. Currently beriberi is much less common in Asia than it used to be.

Evaluation of thiamin status

Specific test to know the deficiency of thiamin is the measurement of the transketolase activity in the red blood corpuscles with and without the addition of TPP *in vitro*. If TPP increases activity by more than 25 per cent indicates thaimine deficiency. Normal individuals have an erythrocyte transketalase activity of 850–1000 µg hexose/ml hydrolysate/hr.

Recommended dietary allowance

Since thiamin is involved in carbohydrate metabolism its requirement is related to energy derived from carbohydrate. Nutrition Expert Group of ICMR suggested an allowance of 0.5 mg per 1000 kcal which applies to adults, pregnant women, lactating women and children. For infants 0.3 mg/1000 kcal is suggested since there are no dietary losses.

Table 16.2: ICMR recommended dietary allowances of thiamin

Group		Thiamin mg/day
Man		
Sedentary	:	1.2
Moderate	:	1.4
Heavy work	:	1.6
Woman		
Sedentary	:	0.9
Moderate	:	1.1
Heavy work	:	1.2
Pregnant Woman	:	+0.2
Lactation		
0–6 months	:	+0.3
6–12 months	:	+0.2
Infants		
0–6 months	:	55 µg/kg
6–12 months	:	50 µg/kg

Contd....

Group		Thiamin mg/day
Children		
1–3 years	:	0.6
4–6 years	:	0.9
7–9 years	:	1.2
Boys		
10–12 years	:	1.1
13–15 years	:	1.2
16–18 years	:	1.3
Girls		
10–18 years	:	1.0

Parmacological uses of Thiamin

Apart from children with thiamin-responsive maple syrup urine disease and thiamin-responsive megaloblastic anaemia, there are no established pharmacological uses of thiamin other than the treatment of deficiency. Because of the neurological involvement in thiamin deficiency, the vitamin has been used in nerve tonics, although there is no evidence that it has any effect except in cases of deficiency. Also there is no evidence of beneficial effects of thiamin supplementation in Alzheimer's disease.

Sources

Diets based on whole wheat, any of the millets, raw hand pounded rice or parboiled rice (hand pounded) usually supply adequate amounts of thiamin. Bran contains most of the thiamin of the rice grain. Polished rice contains negligible amounts of thiamin. Inclusion of pulses in the diet can improve the thiamin content. Wheat bran and wheat germ are very rich sources of thiamin while white flour is devoid of the vitamin. Thiamin deficiency can be prevented by including atleast 100 g of parboiled rice or undermilled raw rice or wheat or any millets. This can also be achieved by including 60–70 g pulse in the diet based exclusively on raw milled rice. Table 16.3 shows the thiamin content of foods.

Table 16.3: Thiamin content of foods

Name of the foodstuff	Thiamin mg/100g
Gingelly seeds	1.0
Groundnut	0.9
Lotus stem, dry	0.8
Soya bean	0.7
Cashewnut	0.6
Pork	0.5
Cow pea	0.5
Bengal gram	0.5
Rice, parboiled	0.2

As per the Indian Government regulations the extent of polishing should not exceed 5 percent. If rice is milled beyond 10 percent then most of the thiamin is lost.

Organ meats, pork, liver and eggs also supply thiamin.

Solubility of thiamin in water and its sensitivity to heat result in some loss during usual cooking practices. Electronic cooking results in minimal losses.

Washing rice may remove 40 per cent of thiamin. Boiling rice in excess water and discarding the water (kanjee) also result in loss of thiamin. In parboiled rice, loss of thiamin due to washing and discarding kanjee is much less.

Thiamin is relatively stable to temperatures upto boiling point, provided that the medium is slightly acid, as in baking with yeast. But if baking powder is used or if soda is added during cooking vegetables, almost all the vitamin may be destroyed. The loss of thiamin in cooking of an ordinary mixed diet is usually about 25 per cent. Modern processes for freezing, canning and dehydrating food result in only small losses.

There are some naturally occurring antithiamin factors in foods which include heat sensitive thiaminase and heat resistant polyphenolic compounds like tannins and caffeic acid. Thiaminase is present in certain varieties of fish. Cooking inactivates this enzyme. Ingestion of large amount of tea or coffee and chewing betel nut which contains heat stable antithiamin factors lead to deterioration in thiamin status.

The thiamin/energy ratios of foods indicate those which protect against beriberi and those which are liable to produce the disease if consumed in excessive amounts. Pulses and most whole cereals have a ratio of about 1.2 mg/1000 kcal and are actively protective against beriberi. Raw polished rice has a value of about 0.15 mg/1000 kcal and is beriberi producing. Most fruits, vegetables and flesh foods have a ratio just above a critical level of about 60 and are weakly effective in preventing beri beri.

RIBOFLAVIN

Riboflavin, B_2 vitamin G, the yellow enzyme was recognized as a vitamin in 1917.

Chemical properties

The chemical structure of riboflavin is given in Figure 16d.

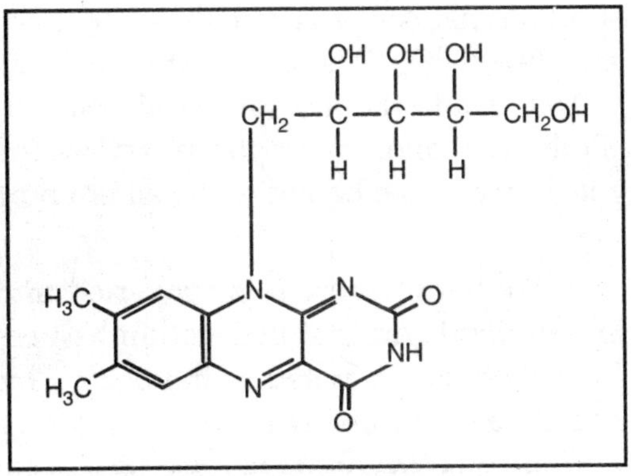

Figure 16d: Riboflavin structure

It is a relatively stable vitamin that is resistant to acid, heat and oxidation. It is unstable in the presence of alkali and light. Because it is slightly soluble in water, some losses occur when small pieces of riboflavin containing food are cooked in large amounts of water for long periods. Major factor causing loss of riboflavin from food is the action of sunlight on milk. Upto 70 per cent of the riboflavin in milk can be destroyed during 4 hours of exposure to sunlight.

Functions

Riboflavin is used to produce two co-enzymes, Flavin Mono Nucleotide (FMN) and Flavin Adenine Dinucleotide (FAD). These co-enzymes function primarily in oxidation reduction reactions in electron transport chain link cycle because of their ability to accept and transfer hydrogen atoms. The proteins to which they become attached are known as flavoproteins.

Reactions dependent on the co-enzymes derived from riboflavin are:

- the release of energy from glucose, fatty acids and amino acids.
- the conversion of amino acid tryptophan into the active form of the vitamin niacin.
- the conversion of vitamin B_6 and folate into their active coenzyme and storage forms. Because vitamin B_6 and folate are required for DNA synthesis, riboflavin has an indirect effect on cell division and therefore growth.
- It has been observed by NIN that respiratory infections result in significantly higher riboflavin excretion and lower blood levels of riboflavin. Saturation of FAD-dependent enzyme erythrocyte glutathione reductase with the coenzyme FAD is increased possibly to meet the demand for reduced glutathione to mount phagocytic response.
- Other biochemical roles of riboflavin include its role in dehydrogenation reactions. It is involved in the production of hormones in the adrenal gland, the formation of red blood cells in bone marrow, the synthesis of glycogen and the catabolism of fatty acids.

Absorption, transport and metabolism

Riboflavin occurs in food in three forms: riboflavin itself, FMN, FAD coenzyme forms of the vitamin. All three forms can be used to meet the body's need. In the intestinal lumen, FMN and FAD are converted into free riboflavin before absorption. The riboflavin is then absorbed by a regulated active transport mechanism largely in the upper portion of the gastro-intestinal tract. More riboflavin is absorbed, when it is taken with meals (about 70%) than when it is taken alone (about 15%). Once inside the intestinal cells the riboflavin is combined with phosphate to form FMN. Both FMN and any unphosphorylated riboflavin are released into the circulation where they largely become bound to the albumin protein and are transported to the body's cells.

Most FMN is released into the liver, where it is converted into FAD by the addition of adenosine diphosphate. Excess riboflavin is stored within tissues as FMN and FAD rather than as free riboflavin. Little riboflavin is stored in the body. Thyroid hormone appears to stimulate the absorption and storage of riboflavin and the synthesis of FMN and FAD.

Riboflavin is excreted mainly in urine, after the kidneys have reabsorbed enough of the vitamin. Normal urinary excretion is 200 mg/24 hr. In deficiency it is reduced to 40 to 70 mg/24 hrs.

Deficiency

Riboflavin deficiency is widely prevalent among the low income groups of the population in all age groups particularly in vulnerable groups and geriatric group. Cereal-based diets without the protective pulses and milk lead to riboflavin deficiency. Riboflavin deficiency is seen associated with tuberculosis, prolonged fevers, malabsorption, hyperthyroidism and malignancy. In fact, riboflavin deficiency can occur whenever there are chronic infections, trauma and negative nitrogen balance. Even simple exercises can increase urinary riboflavin excretion. Ariboflavinosis can be seen with other B vitamin deficiences.

Riboflavin deficiency is characterised by orolingual, dermal, haematological and corneal manifestations.

Orolingual manifestations: Angular stomatitis/glossitis, cheilosis are characteristic features of ariboflavinosis. Early symptoms of ariboflavinosis are soreness and burning of mouth and tongue. The lesions at the angles of mouth are termed as angular stomatitis (Figure 16e). The lesions may progress to small cracks at mucocutaneous junction producing fissures and may get covered by white or yellow crusts. The tongue in general is acutely inflamed called glossitis (Figure 16f). Hypertrophic papillae produce the classical magenta red tongue with pebbled appearance and when the disease progresses, they get atrophic with denudation of the papillae producing a typical bald tongue.

Dry chopped appearance of the lips with superficial ulcers terms as cheilosis is one of the classical features of severe riboflavin deficiency (Figure 16e).

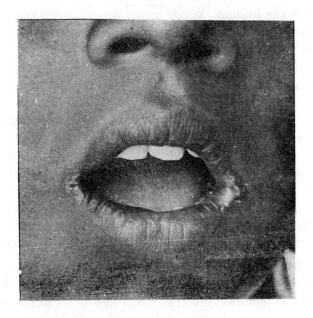

Figure 16e. Angular Stomatitis. This is not specific for lack of riboflavin. Deficiencies of niacin, pyridoxine and iron can all produce it.

Source: *Courtesy:* National Institute of Nutrition, Hyderabad, 500 007.

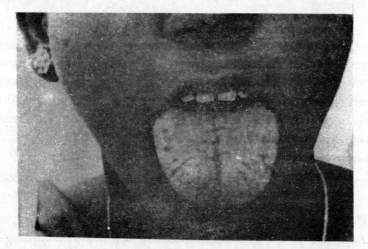

Figure 16f. Tongue changes characteristic of glossitis.

Source: *Courtesy:* National Institute of Nutrition, Hyderabad, 500 007

Dermal lesions: Seborrhoeic dermatitis involving the facial and scrotal skin is common in riboflavin deficiency. It is encountered over the nasolabial folds and on the ears as shown in Figure 16g – Appendix 10. Skin lesions may be due to reduced skin collagen content and maturity. Cross-linked collagen is essential for epidermal integrity.

In riboflavin deficiency, there is biochemical defect of rise in homocysteine which may impair the process of collagen cross-linking.

Ocular manifestations: In humans, visual symptoms photophobia, lacrimation, burning, visual fatigue are reported in riboflavin deficiency. Diminished visual acuity, keratitis can also be attributed to riboflavin deficiency.

Blepharo-conjunctivitis - inflammation of eye lid-epithelial keratitis and nutrition amblyopia can be treated with riboflavin. Though experimental evidence suggests that cataract can be seen more often in riboflavin deficiency, current clinical studies only give an indication that probably along with other factors it may be important in cataractogenesis. A syndrome of oral lesions with diminished visual acuity and temporal pallor of the fundi with neuritis and optic atrophy has been described in prisoners of war. Recent studies in school children suffering from oral lesions suggest that vitamin B_2 is an important component for improving visual acuity.

Neurological manifestations: Current reports stress on behavioural abnormalities in riboflavin deficient children. Reaction time, hand grip strength and steadiness and motor coordination have been reported to be affected and respond to riboflavin supplement.

Haematological manifestations: Normocytic anaemia has been reported in riboflavin deficiency. Riboflavin stimulates reticulocytosis and increases haemoglobin concentration.

Effect on respiratory infections: Infections resulted in significantly higher riboflavin excretion and blood levels of riboflavin. Saturation of FAD-dependent enzyme erythrocyte glutathione reductase with the coenzyme FAD was increased possibly to meet the demand for reduced glutathione to mount phagocytic response. Adverse effects of respiratory infections are likely to be more in riboflavin deficient individuals.

Secondary Nutrient Deficiencies in Riboflavin Deficiency

Riboflavin deficiency is associated with hypochromic anaemia as a result of secondary iron deficiency. In addition to the role of flavo proteins in iron metabolism, it is possible that the anaemia associated with riboflavin deficiency is a consequence of the impairment of vitamin B_6 metabolism in riboflavin deficiency. Pyridoxine oxidase is a flavo protein and like glutathione reductase very sensitive to riboflavin depletion.

Treatment

Riboflavin in doses of 5 and 10 mg is adequate for curing oral and dermal lesions. Oral administration is satisfactory except in case of malabsorption, acute diarrhoea and severe metabolic trauma. Symptoms disappear in a few days to few weeks.

Riboflavin needs to be supplemented to preterm infants. It is sensitive to photometry and hence during phototherapy in hyperbilirubinaemia, riboflavin is required. Biliary excretion in infants and children is associated with impaired absorption of riboflavin and may require daily supplementation.

Evaluation of riboflavin status

Riboflavin status is determined by measuring the increase in activity of the enzyme glutathione reductase in red blood cells in response to the addition of FAD which is required for the enzyme activity. The activity of glutathione reductase in red blood cells of people with normal riboflavin status rises by less than 20 per cent in response to the addition of FAD. In riboflavin deficiency an activation of more than 40 per cent is observed.

Recommended dietary allowances

Riboflavin requirement is related to energy intake – 0.6 mg/1000 kcal. The RDA of ICMR for riboflavin is given in Table 16.4.

Table 16.4: ICMR Recommended Dietary Allowances of riboflavin

Group	Riboflavin mg/day
Man	
Sedentary work	1.4
Moderate work	1.6
Heavy work	1.9
Woman	
Sedentary work	1.1
Moderate work	1.3
Heavy work	1.5
Pregnant woman	+0.2

Contd....

Group	Riboflavin mg/day
Lactation	
0–6 months	+0.3
6– 12 months	+0.2
Infants	
0–6 months	65 µg/kg
6–1 2 months	60 µg/kg
Children	
1–3 years	0.7
4–6 years	1.0
7–9 years	1.2
Boys	
10–1 2 years	1.3
13–15 years	1.5
16–18 years	1.6
Girls	
10–12 years	1.2
13– 15 years	1.2
16–18 years	1.2

Sources

Good sources of riboflavin are milk and milk products (including skimmed milk, butter milk, curds, cheese and whey), eggs, liver and green leafy vegetables. Tender leaves and buds contains more riboflavin than the mature ones. Wheat, millets and pulses are fair sources of riboflavin while rice particularly is a poor source. Riboflavin is the most limiting of all B vitamins in cereal based diets of the poor. It is rather difficult to ensure adequate supply of this vitamin in a predominantly vegetarian diet. Inclusion of milk, greens and pulses in a cereal diet improve the dietary supply of this vitamin. The important sources of riboflavin are given in the Table 16.5.

Table 16.5: Riboflavin content of foods

Name of the foodstuff	Riboflavin mg/100g
Liver sheep	1.70
Skimmed milk powder	1.60
Whole milk powder	1.30
Lotus stem	1.20
Gingelly seeds	0.60
Manthakali leaves	0.50
Almond	0.50
Beet greens	0.50
Egg	0.40
Soyabeen	0.30
Milk Cows	0.19
Milk buffalo	0.10

Polished rice and other refined cereals contain very little riboflavin. Ordinary methods of cooking do not destroy the vitamin apart from losses that occur when the water in which green vegetables have been boiled is discarded. If foods, especially milk are left exposed to sunshine, large losses may occur. Especially good sources of the natural vitamin are yeast extract and meat extract.

NIACIN

Niacin, formerly known as nicotinic acid was originally obtained by the oxidation of nicotine. In 1937 it was recognised as the nutrient able to prevent or cure pellagra in humans and black tongue in dogs. Niacin is used as a generic term, to include derivatives such as nicotinamide.

Chemistry

Nicotinic acid is a simple derivative of pyridine. It is a white crystalline substance readily soluble in water and resistance to heat, oxidation and alkalis; it is infact one of the most stable of the vitamins. It can be easily synthesised commercially.

Figure 16h shows the structure of nicotinic acid.

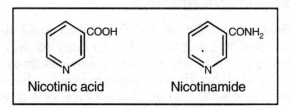

Figure 16h: Structure of nicotinic acid and nicotinamide.

Functions

Niacin is required by all cells. Like thiamin and riboflavin, it plays a vital role in the release of energy from all the energy yielding nutrients-carbohydrate, fat, protein and alcohol. It is also required for the synthesis of protein, fat and the five-carbon sugars (pentoses) needed for the formation of DNA and RNA. The biochemical role of niacin is to form part of the coenzymes Nicotinamide Adenine Dinucleotide, NAD, Nicotinamide Adenine Dinucleotide Phosphate NADP. These coenzymes are required by many of the key pathways of metabolism with NAD being primarily involved in catabolic reactions and NADP functions mainly in anabolic reactions.

Niacin is a partner with riboflavin in the cellular coenzyme systems that convert proteins and the small amount of glycerol from fats to glucose and that oxidise glucose to release controlled energy. In these systems the oxidation of glucose often takes place in the absence of free oxygen simply by the removal of hydrogen ions. These ions are passed down the line between the successively simpler compounds and comprise these systems to the eventual receiver, oxygen with the end products water and carbon dioxide. NAD and NADP operate in these systems. These two coenzymes act in a large number of reversible oxidation reduction reactions.

NAD and NADP participate in more than 200 enzyme reactions. Some of the reactions where niacin in the form of NAD is involved are :

- Conversion of lactate to pyruvate in glycolytic pathway.
- Glyceradehyde – 3-PO4 to 1,3 biphospho glycerate in glycolytic pathway.
- In biological oxidation reduction complex.
- α-ketoglutarate to succinyl CoA in TCA cycle.
- Malate to oxaloactetate in TCA cycle.

Niacin in the form of NADP is involved in the following:

- Glucose-6-PO4 to 6-Phospho gluconolactone in HMP shunt.
- 6-phospho gluconate to 3 keto-6 phosphogluconate in HMP shunt.

Absorption and metabolism

Niacin is readily absorbed from the stomach and small intestine. It is converted into the coenzymes NAD and NADP within the cells and limited stores of these coenzymes are held in the kidneys, liver and brain. Any excess niacin is excreted in urine in the forms of methyl nicotinamide and methyl carboxamido-pyridone. As niacin deficiency develops, the excretion of methyl-carboxamido-pyridone decreases more rapidly than that of methyl nicotinamide.

Niacin and Tryptophan Interrelationship

In 1945, it was discovered that the amino acid tryptophan could cure pellagra. 60 mg of tryptophan can be converted to 1 mg of niacin or niacin equivalent (NE). Protein has approximately 1 per cent tryptophan, 60 g of protein provides about 600 mg of tryptophan which can give rise to 10 mg of niacin. Thus 600 mg of tryptophan in excess of that needed for protein synthesis can be converted to 10 NE. This conversion is three times more efficient

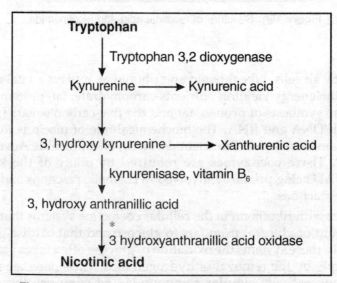

Figure 16i. The conversion of tryptophan to nicotinic acid.

In deficiency of vitamin B$_6$ kynurenic acid and xanthurenic acid appear in the urine in increased amounts.

* Several intermediate steps are involved.

during pregnancy. Changes in hormonal status may result in considerable changes in this ratio between 7 to 30 mg of dietary tryptophan equivalent to 1 mg of niacin in late pregnancy. The intake of tryptophan also affects the ratio. At low intakes, 1 mg of tryptophan may be equivalent to only 1/125 mg of niacin. Niacin equivalent value is preferred than niacin value in food. For the conversion of tryptophan to niacin, thiamin, pyridoxine and riboflavin and perhaps biotin are required.

The steps involved in the conversion of tryptophan to niacin are given in Figure l6i.

$$\text{Niacin Equivalents} = \text{Niacin content (mg)} + \frac{\text{tryptohan (mg)}}{60}$$

Some foods, such as milk that are effective in curing or prevent pellagra are due to their high content of tryptophan, though they are poor in niacin.

Deficiency

Pellagra occurred mainly among poor persons in U.S who used corn (maize) produced in the New World as their dietary staple. It was thought that mould or toxic substance was the cause. Later lack of nitrogen was implicated. Corn diets lack in lysine and tryptophan but were rich in essential amino acid leucine. This led to speculation that an amino acid imbalance was the cause.

The skin symptoms of pellagra are aggravated by exposure to sunlight which led to the belief that it resulted from sun poisoning. It was considered to be an infectious disease because it was common among poor people. The fact that several members of the same family often developed the disease, led some people to suspect hereditary factors were involved. In 1917 a physician named Goldberger working for the United States Public Health Service demonstrated that pellagra was associated with the absence of a specific dietary factor.

Goldberger conducted a series of classic experiments on a group of male prisoners who were put on a diet typical of the areas in which pellagra was prevalent. After five months they developed classic symptoms of pellagra: dermatitis, diarrhoea and depression. Other inmates eating normal prison diet remained healthy. He proved that it was not an infectious disease but implicated the lack of some unknown dietary factor. That factor, niacin was not properly identified until 20 years later.

The efforts to isolate the dietary factor that could prevent pellagra were complicated because many other dietary deficiencies produced similar skin condition. In 1937 Elvehjem at the university of Wisconsin, finally demonstrated that nicotinic acid could cure black tongue in dogs. This led to the use of nicotinic acid to treat pellagra in human beings with dramatic results.

Pellagra is still found in countries where corn is a major staple such as Romania, the former Yugoslavia, some part of Egypt and parts of India where leucine content of sorghum is high. In people developing pellagra because of a sorghum based diet, the addition of isoleucine to the diet can correct the condition. This suggests, that leucine isoleucine balance of a diet could be an additional factor contributing to the onset of pellagra.

Pellagra is not found in Central America, despite the fact that corn provides 80 per cent of kilocalories in this region. This is attributed to the use of alkalis (usually soda lime) in corn preparation which liberates niacin that is bound to proteins in corn and so make it available or absorption.

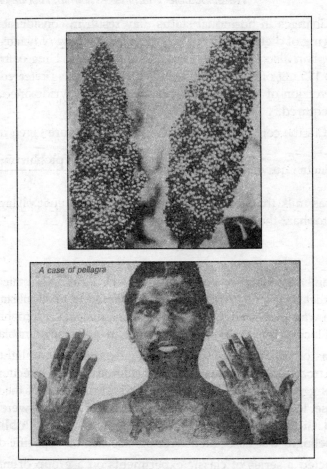

Figure 16j. Jowar and Castle's necklace. People who subsist solely on jowar are likely to develop pellagra. Note dermatitis on the sunlight exposed parts of the body.

Source: Saibaba, A., Jowar, Nutrition, **29**, 1995.

Drug Induced Pellagra

The antituberculosis drug isoniazid can cause pellagra by forming a biologically inactive complex with pyridoxal phosphate, the metabolically active form of vitamin B_6 and hence reducing the activity of kynureninase. This isoniazid induced pellagra responds to the administration of niacin supplements.

The anti-parkinsonian drugs benserazide and carbidopa inhibit the oxidative metabolism of tryptophan and cause reduced excretion of N'-methyl nicotinamide.

Leucine in addition to inhibiting quinolinate also inhibits tryptophan uptake resulting in diminished supply of precursors for nicotinamide nucleotide synthesis. Pellagra is also secondary to alcoholism and malabsorption, genetic disorder defects in the absorption of tryptophan. Pellagra occurs in the middle aged population 20–50. Both sexes are equally affected.

The typical clinical features are loss of weight and increasing debility. Pellagra has been called the disease of the three Ds: dermatitis, diarrhoea and dementia (irreversible organic deterioration of mental faculties) leading to death, the fourth D.

Diarrhoea and mental changes are not present in mild deficiency. Mental symptom is usually depression and not dementia.

Nonspecific signs such as anorexia, nausea, digestive disturbances and emotional changes like anxiety, irritability and insomnia may precede the onset of the disease.

Dermal lesions: These are photo sensitive rash and is seen on exposed extensor surface of the body like the upper and lower extremities, face and neck and is usually bilateral and symmetrical. The lesions are hyperkeratotic and hyperpigmented. The lesions are precipitated by exposure to sunlight, fire and radiant heat. On the neck, the lesions appear in the form of a necklace called Casal's necklace. Other areas such as groin, axilla and lower surface of breasts may be affected. The skin changes have been attributed to decreased collagen content and alterations in copper metabolism (Figure 16k).

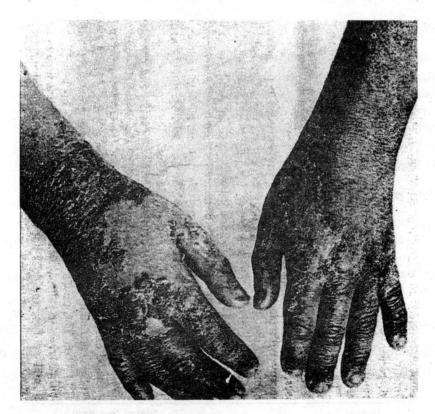

Figure 16k. Dermal lesions of pellagra.
Source: Proudfit T.F., Corinne H. Robinson, 1957, Nutrition and diet therapy, the Macmillan Company, New York.

Gastrointestinal changes: The mucous membrane is inflammed resulting in severe glossitis, stomatitis, oesophagitis, gastritis and enteritis. The inflammation can produce bloody diarrhoea. Diarrhoea is not common among sorghum eaters.

Neurological manifestation: Higher mental functions are deranged in pellagra. Insomnia occurs. As the disease progresses it can manifest in disorientation, hallucination and delirium. Acute encephalopathy characterised by clouding of conciousness occurs. The peripheral nerve may also be affected with paraesthesia and decreased nerve conduction, incoordination and tremors may occur. Spastic paraplegia has been reported. Exaggerated deep tendon reflexes are observed. Serotonin or 5-hydroxy tryptamine is decreased in pellagra and is responsible for mental depression.

Treatment

Pellagra can be cured by a good diet containing adequate amounts of protein, tryptophan and/or niacin as well as other members of B-complex group of vitamins. A moderately severe case requires nicotinic acid or amide in doses of 100–300 mg/day orally. Mental symptoms respond within 24–48 hours and the dermal lesions require 3–4 weeks of therapy. Most cases of pellagra require riboflavin and pyridoxine particularly for neurological manifestations. Oral therapy is satisfactory in all cases except in those with very severe diarrhoea.

Prevention

Pellagra can be prevented by the following measures:
- Replacing sorghum with other cereals.
- Consuming sorghum with good quality proteins.
- Fortifying bread with nicotinic acid.
- Distribution of yeast and niacin tablets as public health programme.
- Developing low leucine strains of sorghum.
- Including groundnuts in every day diet.

Evaluation of niacin status

Measurement of two urinary metabolites, methyl-carboxamido pyridone and methyl nicotinamide and their ratio have been used to measure niacin status. Urinary excretion of less than 0.8 mg/day of methyl nicotinamide is indicative of niacin deficiency. A ratio of less than 1 suggests latent niacin deficiency. Clinical symptoms, however, do not appear until the pyridone has been absent from the urine for several weeks.

Recommended dietary allowances

Niacin requirement is related to energy intake – 6.6 mg/1000 kal. The RDA of ICMR for niacin is given in Table 16.6.

Tables 16.6: ICMR Recommended dietary allowances of niacin

Group	Niacin (mg/day)
Man	
Sedentary work	16
Moderate work	18
Heavy work	21

Contd...

Group	Niacin (mg/day)
Woman	
Sedentary work	12
Moderate work	14
Heavy work	16
Pregnant woman	+2
Lactation	
0–6 months	+4
6–12 months	+3
Infants	
0–6 months	710 µg/kg
6–12 months	650 µg/kg
Children	
1–3 years	8
4–6 years	11
7–9 years	13
Boys	
10–12 years	15
13–15 years	16
16–18 years	17
Girls	
10–12 years	13
13–15 years	14
16–18 years	14

Megavitamin Therapy

Large pharmacological doses of niacin have been used in attempts to reduce high blood cholesterol and triglyceride levels and to treat schizophrenia. Under strict medical supervision, doses of 1.5 to .3 g of niacin (as nicotinic acid) three times a day may reduce total and low-density lipoprotein cholesterol levels and increase high-density lipoprotein cholesterol level in plasma. This may be beneficial in protecting against recurrent non-fatal heart attacks.

Sources

Whole cereals, pulses, nuts and meat are good sources of nicotinic acid. Groundnut is particularly rich in nicotinic acid. Although poor in nicotinic acid, milk is also effective in preventing pellagra because it is rich in tryptophan. Table 16.7 gives some rich sources of niacin.

Table 16.7: Niacin content of foods

Name of Foodstuff	Niacin mg/100g
Groundnut	22
Liver sheep	18
Garden cress seeds	14
Beef muscle	6
Wheat whole	6
Barley	5
Radish leaves	5
Prawn	5
Almond	4
Bengal gram whole	3

In many cereals, especially maize and perhaps also in potatoes, the greater part of the vitamin may be in a bound unabsorbable form. Nicotinic acid can be liberated from the bound form, niacytin, by treatment with alkali. In Mexico, tortillas have been made from maize treated with lime water. This practice may account for a low incidence of pellagra in Mexico.

Cooking causes little destruction of nicotinic acid but it may be lost in the cooking water and 'drippings' from cooked meat if these are discarded. In a mixed diet, from 15 to 25 per cent of the nicotinic acid of cooked food stuffs may be lost in this way. Commercial processing and storage of food stuffs cause little loss.

QUESTIONS

1. Explain the causes of pellagra.
2. Distinguish the following:
   (a) Infantile beriberi
   (b) Wet beriberi
   (c) Dry beriberi
3. What can cause Wernicke's syndrome?
4. How can we prevent losses of thiamin and riboflavin during cooking?
5. Explain the following terms:
   (a) Glossitis
   (b) Cheilosis
   (c) Angular stomatitis.
6. Discuss the role of B-vitamins in carbohydrate, protein and fat metabolism.
7. Give five sources of riboflavin.
8. Give the interrelationship between niacin and tryptophan.
9. Discuss the 3'D's of pellagra.
10. Give the relationship between calories and B-vitamin requirements.
11. Give the RDA of thiamin for all age groups.

12. Give the specific functions of thiamin and riboflavin.
13. How was antiberiberi vitamin discovered?

SUGGESTED READINGS

- Bender A. David, 2002, Nutritional Biochemistry of the vitamins, Cambridge University Press, United Kingdom.
- Shintre Kishore, 2000. 'Micronutrient fortification of cereal flours' Proceedings of the Nutrition Society of India, **48**.
- Information on vitamins : www.eatright.org
- Information on 'Vitamin deficiency' : www.who.int/home/search

CHAPTER 17

WATER SOLUBLE VITAMINS: FOLIC ACID AND VITAMIN B$_{12}$

FOLIC ACID

In 1931 Lucy Wills in Mumbai drew attention to the importance of nutritional megaloblastic anaemia in pregnant women. This anaemia was cured by yeast which contained antianaemic principle — the 'Wills factor' which was later termed as folic acid.

The term folic acid was coined in 1941 by Mitchell et al. because they found this material in leafy vegetable spinach.

Folic acid is a generic term for the chemical pteroylglutamic acid (PGA) and related chemicals with the same biological activities as PGA. PGA itself is rarely found in significant amounts either in food or in the human body. Instead, food contains a variety of chemically related substances that all have the biological activities of folic acid. The term folate is commonly used to describe any compound or mixture of compounds with the activities of pteroylmonoglutamic acid.

Figure 17a shows the structure of pteroylmonoglutamic acid.

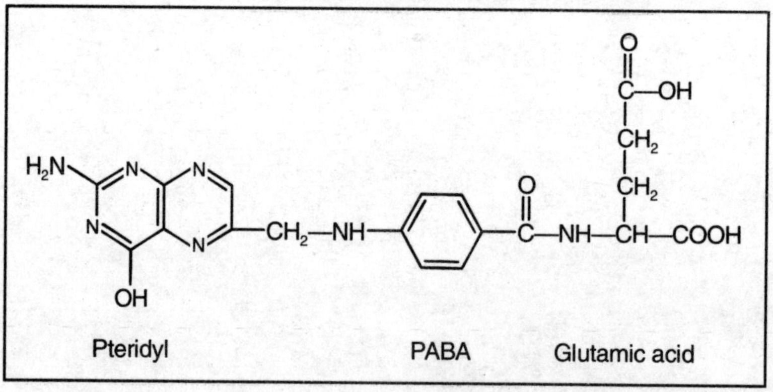

Figure17a: Pteroylmonoglutamic Acid (PGA)—Folic Acid.

Functions

Folate is now known to be required for the normal growth and division of all cells.

The specific biochemical function of folate is to act as a coenzyme in reactions involving the transfer of one-carbon unit such as the methyl group (CH_3) from one metabolite to another. Examples of processes requiring the presence of folate are the following:

- Along with vitamin B$_{12}$, folic acid helps in the transmethylation of homocysteine to methionine, ethanolamine to choline and uracil to thymine.

- The conversion of the amino acid phenylalanine into the amino acid tyrosine.
- The formation of the haeme group of haemoglobin.
- The synthesis of the purine and pyrimidine bases needed for the synthesis of deoxyribonucleic acid (DNA) and ribonucleic acid (RNA).
- The formation of the vitamin like compound choline from ethanolamine.
- The conversion of the vitamin niacin to N-methyl nicotinamide, the from in which it is excreted.
- Folic acid is required for the normal metabolic pathway of histidine, particularly in the conversion of formimino glumatic acid to glumatic acid.

Cells whose activities require rapid cell growth and division are particularly sensitive to folate deficiency because folate is required for the formation of amino acids (and therefore proteins) and nucleic acids, some of the key compounds of the cell. Examples of such cells are red blood cells and the cells lining the gastrointestinal tract. The involvement of folate in haemoglobin synthesis is another factor that makes red blood cell formation particularly sensitive to folate deficiency. A substantial interrelationship exists between folate and B$_{12}$.

Both vitamins help in the development of red blood cells beyond the megaloblastic stage. Thus deficiency of these two vitamins leads to accumulation of megaloblasts and myeloblasts.

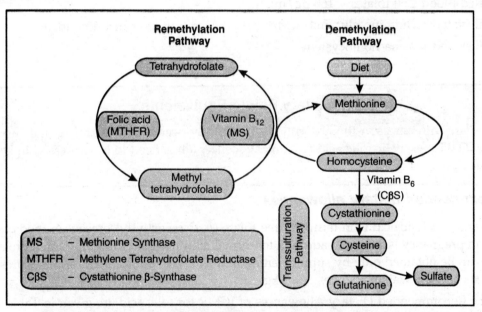

Figure17b: Role of folic acid, vitamin B$_{12}$ and vitamin B$_6$ in metabolic pathway of homocysteine. Deficiency of these vitamins increase homocysteine levels which may be a contributary factor to atherosclerosis.

Absorption, transport and metabolism

About three-quarters of the folate in foods is in polyglutamyl forms. These are normally hydrolysed to free folate by a conjugases (γ-glutamyl carboxypeptidase) present in small intestinal epithelium. Free folate is actively absorbed from the upper small intestine.

Once absorbed into the intestinal cell walls, folate is transported in the blood to all cells of the body. Any excess is stored in the liver. The main form in which folate is transported around the body is N^5 - methyl tetrahydrofolate.

Most adults excrete upto 40 μg of folate in their urine each day. Losses in faeces amount to about 200 μg/day. This total includes folate synthesised by bacteria in the large intestine and so can often be higher than the total dietary intake of folate. Pregnant women excrete increased quantities, requiring an additional 200 to 300 μg of folate intake each day to compensate for this increased loss. This may explain why pregnant women are at increased risk of folate deficiency.

Impaired absorption of folate is seen in malabsorptive states (regional enteritis, crohn's disease, celiac disease).

Evaluation of Folate Status

The following criteria are used to evaluate folate status provided there is no vitamin B_{12} deficiency.

- Positive megloblastic anaemia.
- Plasma folates < 3 ng/ml.
- Red Blood Cell folates < 160 ng/ml.
- Elevated formimino glutamic acid (FIGLU) excretion after histidine load.
- Elevated plasma homocysteine.

Dietary Folate Equivalents

There are differences in the absorption of naturally occurring food folate and the more bioavailable synthetic folic acid (1.7 times). Hence, folate need to be expressed in Dietary Folate Equivalents–DFEs.

Recommended dietary allowances

Allowance for folic acid is in terms of free folate (*L. Casei* activity) present in foods. RDA of folate in pregnancy is 300 μg in addition to normal requirement of 100 μg. Such high levels of folate can be obtained only by supplementation. Folic acid requirement can be expressed on the basis of body weight also i.e., 3 μg/kg.

The Recommended Dietary Allowances of ICMR for folic acid are given in Table 17.1.

Table 17.1: ICMR Recommended Dietary Allowances of folic acid

Group	Folic acid µg/day
Man	100
Woman	100
Pregnancy	400
Lactation	150

Contd....

Group	Folic acid µg/day
Infants	25
Children	
1–3 years	30
4–6 years	40
7–9 years	60
Boys and girls	
10–12 years	70
13–15 years	100
16–18years	100

Sources

Folic acid is present both in animal and plant foods. Fresh green vegetables, liver, pulses are good sources of this vitamin. The important sources of folic acid are given in Table 17.2.

Table 17.2: Folic acid content of foods

Name of the foodstuff	Free folic acid µg/100g
Liver Sheep	65.5
Spinach	51.0
Gingelly seeds	51.0
Cluster beans	50.0
Amaranth tender	41.0
Ambat Chuka	40.0
Bengal gram whole	34.0
Ladies fingers	25.3
Green gram dal	24.5
Curry leaves	23.5
Wheat whole	14.2
Tomato ripe	14.0

VITAMIN B₁₂

Until 1926, pernicious anaemia was a fatal disease of unknown origin with an unknown cure. In 1926 Minot and Murphy found that pernicious anaemia could be cured by feeding a patient atleast 0.3 kg of raw liver per day.

Also in 1926 Castle noted that patients with pernicious anaemia had a low level of gastric secretion. He suggested that the anti-pernicious anaemia factor had two components; an 'extrinsic factor' found in food and an 'intrinsic factor' within normal gastric secretions. The extrinsic factor is now known as vitamin B_{12}–cobalamine. The intrinsic factor, a mucoprotein, facilitate the absorption of vitamin B_{12}. Deficiency of intrinsic factor can cause pernicious anaemia.

The common pharmaceutical form of vitamin B_{12} used widely in supplements, is cyano cobalamine. The structure of cyano cobalamine is given in Figure 17c. Vitamin B_{12} was isolated in 1948 from liver as a red crystalline compound, containing cobalt. It has derived the names of cobalamine and cyanocobalamine because of the presence of cobalt and cyanide (CN) group respectively in its structure. Other names of vitamin B_{12} are antipernicious anaemia factor and extrinsic factor of Castle.

Functions

Vitamin B_{12}, like folate, is involved in biochemical processes essential for DNA synthesis and therefore for the growth and division of cells. It helps in the transfer of carboxyl group.

Vitamin B_{12} acts as a coenzyme mediating the conversion of homocysteine to the amino acid methionine.

In the bone marrow, where the erythroblast precursors of red blood cells are formed both vitamin B_{12} and folate are needed. $N^{5,10}$ methylene tetra hydrofolate provides the methyl groups needed for the synthesis of DNA. If DNA cannot be produced in adequate amounts, the erythroblasts cannot divide and mature properly. Instead, they simply grow in size to produce abnormally large megaloblastic red blood cells characteristic of the anaemia found both in pernicious anaemia and when folate is merely deficient. Although vitamin B_{12} is required for

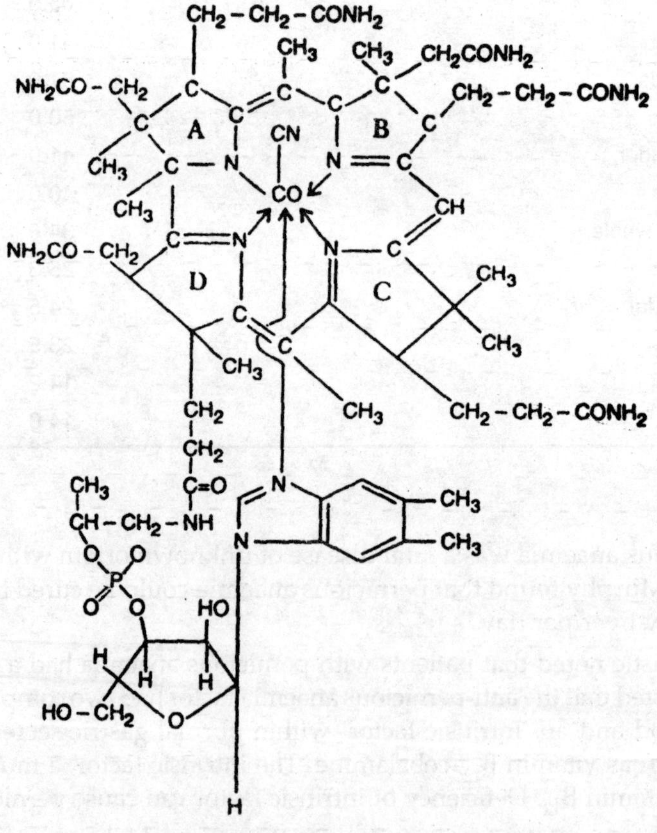

Figure 17c. Structure of Vitamin B_{12}

the synthesis of DNA in all human cells, the erythroblasts are particularly vulnerable to vitamin B$_{12}$ deficiency because of the extremely rapid rate at which they normally divide. New red blood cells are normally produced at a rate of atleast 200 million per minute.

Vitamin B$_{12}$ is also required for the synthesis of myelin, the white sheath of lipoprotein that surrounds many nerve fibres. During vitamin B$_{12}$ deficiency, progressive demyelination of nerve fibres occurs, leading to a variety of neurological symptoms.

Vitamin B$_{12}$ is involved in the conversion of methylmalonyl-CoA to succinyl CoA, which is involved in the degradation of fatty acids containing an odd number of carbon atoms.

Absorption, Transport and Metabolism

Vitamin B$_{12}$ is absorbed primarily in the terminal ileum. The absorption of vitamin B$_{12}$ is mediated by the intrinsic factor, which is a heat labile mucoprotein secreted from parietal cells in the walls of the stomach. If intrinsic factor is deficient, intramuscular injection of B$_{12}$ should be given. The proportion of dietary vitamin B$_{12}$ that is absorbed decreases as the amount consumed increases. Absorption declines with age.

After absorption, vitamin B$_{12}$ passes into the circulation, where it becomes bound to one of three transport proteins known as transcobalamins I, II and III. These proteins carry vitamin B$_{12}$ to the various tissues of the body, particularly the liver and bone marrow.

Excess vitamin B$_{12}$ is stored in the liver, largely bound within a vitamin B$_{12}$ protein complex. The total amount stored in the liver can be as high as 2000 to 2500 μg which is sufficient to last for 6-10 years.

Any condition that alters intrinsic factor production, interferes with intestinal absorption in the terminal ileum or reduces transcobalamin level, reduces the availability of vitamin B$_{12}$.

Recommended Dietary Allowances

The Recommended Dietary Allowances prescribed by ICMR for B$_{12}$ are given in Table 17.3.

Table 17.3: ICMR Recommended dietary allowances for vitamin B$_{12}$

Group	Vitamin B$_{12}$ µg/day
Man	1.0
Woman	1.0
Pregnancy	1.0
Lactation	1.5
Infants	0.2
Children Boys and Girls 1-18 years	0.2-1.0

Sources

Vitamin B$_{12}$ is synthesised by bacteria and is present only in animal foods. Although a majority of Indians live on a diet predominantly based on foods of vegetable origin, B$_{12}$ deficiency perse is not wide spread. Some B$_{12}$ may be provided by the bacterial contamination and by using fermented food. B$_{12}$ content foods is given in Table 17.4.

Table 17.4: Vitamin B$_{12}$ content of foods

Name of the foodstuff	Vitamin B$_{12}$ µg/100g
Liver Sheep	91.9
Liver goat	90.4
Shrimp	9.0
Goat meat	2.8
Mutton	2.6
Egg hen	1.8
Milk buffalo	0.14
Milk cow	0.14
Skimmed milk powder	0.80

MEGALOBLASTIC ANAEMIA AND FOLIC ACID AND B$_{12}$ DEFICIENCY

Haemopoietic tissue is one of a number of rapidly proliferating tissues in which DNA synthesis is intense. Both vitamin B$_{12}$ and folate are essential for DNA synthesis and deficiency of either or both causes a failure of DNA synthesis and disordered cell proliferation. Haemopoiesis is particularly susceptible and division of cells is delayed and eventually halted. Morphological changes appear in the marrow cells. In the erythrocyte series these changes are described as megaloblastic because the cells appear abnormally large. They are nucleated red cell precursors. Megaloblasts appear in bone marrow as well as in peripheral blood.

FOLATE DEFICIENCY

Causes

Poor dietary intake: Megaloblastic anaemia is common among poor vegetarians. This is due to poor intake of milk, fresh fruits and vegetables. As such the Indian diet is a poor source of folic acid and cooking practices commonly encountered tend to destroy the folic acid to a considerable extent.

Low absorption: This anaemia in babies is more frequent in those born to mothers who also have a folic acid deficiency. Anaemia is present in infants whose diet lacks in vitamin C because folic acid cannot be converted to its active form folinic acid. Low folic acid absorption can occur in coeliac disease and in tropical sprue. Folate absorption is impaired in pregnancy.

Vitamin B$_{12}$ deficiency can result in folic acid deficiency by causing folate entrapment in the metabolically useless form of 5 methyl tetrahydrofolate.

Increased losses: In haemodialysis increased losses of folic acid may occur.

Increased requirement: Increased requirements due to growth and pregnancy are believed to be the most frequent causes. In haemolysis, when there is cell proliferation there is folic acid deficiency.

Infestation and infection: Malarial infection may play a part in pathogenesis of megaloblastic anaemia. Chronic infections and parasitic infestation may impair absorption of folate.

Drugs: Anticonvulsant drugs and oral contraceptives may impair folate absorption in some women. Patients taking anticonvulsant drugs for treatment of epilepsy tend to become folate deficient. Increased folate catabolism has been proposed. Methotrexate can cause malabsorption of folic acid.

Alcoholics comprise the only group that generally has all metabolic defects leading to folic acid deficiency. Less utilisation and increased excretion, increased requirement and increased destruction of folic acid results in deficiency state in alcoholics.

Prevalence

In tropical countries most cases of megaloblastic disease are due to folate deficiency associated with malnutrition, infection and pregnancy. It is common in the age group 20–30 years.

Clinical Features

General symptoms of iron deficiency are present in folic acid deficiency. Symptoms like weakness, tiredness dyspnoea, sore tongue, diarrhoea irritability and forgetfulness, anorexia, headache and palpitation are observed in folic acid deficiency. There is weight loss. Glossitis is less common than in vitamin B$_{12}$ deficiency. Neurological problems are very rare.

Localised Deficiency

Localised folate deficiency causes megaloblastic changes in the cervix in women taking oral contraceptives. Other localised folate deficiencies have since been found in the bronchial and oral tissues of smokers and the colonic tissue of patients with ulcerative colitis. Localised folate deficiencies may have a cocarcinogenic effect, meaning that the affected tissues are at increased risk of cancers produced by specific carcinogens.

Folate Deficiency During Pregnancy

Normal adult woman requirement of folic acid is 100 μg/day. ICMR recommendations during pregnancy are 400 μg/day. The recommended intake of folacin is based on its role in promoting normal foetal growth and preventing macrocytic anaemia of pregnancy. Folic acid is needed for the synthesis of essential components of DNA and RNA which increase rapidly during growth, there by, increasing the requirements . Also folacin is essential for the development of RBCs which must increase as the mothers blood volume increases.

There is notable decrease in folate absorption and an increase in urinary excretion during pregnancy which may contribute to maternal store depletion .

Folate deficiency produces its first effects in tissues with a high rate of cell division, such as intestinal cells and red blood cells. It has also been implicated in pregnancy induced hypertension, a condition of late pregnancy with symptoms of high blood pressure, proteinuria and oedema. Folate deficiency during pregnancy has been firmly linked to various forms of damage to the developing foetus.

Folic acid and its potential influence on pregnancy outcome is its role in preventing neural tube defects such as spina bifida and anencephaly.

Studies showed that folic acid supplementation is associated not only with a significant reduction in birth defects, but also an increase in recognized spontaneous abortions. It may be that folic acid acts through an unusual mechanism-terathanasia—the selective promotion of spontaneous abortion of defective foetuses.

Studies have shown that red cell folate levels exceeding 906 m Mol/L (400ng/ml) are best for preventing neural tube defects.

It is crucial to note that because the neural tube closes by 28 days of gestation (before most women realise they are pregnant) supplementation with folic acid should ideally occur with 400–800 µg/day prior to conception. Increased intake of foods rich in folic acid throughout child bearing years, e.g., dark green leafy vegetables, legumes, orange juice, soya and fortifying food with folic acid may prevent neural tube defects.

Diagnosis

Haemoglobin levels may be as low 4 g/dl. Glossitis is often present. Paraesthesia is a common complaint. The excretion of formimino glutamic acid (FIGLU) after a histidine load as an index and found consistant evidence of a deranged metabolism of folic acid. Demonstration of FIGLU in the urine is a test of folic acid deficiency. Plasma folate is less than 3 µg/ml. There is free hydrochloric acid in the gastric juice.

Treatment

Folic acid in dose of 5 to 10 mg daily is effective. Patients who have less than 5 g/dl of haemoglobin need blood transfusion. Iron and B_{12} are often required before a full haematological response can occur.

Dietary Considerations

Foods rich in folic acid like pulses, green leafy vegetables, cluster beans, ladies finger, gingelly seeds, liver and eggs should be included in the diet.

VITAMIN B_{12} DEFICIENCY

Vitamin B_{12} must be bound to intrinsic factor, produced by the parietal cells of the stomach, before it is absorbed in the terminal ileum. Inability to produce intrinsic factor results in pernicious anaemia. The red cell count is often less than 2.5 million and a large proportion of the cells are macrocytic. The anaemia occurs chiefly in middle aged and elderly persons and may be a genetic defect. Antibodies against gastric mucosa can probably be responsible for destroying the mechanism of producing intrinsic factor. The disease thus arises as an autoimmune disorder.

Nutritional vitamin B_{12} deficiency is not very common, even in populations where intake of the vitamin B_{12} is far below the daily requirement of 0.5 µg-1 µg. Vitamin B_{12} deficiency takes atleast 3 years to appear (vitamin B_{12} is stored in the liver where there may be upto 3 years supply).

Causes of Pernicious Anaemia

Inadequate ingestion : A poor diet lacking in micro organisms and animal foods which are the sole source of vitamin B$_{12}$ can lead to pernicious anaemia. Chronic alcoholism, poverty, religious taboos and dietary fads can cause B$_{12}$ deficiency. Infants solely breastfed for long period of time develop anaemia due to dietary vitamin B$_{12}$ deficiency.

Inadequate absorption and utilisation : Inadequate or absence of secretion of intrinsic factor due to heredity or congenital production of defective intrinsic factor gastric atrophy, endocrine disorders associated with gastric damage or due to gastrectomy pernicious anaemia can occur. Bacterial proliferation in stagnant loops and in tropical sprue there is malabsorption of B$_{12}$. Parasitic infestation such as fish tapeworm may remove vitamin B$_{12}$ from the gut.

Inadequate utilisation : This is due to the presence of vitamin B$_{12}$ antagonists.

Increased requirements : During infancy and pregnancy there is increased requirements of vitamin B$_{12}$ as it is essential for nucleic acid synthesis.

Prevalence

The majority of patients with vitamin B$_{12}$ deficiency have Addisonian pernicious anaemia. This appears to be relatively uncommon in tropical countries. Addisonian pernicious anaemia is due to a failure of secretion of intrinsic factor by the stomach. The disease is rare before the age of 30,occurs mainly between 45 and 65 years and affects females more frequently than males.

Clinical Features

Patients with pernicious anaemia have a lemon yellow or pale skin. Anorexia, glossitis, achlorhydria, abdominal discomfort, frequent diarrhoea, weight loss and general weakness can also occur. The surface of the tongue is usually smooth and atrophic but sometimes it is red and inflammed. Gastric secretions are devoid of pepsin, acid and intrinsic factor. Numbness of limbs, coldness of extremities and difficulty in walking are manifestations of neurologic changes. The haemoglobin content may be as low as 8 per cent. Demyelination of white fibers of spinal cord occurs in severe cases. Psychiatric symptoms may occur associated with low levels of vitamin B$_{12}$ in the plasma, but in the absence of other signs of neuropathy. Pernicious anaemia is associated with an increased risk of gastric cancer. Clinical manifestations are mental apathy, pigmentation, growth retardation and megaloblastic bone marrow. In young females there may be infertility.

Diagnosis

The differential diagnosis of pernicious anaemia from other forms of megaloblastic anaemia depends upon the age of the patient (common among females aged between 45 and 65), the finding of histamine-fast or pentagastrin-fast achlorhydria, upon the absence of pregnancy and the lack of evidence of malnutrition, malabsorption of structural change in the small intestine. Plasma vitamin B$_{12}$ is below 160 ng/l while plasma folate is usually normal. The schilling test shows subnormal absorption which is corrected if intrinsic factor is given at the same time.

Treatment

If the haemoglobin level is under 4 g/dl blood transfusion should always be given. Physical activity should be at a minimum until the haemoglobin is above 7 g/dl.

Vitamin B_{12} should be given in a dosage of 1,000 mcg intramuscularly twice during the first week, then 250 mcg weekly until the blood count is normal. Then 1000 mcg every six weeks is given. Folic acid should never be used alone in the treatment of pernicious anaemia as it does not prevent the development of neurological complications and may precipitate them.

Within 48 hours of the first injection of a cobalamin the bone marrow shows a striking change from a megaloblastic to normoblastic state. Within two or three days the reticulocyte count begins to rise, reaching a maximum about the 4th or 7th day.

To cope up with regeneration of blood, ferrous sulphate 200 mg thrice daily is given.

Vitamin B_{12} levels in maternal milk and serum are low in pernicious anaemia. The clinical picture gets corrected by administering a single dose of 50 µg of vitamin B_{12} to the mother or to the infant.

Dietary Consideration

Poor appetite and gastrointestinal discomfort seriously interfere with an adequate food intake so that the patients often present a picture of general nutritional deficiency. A high protein diet of 100 to 150 g of protein with high calorie diet is recommended. Supplementation of liver extracts would be effective in the treatment of pernicious anaemia.

Achlorhydria retards digestion, hence fat in diet should be kept to moderate levels, restricting especially fried foods that may further delay gastric emptying.

A soft or clear liquid diet is preferable until glossitis completely disappears. Spicy food should be avoided. A soft diet is recommended since there is anorexia and irritation of gastrointestinal tract.

Supplementation with ascorbic acid is essential if citrus fruits and other rich sources of vitamin C are not ingested. High protein high calorie beverages, two or three times daily should be given. They may be prepared from milk, non fat dry milk, protein concentrates and fruits.

PREVENTION OF ANAEMIA

Anaemia can be prevented by supplementation, education and fortification.

Supplementation

To prevent anaemia under National Nutritional Anaemia Prophylaxis Programme, distribution of iron and folate tablets to pregnant women during last trimester and for pre-school children is in the operation as part of MCH services. Expectant and nursing mothers are given 180 mg of ferrous sulphate and 0.5 mg of folic acid. Children in the age group 1–5 years are given 60 mg of ferrous sulphate and 0.1 mg of folic acid.

Vegans should take vitamin B_{12} supplementation.

Education

Emphasis should be laid on educating both the health functionaries as well as the general population about anaemia. All medical, health and social workers, horticulture department and voluntary organisations have roles to play in promoting the consumption of foods rich in erythropoietic nutrients. Extensive efforts by community level workers and effective use of modern media are recommended for achieving success in this strategy. Following points need to be considered for promotion of the strategy:

- Promotion of consumption of pulses, green leafy vegetables, other vegetables (which are rich in iron and folic acid) and meat products rich in vitamin B_{12} and iron.
- Creation of awareness in mothers attending antenatal clinics, immunisation sessions, anganwadi centres and creches about the prevalence of anaemia, ill-effects of anaemia and its preventable nature.

Table 17.5 summarises the differentiating characteristics of anaemias.

Table 17.5: Differentiating characteristics of anaemias

Characteristics	Iron deficiency	B_{12} deficiency	Folic acid deficiency
1. Type of anaemia	Hypochromic microcytic		Megaloblasic—Figure 17d, Appendix 11.
2. Pathological changes	RBCs are pale and small in size. MCV < 80	Variation and irregular shape and size of RBC usually larger than normal, have their full complement of Hb normochromic RBC life span reduced to 60 days. MCV < 100	
3. Vulnerable groups	Pregnant and lactating women infants and children.	Vegans (no milk, eggs or animal food or fermented food), Pregnant women, after gastrectomy.	Infants, pregnant women, elderly patients.

4. Causes	A. Blood loss
	    a. Accidental haemorrhage
	    b. Chronic diseases, cancer, ulcer
	    c. Excessive blood donation
	    d. Excessive blood donation
	    e. Parasite like hookworm
	    f. Repeated pregnancy
	 B. Deficiency of iron in diet
	 C. Increased demand Pregnancy lactation and infancy
	 D. Inadequate iron absorption
	    a. Diarrhoea
	    b. Lack of acid secretion by stomach
	    c. Antacid therapy
		A. Less intrinsic factor
		 B. Complete vegetarian diet, with no fermented foods.
		 C. After gastrectomy
		 D. Tape worm infestation
		 E. Malabsorption
			A. Destruction of folic acid during cooking.
			 B. Increased demand (infancy, pregnancy, alcoholism).
			 C. Malabsorption
			 D. Congenital defects
			 E. Prolonged use of antiepileptic drugs, oral contraceptives and folate antimetabolities.
			 F. Loss in haemodialysis.

Contd...

Characteristics	Iron deficiency	B$_{12}$ deficiency	Folic acid deficiency
5. Symptoms	General fatigue, breathlessness, giddiness. dimness of vision, headache, anorexia, palpitation, angular stomatitis, koilonychia glossitis, impaired motor, language and scholastic achievement, decreased physical activity.	Lemon yellow or pale skin, anorexia, glossitis, diarrhoea, weight loss, coldness of entremities, inc. risk of gastric cancer.	Paraesthesia tropical sprue fatigue, diarrhoea glossitis.
6. Diagnosis	Hb level < 12 g/dl in adult women < 13 g/dl in adult men < 7.5 g/dl indicates advanced cases.	Given 1 µg dose of radioactive B$_{12}$, 30% recovered in faeces healthy one, 70% in pernicious anaemia. Schilling test.	A. Folic acid content of Serum. B. Absorption least with tritium labelled folic acid. C. FIGLU excretion test.
7. Treatment	A Oral iron preparation (280 mg of FeSO$_4$FH$_2$O) has 60 mg of elemental iron. B. For infants the dose is about 6 mg/kg (FeSO$_4$ mixture)	1000 µg of vitamin B$_{12}$ given by intramuscular injection twice weekly until Hb is normal. Then injection 100 mg every six weeks is given. If Hb level is 4 g/dl, blood transfusion given.	Folic acid dose of 5-10 mg daily. Hb level is 5 g/dl blood transfusion given for anticonvulsant therapy Fa is 10-5 mg daily 1000 µg vitamin B$_{12}$ weekly.

Source: Srilakshmi, B., 2005, Dietetics, New Age International (P) Limited, Publishers, New Delhi.

QUESTIONS

1. Why is it that folic acid deficiency is common during pregnancy?
2. What is pernicious anaemia?
3. Vitamin B$_{12}$ is present only in animal sources. How are vegetarians meet their requirement?
4. What is the diagnostic test of folic acid deficiency?
5. Give sources of folic acid and B$_{12}$.
6. List the functions of folic acid in the body.
7. List the functions of B$_{12}$.
8. What is FIGLU test?
9. Give RDA of folic acid for different age groups.
10. What is megaloblastic anaemia?
11. Give the interrelationship of folic acid, B$_{12}$ and B$_6$.

SUGGESTED REFERENCES

- Hokin Bevan, D. and Terry Butter, 1999. Cyanocobalamin status in Seventh-day Advertist ministers in Australia, Am. J. Clin Nutr, **70**.
- Relationship between plasma homocysteine level and folate and vitamin B$_6$ status. National Institute of Nutrition, Annual Report, 1999–2000.
- Neural tube defects : www.sbaa.org/

CHAPTER 18

WATER SOLUBLE VITAMINS: VITAMIN B₆, PANTOTHENIC ACID, BIOTIN AND VITAMIN C

VITAMIN B₆

Vitamin B_6 is a generic term for a group of vitamins with similar functions. Three forms of vitamin B_6 occur in nature - pyridoxine, pyridoxal and pyridoxamine. In the body, all three forms are equally active as precursors of the potent pyridoxine coenzyme pyridoxal phosphate. Pyridoxine is water soluble, heat stable and sensitive to light and alkalis. It is easily absorbed in the upper portion of the small intestine and is found throughout the body tissues, evidence of its many essential metabolic activities.

Figure 18a gives the structures of pyridoxine and derivatives.

FUNCTIONS

Co-enzyme in Protein Metabolism

In its active phosphate form pyridoxine is a coenzyme in many types of transamination and decarboxylation reactions in amino acid metabolism.

Decarboxylation: Converts glutamic acid to gamma-amino butyric acid, a substance found in grey matter in the brain. Since aminobutyric acid affects central synaptic activity, it is a regulatory factor for the neurons. Also the pyridoxine co-enzyme converts tryptophan to serotonin, a potent vasoconstrictor, which stimulates cerebral activity and brain metabolism.

Deamination: Renders carbon residues available for energy by removing the amino groups from amino acids such as serine and threonine.

Transamination: Removes the amino group and transfers it to a new carbon skeleton forming a new amino acid or other compound.

Trans-sulphuration: Transfers sulphur from methionine to another amino acid, serine to form the derivative amino acid cysteine.

Nicotinic acid formation: Participates in nicotinic acid formation from tryptophan.

Haemoglobin synthesis: Incorporates the amino acid glycine and succinate, a glucose metabolite in the citric acid cycle into haeme, the essential nonprotein core of haemoglobin.

Amino acid transport: Actively transports amino acids from the intestine into circulation and across cell walls into the cells.

Coenzyme in Carbohydrate and Fat Metabolism

By way of decarboxylation and transamination reactions, the active coenzyme provides metabolites for energy producing fuel in the citric acid cycle and converts the essential fatty acid linoleic acid to another fatty acid, arachidonic acid.

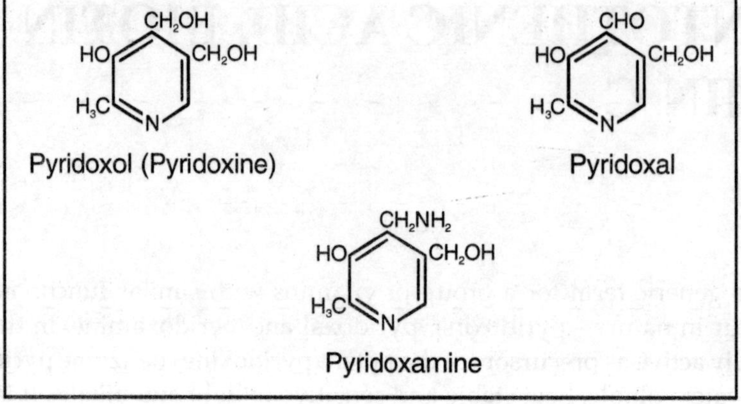

Figure 18a. Pyridoxine and derivatives.

Deficiency

It is usually a part of general deficiency of B-complex group of vitamins and is often seen in association with niacin and riboflavin deficiencies. In cereal-pulse based diets, bioavailability problems might contribute to the deficiency. Malabsorption or losses during chronic dialysis can lead to pyridoxine deficiency. Pregnancy is usually associated with pyridoxine deficiency and that can lead to deficiency in infants. Processed milk formulae or other foods which result in considerable loss of the vitamin produce pyridoxine deficiency in infants. Chronic alcoholism is yet another factor leading to pyridoxine deficiency. Alcohol breaks down pyridoxal phosphate and impairs the ability of liver to store the vitamin.

Pyridoxine deficiency often occurs as a side effect of drugs. Isoniazid used as a chemotherapeutic agent for tuberculosis is an antagonist of pyridoxine. It is believed that isoniazid forms a hydrazone complex with pyridoxal, resulting in inactivation of the vitamin. Also isoniazid inhibits the conversion of glutamic acid to gamma-amino butyric acid, the only amino acid the brain metabolises, thus it causes side effects of neuritis. Treatment with large doses, 50–100 mg daily of pyridoxine prevents this effect.

Anaemia: A hypochromic, microcytic anaemia occurs even in the presence of a high serum-iron level in some persons. A deficiency of pyridoxine has been demonstrated in these persons by a special test and the anaemia subsequently cured by supplying the deficient vitamin.

Central nervous system disturbances: By virtue of its role in the formation of the two regulatory compounds in brain activity, serotonin and gamma-aminobutyric acid, pyridoxine controls related neurologic conditions. In infants deprived of the vitamin, there is increased hyper-irritability that progresses to convulsive seizures. For example, a classic object lesson occurred early in the 1950's. A group of infants who had been fed a commercial milk formula, in which most of the pyridoxine content had inadvertently been destroyed by high-temperature autoclaving, developed convulsions. The seizures ceased when a vitamin B$_6$ supplemented formula was used. Sleep disturbances, irritability and depression have often been attributed to pyridoxine deficiency.

Oral contraceptive associated depressions can be treated with pyridoxine.

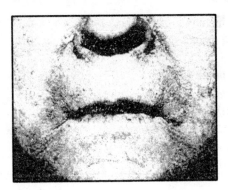

Figure 18b. Dermatitis of vitamin B$_6$ deficiency. The skin is greasy and flaky unlike the skin affected by the dermatitis of pellagra.

Source: Sizer Frances Sienkiewicz and Eleanor Noss Whitney, 2000, Nutrition, concepts and controversies, Wadsworth/Thomson Learning, Belmont.

Oral and Dermal Lesions: Oral lesions like angular stomatitis, glossitis and cheilosis in pregnant and lactating mothers have been described in pyridoxine deficiency. Riboflavin deficiency impairs pyridoxal phosphate synthesis. Recent work in rats at National Institute of Nutrition suggests that both riboflavin and pyridoxine deficiencies affect collagen synthesis and maturation which probably results in varying skin lesions in these deficiencies.

Haematological Manifestations: Pyridoxine responsive hypochromic microcytic anaemia due to genetic failure of incorporation of iron into haemoglobin is characterised by hyperferremia with sideroblasts in the bone marrow. Sideroblastic anaemias of this nature rarely occur due to dietary deficiency.

Treatment

Oral lesions and peripheral neuritis due to dietary deficiency can be treated with 10–20 mg of vitamin given orally or by parenteral route. Pyridoxine has been used in the treatment of side effects of liver disease and alcoholism. Vomiting during pregnancy and depression associated with oral contraceptive therapy are often treated with 20 mg pyridoxine.

An abnormal state of tryptophan metabolism contributes to the increased need.

Recommended Dietary Allowances

The Recommended Dietary Allowances of ICMR for pyridoxine are given in Table 18.1.

Table18.1: ICMR Recommended Dietary Allowances of pyridoxine

Group	Pyridoxine mg/day
Man	2.0
Woman	2.0
Pregnancy	2.5
Lactation	2.5
Infants	
0–6 months	0.1
6–12 months	0.4
Children	
1–6 years	0.9
7–9 years	1.6
Boys and Girls	
10–12 years	1.6
Boys and Girls	
13–18 years	2.0

Sources

The pyridoxine content of Indian foods has not been systematically studied. Meat, pulses and wheat are known to be rich sources while other cereals are fair sources of the vitamin. Fruits and vegetables are relatively poor sources. While cooking and processing meat and milk, considerable amounts of the vitamin are lost. In foods of vegetable origin, however, there are hardly any losses. This appears to be related to the form in which the vitamin is present in foods.

PANTOTHENIC ACID

It is a constituent of Coenzyme A and present in all living matter. It is widely distributed in foods and deficiency is unlikely in man. In 1939 R.J. Williams isolated the vitamin, later synthesised and called it pantothenic acid.

Figure l8c gives the structure of pantothenic acid and Coenzyme A.

Bound pantothenate performs multiple roles in cellular metabolism and regulation. The co-enzyme form of pantothenic acid is Co-enzyme A. Co-enzyme A is essential for the synthesis of fatty acids and their incorporation into membrane phospholipids. It is also required for the synthesis of cholesterol, steroid hormones, vitamin A, vitamin D and all compounds formed from isoprenoid units. It helps in the conversion of pyruvate to acetyl co-enzyme A and -ketogluterate to succinyl co-enzyme A in TCA cycle.

Pantothenate also contributes to the synthesis of amino acids, such as leucine, arginine and methionine. It is essential for the synthesis of B_{12}, haemoglobin and cytochromes.

The degradation of fatty acids through β-oxidation and the oxidative degradation of amino acids also depend on CoA, which then makes the products of catabolism available for energy extraction through TCA cycle.

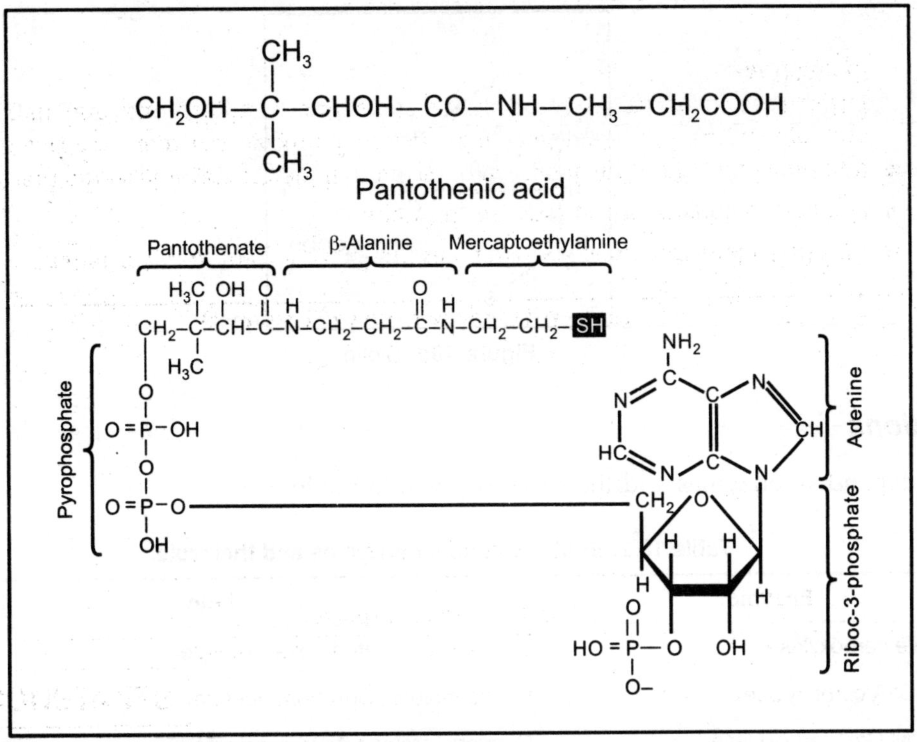

Figure 18c. Structure of pantothenic acid and Coenzyme A.

Pantothenic acid deficiency affects the adrenal cortex, the nervous system, skin and hair. In rats, deficiency leads to impaired antibody formation, inflammation of the respiratory tract, anaemia, loss of hair, pigmentation and reproductive failure. Pantothenic acid deficiency is rare in humans.

Some physicians use pantothenic acid for relieving the 'burning foot' syndrome though the relationship is not confirmed. Burning feet syndrome is characterised by abnormal skin sensations, exacerbated by warmth and diminished with cold of the feet and lower legs. Though administration of the vitamin bring back the pigment to the grey hairs of experimentally deficient rats, this has not been proven in humans.

Most human diets provide 3-10 mg daily derived from a variety of natural foods and this is ample to meet the needs. For adult patients on total parenteral nutrition 15 mg is an adequate daily dose and 1 mg daily is sufficient for infants.

The best sources of pantothenic acid are liver, kidney, egg-yolk, yeast and fresh vegetables. Milk and meat are fairly good sources.

BIOTIN

Biotin deficiency does not occur in man except under extraordinary circumstances.

Figure 18d gives the structure of biotin.

Biotin functions in cells covalently bound to enzymes. Acetyl CoA carboxylase is a biotin dependent enzyme. It helps in the biosynthesis of fatty acid from acetyl CoA.

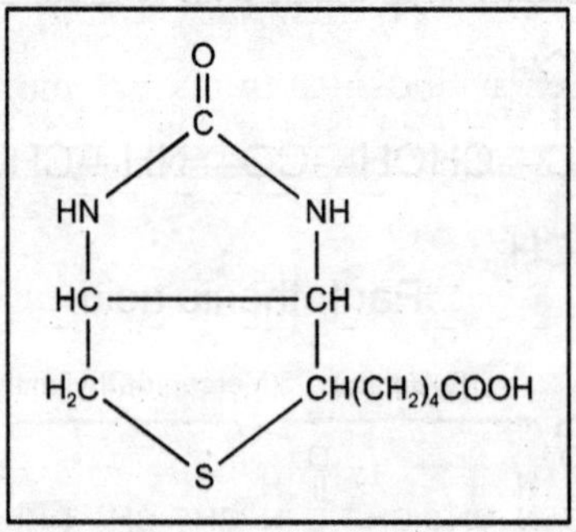

Figure 18d. Biotin

Functions

Biotin-dependent enzymes and their role is given in Table.

Table 18.2: Biotin-dependent enzymes and their role.

Enzyme	Role
Pyruvate carboxylase	Converts pyruvate to oxaloacetate
Acetyl CoA carboxylase	Forms malonyl CoA from acetate
Propionyl CoA carboxylase	Converts propionate to succinate
β-methyl crotonyl CoA carboxylase	Converts β-methyl crotonyl CoA to β-methyl glutaconyl CoA

Deficiency

Biotin deficiency in humans is characterised by depression, hallucinations, muscle pain, localised paresthesia, anorexia nausea, alopecia and scaly dermatitis. Deficiency in rats is associated with decreased hepatic ornithine transcarbamylase mRNA and activity; this enzyme is important in the urea cycle. People ingesting raw eggs in excess amounts are likely to develop biotin deficiency due to impaired biotin absorption. Impaired biotin absorption may occur also with gastrointestinal disorders such as inflammatory bowel disease and achlorhydria or with people on anticonvulsant drug therapy. Excessive alcohol ingestion and sulphonamide therapy also increase the risk of deficiency.

Sources

Biotin is found widely distributed in foods. Good food sources of the vitamin are liver, soyabeans and egg yolk. Cereals, legumes and nuts also contain relatively high amounts of biotin. Within many foods, biotin is found bound to protein or as biocytin, which is also called biotinyllysine. Biotin is also produced by bacteria within the colon.

Avidin, a glycoprotein in raw egg whites, may irreversibly bind biotin in a non-covalent bond and prevent biotin absorption. Because avidin is heat-labile, ingestion of cooked egg whites does not compromise biotin absorption.

ROLE OF B VITAMINS IN ENERGY METABOLISM

Various vitamin cofactors and their action sites in energy metabolism is summarised in figure 18e.

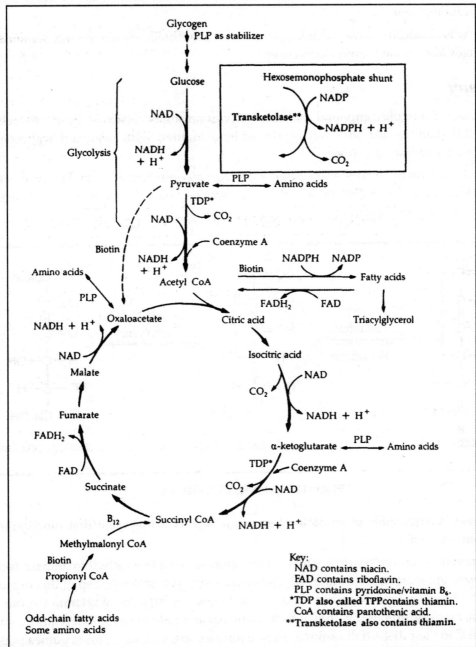

Figure18e. Various vitamin cofactors and their action sites in energy metabolism. The role of thiamin as TDP is shown by an asterisk.

Source: Groff L. James and Sareen S. Gropper, 1999, Advanced Nutrition and Human Metabolism, Wadsworth, Thomson Learning, Belmont.

VITAMIN C

The chemical name for vitamin C is ascorbic acid and it is also known as hexuronic acid and antiscorbutic nutrient.

Scurvy was classically a disease of sailors. In 1747, the British physician Lind demonstrated that oranges and lemons could cure scurvy.

Chemistry

Ascorbic acid is a simple compound containing six carbon atoms, related to the monosaccharide glucose. It is stable to acid but easily destroyed by oxidation, light, alkali and heat especially in the presence of iron or copper,

The oxidised form of ascorbic acid known as dehydroascorbic acid also has vitamin C activity. The oxidation products of dehydroascorbic acid have no vitamin C activity. The structure of vitamin C is given in Figure 18f.

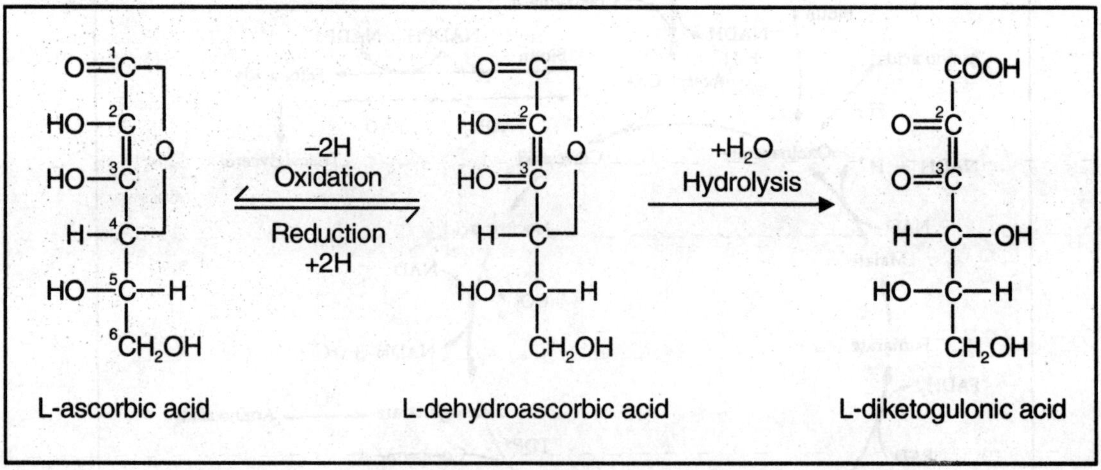

Figure18f. Metabolism of vitamin C

Vitamin C is susceptible to oxidation because it is a reducing agent that function in the body as antioxidant.

Most mammals can synthesise vitamin C from glucose but a few including humans lack the liver enzyme gulonolactone-oxidase, which is required to catalyse one step of this process. It is the lack of this enzyme that forces humans to depend on supplies of vitamin C from their food. Man, monkey, guinea pig, Indian fruit eating bat and red vented bulbul require a supply of vitamin C in their diet. Of the animals that require a supply of the vitamin, guinea pigs and monkeys are most widely used in research. Now fish are also used in research of vitamin C. In plants vitamin C accumulates during the ripening process and is presumably synthesised within the plant cells from naturally occurring glucose.

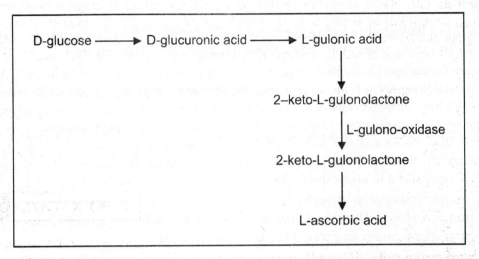

Figure18g. Biosynthesis of vitamin C. Species that require a dietary source of vitamin lack the enzyme L-gulonoxidase which converts L-gulonolactone to 2-keto-L-gulonolactone.

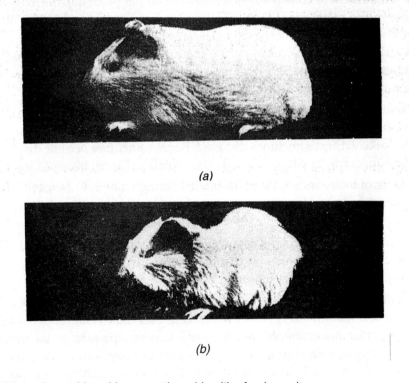

Figure18h. Effect of ascorbic acid on growth and health of guinea pigs.

(a) Deficient animal (b) Supplemented animal.

Source: Proudfit T.F; Corinne H. Robinson,1957, Nutrition and diet therapy. The Macmillan Company, New York.

Functions

Vitamin C is a biological reducing agent especially during hydroxylation reactions and it is an antioxidant that protects the body against damaging oxidizing agents.

Collagen formation: Collagen is a major structural protein of connective tissue (which binds cells and tissues together), bone, teeth, cartilage, skin and scar tissue. Vitamin C is specifically required by the fibroblast cells of connective tissue (responsible for collagen synthesis) and the boneforming osteoblasts within bone. It is estimated that collagen constitutes about one quarter of all the protein in the body. Collagen is formed from a precursor protein known as tropocollagen by the hydroxylation of the amino acids proline and lysine within tropocollagen. Vitamin C is required to allow these essential hydroxylation reactions to proceed.

The enzymes that catalyse these hydroxylation reactions require the direct participation of ferrous iron and oxygen. The role of vitamin C is to act as a reducing agent that keeps the iron in the ferrous state, preventing its oxidation to the ferric state.

Any deficiency in vitamin C results in defective collagen synthesis, associated with impaired wound healing, disruption of capillaries and faulty bone and tooth formation. One of the first effects of any impairment of collagen synthesis are small pin point haemorrhages which result from weakness in the membranes that line the blood capillaries and in the fibres that hold cells together under the surface of the skin. These weaknesses allow blood to escape into the enlarged intercellular spaces, accounting for the capillary bleeding associated with scurvy. These subcutaneous haemorrhages appear most often in areas subjected to mechanical stress, such as the gums, which become soft, spongy and prone to bleeding.

If collagen synthesis is impaired, the matrix formation is defective and it becomes less able to accumulate the calcium and phosphorus required for proper bone mineralisation. As a result the bone becomes weakened and sometimes distorted. Bones sometimes become displaced from their joints when the supporting cartilage, which is also mainly collagen, becomes weakened.

The dentin layer of tooth does not form normally during vitamin C deficiency. This results in teeth that are structurally weak and more prone to mechanical injury and decay. Skin grafts to repair burned tissue have been found to heal more quickly when adequate vitamin C is present.

Carnitine synthesis: Vitamin C is required for the synthesis of carnitine. Carnitine is a small nitrogen-containing organic compound involved in the transport of fatty acids into mitochondria to be oxidised to release energy for use by cells.

Neurotransmitter synthesis: Vitamin C is required to sustain the activity of the copper-containing enzyme dopamine oxygenase, which catalyses the oxidation of dopamine to form the neurotransmitter norepinephrine. Vitamin C also appears to be involved in the hydroxylation of tryptophan during the biosynthesis of serotonin (5-hydroxy tryptamine). The involvement of vitamin C in the synthesis of neurotransmitters probably explains the presence of high concentration of vitamin C in brain and adrenal tissues.

Activation of hormones: Many peptide hormones and hormone releasing factors are synthesised as precursor molecules that are enzymatically modified into their active forms. Vitamin C is essential for the activation of bombesin (human gastrin-releasing peptide) calcitonin, gastrin, oxytocin, thyrotropin, corticotropin, vasopressin, growth hormone-releasing factor.

Drug detoxification: Vitamin C is required for the optimal activity of various drug-detoxifying metabolic systems within the body. These include the mixed-function oxidase system and the flavin-monooxygenase system in the liver.

General Antioxidant: A variety of damaging oxidising agents occur in the body, as a result of both normal metabolic processes and exposure to drugs and environmental pollutants. A range of enzymes and antioxidant reducing agents (including vitamin E, -β carotene and vitamin C) are able to convert these oxidising agents to harmless substances that can be excreted. Vitamin C can combine with and so "scavenge" many types of oxidising free radicals. It can also regenerate the reduced form of vitamin E converting that vitamin back into the form in which it can act as an antioxidant.

Vitamin C is known to be involved in regulating cholesterol metabolism and in maintaining the structure of blood vessels and the antioxidant effects of the vitamin might prevent tissue damage that leads to cardiovascular disease.

Iron metabolism: Vitamin C acts as a reducing agent, that is, able to keep ferric ions in ferrous form and facilitate absorption. Vitamin C forms soluble complexes with ferric ions, which preserve the iron solubility on the more alkaline duodenal pH. Vitamin C also assists in the transfer of iron from blood plasma into ferritin for storage in the liver as well as the release of iron from ferritin when required. The role of ascorbate in iron metabolism is related not only to enhanced absorption but also to intracellular metabolism of iron binding protein.

Vitamin C also aids calcium absorption by preventing the incorporation of calcium into insoluble complexes. Vitamin C converts inactive form of folic acid into its active form dihydrofolic acid and tetra hydrofolic acid and also stabilises the active form. Vitamin C alleviates allergic reactions, enhances immune function, stimulates formation of bile and facilitate the release of some steroid hormones. Vitamin C is necessary for the conversion of cholesterol to bile acids and has been reported to be involved in the detoxification of many chemical carcinogens.

Absorption, Transport and Metabolism

Ascorbic acid is absorbed in the jejunum, principally by a sodium dependent active transport mechanism. Dehydroascorbic acid is passively absorbed.

As intake increases, the efficiency of absorption falls. While vitamin C is filtered through the kidneys, enough is reabsorbed to maintain a plasma concentration of 1.2 to 1.5 mg /dl and a total body pool of 1.2 to 2.0 g. All vitamin C in excess of the amounts needed to maintain these plasma and body levels, is excreted in urine.

Since vitamin C is metabolised to oxalic acid, patients with kidney stones or renal insufficiency are currently advised to avoid excessive intake of vitamin C.

Deficiency

Scurvy, the most severe form of vitamin C deficiency is relatively rare throughout the world. Faulty cooking habits and inadequate intake of fresh vegetables and fruits are the major causes of dietary deficiency of vitamin C.

The early symptoms are non specific, including listlessness, fatigue, weakness, shortness of breath, muscle cramps, aching bones, joints and muscles and loss of appetite.

The clinical features of scurvy are characterised by gingivitis (bleeding gums), petechiae (small haemorrhagic spots), arthralgia (pain in the joint), depression, postural hypotension and a marked limitation to perform strenuous work. Delayed wound healing occurs due to reduced synthesis of connective tissue. Haemorrhages can cause anaemia of vitamin C. Pinpoint haemorrhages under the skin causing the reddish-blue spots occur when the total vitamin C reserves in the body falls below 300 mg. Intakes of 6.5 to 10 mg of ascorbic acid per day are effective in eliminating the clinical symptoms of scurvy.

Breastfed infants are not susceptible to scurvy as it contains adequate amounts of vitamin C and as there is no need for heat processing.

The main deficiency symptoms of vitamin C in infants are as follows:

Tender bones: There is evidence of general tenderness especially noticeable in the legs. The legs assume the typical frog like position.

Petechial haemorrhages: The capillaries become brittle and burst thus giving rise to red and purple spots over the body.

Gingivitis: This is also known as bleeding gums. There is spongy swellings of the mucous membrane.

Delayed wound healing: The wound healing is delayed due to failure of the cells to deposit collagen fibrils.

Cessasation of bone growth: The bones cease to grow. The cells of growing epiphyses continue to proliferate but no new matrix is laid down between the cells. Consequently, bones fracture easily at the point of growth because they fail to ossify.

Children may also develop anaemia and pyrexia.

Scurvy in infants and children is treated by giving 10-25 mg vitamin C, 2-3 times a day. Spontaneous bleeding decreases within 24 hours. Muscle and bone lesions take 2-3 weeks time to heal. Large ecchymosis heal in 10-12 days. Anaemia gets corrected within 2-4 weeks.

The typical symptoms are seen in Figure 18i – Appendix 10.

EVALUATION OF VITAMIN C STATUS

Measurements of vitamin C levels in blood plasma and within leukocytes are currently used to evaluate vitamin C status in humans.

RECOMMENDED DIETARY ALLOWANCES

The Recommended Dietary Allowances of ICMR for ascorbic acid are given in Table 18.2.

Table 18.2: ICMR recommende dietary allowances of vitamin C

Group	Vitamin C mg/day
Man	40
Woman	40
Pregnant woman	40

Contd....

Group	Vitamin C mg/day
Lactation	80
Infants	
0-12 months	25
Children	
Boys	40
Girls	

SOURCES

Ascorbic acid occurs widely in plant foods, particularly in fresh fruits and vegetables especially green leafy vegetables. Amla is the richest source of vitamin C. Guava, orange and lime are also good sources of vitamin C. Green leafy vegetables like drumstick leaves and agathi are good sources of vitamin C. Meat, milk, cereals and pulses are poor sources of ascorbic acid.

Of all the vitamins, ascorbic acid is the most susceptible to destruction by atmospheric oxidation. One of the characteristic properties of this vitamin is its intense reducing action and hence it is oxidized rapidly in air. It is for this reason that when vegetables become dry and stale or cut and exposed to air most of the vitamin C originally present is destroyed.

However, when dry pulses and beans are allowed to germinate vitamin C is formed in the grain and the growing sprout, about 85 per cent being present in the former and 15 per cent in the latter part. During famine situations namely, prolonged drought where fresh vegetables or fruits cannot be obtained, sprouted grains can be used as a source of vitamin C. Sprouted green gram contains about 3 times more vitamin C than does sprouted bengal gram. 17-20 mg of vitamin C is produced during germination per 100 g of pulses.

Heating or drying of fresh fruits or vegetables usually leads to destruction of most of the vitamin C. Amla is an exception among fruits not only because of its high acidity, high vitamin C content but also because it contains substances which partially protect the vitamin from destruction on heating or drying.

The vitamin C content of food is maximised by the following processes:

- Harvesting at the peak of maturity.
- Storing in a cool, moist place.
- Limiting exposure to air and sunlight.
- Avoiding soaking food in water.
- Cooking food in the minimal amount of water or even better, cooking by microwave.
- Cooking the food in pieces as large as possible.
- Eating fruits immediately after cutting.
- Avoiding making juices or macerating.
- Eating vegetable preparations immediately after cooking.
- Wherever possible fresh raw vegetables should be used for obtaining enough vitamin C.

Table 18.3: Ascorbic acid content of foods

Name of the foodstuff	Ascorbic acid mg/100g
Amla	600
Drumstick leaves	220
Guava	212
Cashew fruit	180
Agathi	169
Capsicum	137
Cabbage	124
Bitter gourd	96
Zizypus jujuba	76
Orange juice	30
Tomato ripe	27

VITAMIN C AND DISEASES

The present evidence suggests the theory that vitamin C supplementation significantly decreases the duration of an episode of cold and reduced severity of the symptoms. During an infection phagocytes become activated to fight the infection and produce free radicals, which are released from the cells. By combining with these 'free radicals', vitamin C may decrease their inflammatory effects. Large doses of vitamin C are prescribed during infections to increase the capacity of healing and immunocompetence.

Epidemiological studies suggest that consumption of vitamin C rich foods is associated with a lower risk of stomach and oesophageal cancers. Possible mechanisms of ascorbate action against cancer development include a role in immuno competence, an ability to act as a free radical scavenger or antioxidant and an ability to detoxify carcinogens or to block carcinogenic processes.

Vitamin C is a potent antioxidant and hence large doses have been advocated for prevention of cancers and cardiovascular disease. It can lower blood concentrations of cholesterol and triglycerides. Cholesterol is converted to cholic acid by ascorbic acid.

Vitamin like substances

Some of the compounds are not classified as vitamins because they may occur in plants and animals in much larger quantities than vitamins and have no catalytic action.

Lipoic acid — Oxidative decarboxylation of α-keto acids

Choline — Lipotropic factor

Inositol — Due to its alcoholic nature, inositol forms esters with acids. The most important of these is phytic acid, the hexa phosphate ester, formed with phosphoric acid. Phytic acid forms insoluble salts with calcium and magnesium preventing the absorption of these minerals. Inositol among with choline is considered to have lipotropic action is animals.

Carnitine — Transports long chain fatty acids into mitochondria for subsequent oxidation.

QUESTIONS

1. Why is the body's need for vitamin B$_6$ related to protein intake?
2. Discuss deficiency symptoms of pyridoxine.
3. As part of the treatment of tuberculosis, B$_6$ is prescribed in high doses. Why?
4. Give the functions of vitamin C.
5. Discuss the typical deficiency symptoms of vitamin C.
6. Describe the best sources of vitamin C.
7. How can you prevent losses of vitamin C during cooking?
8. What is meant by 'mega doses' of vitamins? Are they really useful to us?
9. Write short notes on pantothenic acid and biotin.
10. Write a note on antioxidant property of vitamin C.

SUGGESTED REFERENCES

- Phagocytosis and wound healing in riboflavin and pyridoxine deficiencies, 1991-92, Annual report, NIN, Hyderabad.
- Water soluble vitamins : www.ncbi.nlm.gov/science 96
- Bhaskaram P, 2002, Micronutrient malnutrition, infection and immunity. An overview. Nutrition **60.**

CHAPTER 19

ANTIOXIDANTS

The normal functioning of cells is dependent on a proper balance of prooxidants and antioxidants. The former promote the release of oxygen to provide energy needed for cell functioning. In this process, different biochemical reactions take place, which continuously produce various free radicals. If these free radicals are not quenched by antioxidants, they cause damage to the cells, proteins, DNA and RNA. Cumulative tissue injury thus caused by free radicals is now known to underlie the pathogenesis of such diverse conditions as cancer, atherosclerosis, radiation damage and accelerated ageing.

Thus the USDA definition of an antioxidant can be extended in a nutritional context to include 'compounds that protect biological systems against the potentially harmful effects of processes or reactions that can cause excessive oxidations'.

Free radicals are chemical species with one or more unpaired electrons. Paired electrons spin in opposite directions and their energy is neutralized, while a molecule or radical with an unpaired electron has unbalanced energy and becomes unstable and highly reactive. It can either lose an electron and get "oxidized" or lose an electron and get reduced.

In biological systems, removal or addition of electrons is the most frequent mechanism known as Redox (Reduction oxidation) reaction. The reduction is the addition of an electron (e^-) to an acceptor molecule, which stores energy, while oxidation is removal of an electron from a molecule to release energy. During the process of release of energy to perform normal activities of life, electrons are transferred between the molecules resulting in many Reactive Oxygen Species and the non-oxygen free radicals in the body.

FREE RADICALS OF OXYGEN

There are three known free radicals, the superoxide, the hydroxyl and the peroxide. When molecular oxygen accepts one electron at a time, superoxide radical is formed.

$$O_2 + e^- \longrightarrow O_2^-$$

Superoxide can accept a proton H^+ to form a perhydroxy radical (HOO) which is also a free radical. Perhydroxy radical has greater solubility in fat solvents and are highly toxic to the cell membranes which are rich in lipids.

$$O_2^- + e^- + 2H^+ \longrightarrow H_2O_2$$

In the second step, superoxide takes up another electron, forming peroxide, which combines with hydrogen ions in the cellular fluid to form hydrogen peroxide. Hydrogen peroxide is more stable and hence less toxic than superoxide. But hydrogen peroxide survives longer and can move considerable distance from the site of its origin, by entering the circulating body fluids, causing damage along its route. Hydrogen peroxide is not a free radical but a free radical inducer.

The toxicity of hydrogen peroxide is further enhanced in cells rich in transition metals iron and copper as in red blood cells. Iron and copper are present in the respiratory components of all tissues and are sites for splitting hydrogen peroxide into a highly toxic hydroxyl radical and hydroxyl ion. This reaction in known as Fenton's Reaction.

Hydroxyl radical is highly toxic but has a short life span, cannot diffuse across cell membranes and cannot spread its toxic effect to neighbouring tissues. Superoxide, hydrogen peroxide, hydroxyl radicals and singlet oxygen (molecular oxygen with an electron lost) are known as Reactive oxygen Species.

SOURCES OF FREE RADICALS AND REACTIVE OXYGEN SPECIES

During respiration, very minute quantities of reactive oxygen species are formed in the cells and get inactivated. Red blood cells, with high oxygen and iron content is a major site of reactive oxygen species formation and their inactivation.

'Respiratory Burst' is a process triggered by the appearance of particulate or non-particulate foreign body. Bacteria from contaminated water or food in the gastro-intestinal tract, or fumes or smoke from tobacco, gaseous or aerosolic pollutants from automobile exhaust, industrial chimneys or dust particles inhaled into the lungs can stimulate Respiratory Burst. It is a process by which white blood cells, specifically the neutrophils move into the site, engulf the foreign matter, phagocytise them and digest them in a swift move to prevent and contain their damage potential. During this process, reactive oxygen species are formed in excessive quantities together with another toxic radical hypochlorite. The process occurs frequently in the mucosal surfaces of gastro intestinal tract and the respiratory tract and the toxins are spread through blood circulation.

Table 19.1: Factors that increase Free-Radical Formation

Body factors	Environmental factors
Energy metabolism	Air pollution
Diabetes	Asbestos
Exercise	High levels of vitamin C
Acute illness	High levels of oxygen
Immune response	Radioactive emissions (for example, from radon gas)
Injury	Some herbicides
Obesity	Tobacco smoke
Other diseases	Trace minerals (iron, copper)
Other metabolic reactions	Ultraviolet light rays
Xenobiotics	

Detoxification of xenobiotics is yet another avenue for free radical generation in the body. A variety of drugs like antibiotics, antimicrobials, anticancer drugs, analgesics, pesticide residues contaminating the food and drug sources and chemicals like benzene and hexane are detoxified in the body by a system known as cyt P_{450} mediated mixed function oxidases, especially in the liver cells. This system is induced by the exposure to toxins and provides great protection. However, during this process large quantities of reactive oxygen species are formed causing damage to the liver cells.

Under ischaemic conditions (oxygen inadequacy) reactive oxygen species are generated in excessive amounts. Autooxidation of small molecules like adrenaline, ferredoxin and even the life sustaining glucose - when present in high levels - produce free radicals and endanger the cells and tissues. Several commonly used drugs like paracetamol and dietary constituents like nitrate are metabolized to toxic components and free radicals.

Nitrate is present in water and foods. In the acid environment of the stomach, nitrate is reduced to nitrite. The latter is a reactive radical and combines with amines and amides of proteins to form N-nitros derivatives which are free radical generators. Nitrosated proteins are found abundantly in cured and smoked meat, fish and milk products. Nitrates are present in vegetables like beet root, celery and spinach.

400 different compounds have been identified in tobacco tar, capable of inducing respiratory burst in the alveoli. Carbon monoxide, cyanide, tobacco specific nitrosamines, superoxide and nitric oxide have also been identified as contributors to tobacco toxicity.

DISEASE PROCESSES BY FREE RADICALS AND REACTIVE OXYGEN SPECIES

Free radicals and reactive oxygen species abstract hydrogen from membrane phospholipids which contain polyunsaturated fatty acid chains, producing reactive free radicals. Oxygen adds on to the site of free radicals formation to produce a peroxide in the second step. Fatty acid peroxide now abstracts a hydrogen from a second fatty acid on the membrane producing a second free radical. This can proceed as a chain reaction, with increasing free radical as well as peroxide formation on the cell membrane. Membrane peroxidation leads to fragmentation of the membrane and release of free radicals in the tissues, affecting the structural integrity and permeability. While lipid peroxidation is the first step on the membrane, proteins on the membrane as well as the cytoplasm are acted upon by free radicals and reactive oxygen species in several ways like modification, oxidation, hydrolysis and fragmentation and inactivation. Oxidatively modified protein of the lipoprotein LDL is known to be the mediator in cholesterol deposition in the blood vessels causing heart attack and stroke.

Free radicals and reactive oxygen species react with DNA, producing strand breakage, mutations leading to cancer and also interfere in the regulatory control of growth differentiation, cell division and cell death.

Table 19.2: Free radicals and reactive oxygen species mediated damage to cells and tissues.

Site of damage	Pathological changes
DNA	Strand breaks leading to mutation and cancer.
Nucleotides, thiol dependent enzymes, protein cross linking	Metabolic disturbances, leading to inflammation. diabetes mellitus, heart disease, asthma.
Extracellular macromolecules, e.g., hyaluronic acid, membranes lipid peroxidation	Joint diseases, allergy, inflammation, oedema and degenerative changes and reduced immunity.

MARKERS OF OXIDATIVE STRESS

There are two assays that are used as markers of oxidative stress. The first of these is the immunoassay of oxidatively modified LDL particles. This is specific to CVD risk with dietary and supplemental antioxidant consumption.

The second assay is the measurement of the compound isoprostane F_2a. It measures the presence of a continuously formed free radical compound that is produced by free radical oxidation of specific polyunsaturated fatty acids. Isoprostane F_2a has a structure similar to that of the prostaglandins. It is used to assess the oxidative stress of infants receiving therapeutic levels of oxygen.

ANTIOXIDANT DEFENCE SYSTEMS

Antioxidant defence system of the body consists of endogenous and exogenous antioxidants which work together at the molecular level to protect cell membranes, lipoproteins, DNA and RNA from the damaging effects of free radicals. Exogenous antioxidants are nutrients such as ascorbic acid, tocopherols and β-carotene and nonnutrients obtained through intake of different diets.

Compounds regarded as a first line of defence, i.e., primary antioxidants or as secondary antioxidants are listed in Table 19.3. Some are synthesized by cells (endogenous), and others need to be provided by the diet. For example, a number of enzymes with antioxidant function require trace elements from the diet as cofactors. Cytoplasmic and mitochondrial superoxide dismutases require copper, zinc and manganese to catalyse the removal of superoxide radicals (O_2^-) produced by the cell. Hydrogen peroxide (H_2O_2) is removed by catalase which requires iron and also by cytosolic glutathione peroxidase (GSHPx). This enzyme also removes potentially toxic lipid hydroperoxides from the cell and is dependent on selenium for optimal function.

Table 19.3: Compounds with established or proposed antioxidant activity in vivo

Primary antioxidant	Secondary antioxidant
Vitamin E*	Copper*
Vitamin C*	Glutathione reductase
Carotenoids*	Ascorbate reductase
Flavonoids*	Glucose-6 phosphate dehydrogenase
Polyamines	Ceruloplasmin
Melatonin	Transferrin
Oestrogen	Metallothionein
Ubiquinone	Albumin
Lipoic acid	Bilirubin
Uric acid	N-acetylcysteine
Glutathione	
Superoxide dismutase	
Glutathione peroxidase	
Catalase	

*Needed in the diet
Endogenous but possibly also needed in the diet (all the other compounds are endogenous)
Source: Garrow, J.S. et al, 2000, Human Nutrition and Dietetice, Churchill, Livingstone, Edinburgh.

Non-enzymic antioxidants are small molecular weight compounds. Endogenously produced examples include glutathione and uric acid. Micronutrients of dietary origin with antioxidant functions include the following.

- Vitamin E is an example of a phenolic antioxidant. Such molecules readily donate the hydrogen from the hydroxyl (HO) group on the ring structure to free radicals which then become unreactive.

Vitamin E is particularly effective in preventing lipid peroxidation, a series of chemical reactions involving the oxidative deterioration of polyunstaturated fatty acids. On donating the hydrogen, vitamin E becomes a relatively unreactive free radical which is unable to attack adjacent fatty acids because the unpaired electron on the oxygen atom becomes delocalised into the aromatic ring structure.

Lipid peroxidation may cause disruption of cell structure and function and thus play an important role in the aetiology of many diseases.

Although vitamin E is primarily located in cell and organelle membranes where it can exert its maximum protective effect, its concentration may only be one molecule for every 2000 phospholipid molecules. This suggests that it is rapidly regenerated possibly by vitamin C.

Table 19.4: Optimal plasma levels of antioxidants micromol/litre

Vitamin	Plasma level
Vitamin C	> or = 50
Vitamin E	> or = 30
Vitamin A	> or = 22
Beta-carotene	> or = 0.4
α-plus β-carotene	> or = 0.4–0.5

Source: Cited from: Joseph Maria 1999, M. Antioxidants and Cancer. "A manual of second regional workshop on planning diet for health" Indian Dietetic Association.

- Vitamin C (L-ascorbic acid) is one of the most important water-soluble antioxidants in cells. It is synthesized in the liver by most animals, but not by man who depends on dietary sources for adequate supply. Ascorbic acid is a strong reducing agent and serves as an antioxidant and as a cofactor in hydroxylation reactions. Vitamin C efficiently scavenges a range of reactive oxygen species such as O_2^-, OH^-, peroxyl radicals and singlet oxygen and can also chelate trace elements such as Fe and Cu, thus inhibiting the catalytic decomposition of hydroperoxides to potentially damaging products.

- β-carotene is effective at scavenging singlet oxygen. It is also an effective antioxidant at low partial pressures of oxygen under conditions where singlet oxygen is not formed, and therefore may be important at the physiological oxygen tensions in tissues. There are many other carotenoids in foods that are also found in tissues. Their nutritional and biochemical significance is poorly understood but may be highly specific as some tissues accumulate particular carotenoids. For example, lycopene is the major carotenoid in the testes and the macula of the retina contains high concentrations of zeaxanthin and lutein.

- Ubiquinone is a lipophilic quinone which functions as an electron carrier in the mitochondrial electron transport chain of the cell. However, it also has antioxidant properties *in vitro*.

Ubiquinone is synthesized in the body from precursors of cholesterol. For this reason it is not classed as a vitamin. However, the ability to synthesize ubiquinone decreases with age and there may be an increasing dependence on food to supply the nutrient.

Table 19.5: Dietary antioxidants

Nutrient	Non-nutrients
β-carotene-Provitamin A,	Carotenoids (Lycopene,
Ascorbic acid-Vitamin C	Xanthophylls)
Tocopherols	Lutein, α-and γ-carotenes
Tocotrienols	(cryptoxanthine, zeaxanthine)
Riboflavin	Flavonoids (quercetin, myricetin,
Sulphur amino acids: Cysteine	quercetagatin, gossypetin)
and methionine	Anthocyanins
Selenium	Isoflavones
	Phenolic compounds (catechin)
	Indoles

Source: Mani Bhooma N.et al. 1999. Your Doctor in the Kitchen, Nutrition 33,1.

- Food polyphenols, such as the flavonoids, chalcones, cinnamic acids, coumarins and antho-cyanins, are ubiquitous dietary components. Originally regarded as being nutritionally inert, there is now increasing interest in their antioxidant properties. Indeed low intakes of flavonoids such as quercetin, myricetin and kaempferol have been associated with increased risk of coronary heart disease.

The endogenous antioxidants are detoxifying enzymes which are primarily physiological in origin.

In phase I, drug metabolising enzymes such as Mixed Function Oxidases, MFO, play a major role in detoxifying the toxic chemicals. In Phase II, many non-enzymatic organic molecules such as glucuronic acid, glutathione, glycine bind to the functional groups of the toxic chemicals or to the resultant Phase I metabolic products and form polar compounds in order to facilitate their excretion from the body. Different antioxidant enzymes are involved in Phase II metabolism such as glutathione S-transferase, NADPH, quinone reductase, UDP glucuronysyl transferase and epoxide reductase. The activity of these enzymes is enhanced by several non-nutrient phytochemicals that are present in different foods which are useful in detoxifying the toxins. In this phase, the balance between glutathione S-transferase and quinone reductase determine the toxicity of chemical carcinogens. These enzymes require certain trace elements such as Se, Zn, Cu and Fe that can be obtained through dietary sources.

Major antioxidant mechanisms involved in fighting free radical damage are:

- Interaction of ascorbic acid and glutathione (GSH) with oxidants and oxidising agents.
- Scavenging of free radicals and singlet oxygen by vitamin E, ascorbic acid, β-carotene and superoxide dismutase (SOD).

- Reduction of hydroperoxides by glutathione peroxidases (GSHPx) and catalase enzymes.
- Binding of transition metal by various chelators and repair of cellular damage by various metabolic activities.

COMBATING FREE RADICALS AND REACTIVE OXYGEN SPECIES

Potentially injurious effects of free radicals and reactive oxygen species are prevented by a well organized antioxidant defence system.

- The first line of defence is prevention. The multistep reduction of oxygen to water in the mitochondria is carried out by cytochromes and other metalloenzymes held together so that the intermediates like superoxide are not released into the cell. Similarly ions of the transition metals like iron and copper which can trigger reactive oxygen species formation are bound or sequestered by proteins like transferrin and ceruloplasmin, to keep them out.

- The second line of defense is provided by the antioxidant enzymes present in all cells. They speedily attack the reactive oxygen species and inactivate them. Superoxide dismutase reacts with superoxide to give less toxic hydrogen peroxide.

$$2O_2^- + 2H^+ \longrightarrow H_2O_2$$

Hydrogen peroxide is inactivated by two distinct enzymes. Catalase acts on the molecule and splits it to water and oxygen.

$$2H_2O_2 \longrightarrow H_2O + O_2$$

A second enzyme glutathione peroxidase – GPx – detoxifies hydrogen peroxide, using a donor of antioxidants known as glutathione (GSH). GSH can exist in two interconvertible forms.

$$2GSH \rightleftharpoons GSSG$$

It can give hydrogen to combat oxidant stress. It can also take up hydrogen and can be considered as a storage form of antioxidant. While combating free radicals and reactive oxygen species, glutathione gets inactivated to the oxidised form but can be regenerated by the cellular metabolism using another enzyme glutathione reductase.

$$GSSG + \text{Hydrogen donor} \longrightarrow 2GSH \text{ (glutathione reductase)}$$

The hydrogen donor is a nucleotide carrying the vitamin niacin. The enzyme GPx contains selenium. Dietary deficiencies of selenium and niacin also lead to antioxidant deficiency. The enzyme superoxide dismutase contains copper, zinc and manganese. Dietary deficiencies of these minerals also lead to antioxidant insufficiency. Riboflavin is needed for maintaining the niacin containing nucleotide participating step in GSH regeneration making riboflavin also an antioxidant vitamin.

- The third line of defence is the damage control provided by the free radical scavengers. They react rapidly with the free radicals, inactivate them and arrest the chain propagation. In the process, they are inactivated into less toxic radicals. The scavenger active on the cell membrane is vitamin E.

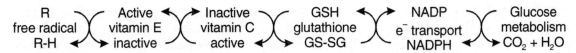

The inactive form of tocopherol on the cell membrane is regenerated on the cytoplasmic side with vitamin C as the hydrogen donor or free radical scavenger, rendering the vitamin oxidised and inactive. This in turn is reduced and regenerated by glutathione. The resultant oxidised glutathione is reduced to provide a continuous supply of GSH by a cellular enzyme glutathione reductase, which in turn needs the coenzymes of the vitamin niacin, NAD and NADP. These cofactors are provided by glucose metabolism with the help of coenzymes of riboflavin and these vitamins also share the work of free radical scavenging.

- The final defence is by repair of the damaged molecules and structures by accelerated removal of damaged molecules. For example, LPO products on the membrane is removed by specific phospholipases which cleave the damaged fatty acyl chain which is followed by replacement with fresh fatty acid.

Damaged proteins are digested by proteases and damaged part of DNA are cleaved and repaired. The repair mechanism is limited and is not exhaustive leading to diseases and disorders.

ANTIOXIDANTS AND DISEASE

Free radical reactions have been implicated as a cause or consequence in the following conditions.

Immunity and Ageing

The body maintains a complex set of defences against illness and infection. Skin, mucous membranes and acidic secretions are among the first line of defence. Cellular immunity modified by the T cells of the thymus gland and antibodies are the next line of protection. Nutrients such as vitamin A (especially β-carotene and other carotenoids) vitamin E, vitamin C and vitamin B_6 and folacin protect the body by supporting antioxidant efforts. Iron, zinc and selenium also have important roles.

Damage from oxidation of cells can impair the body's defences against some types of cancer. Chromosomal damage is directly related to cancer and cell mutation and β-carotene is protective against x-ray damages.

In the ageing process, free radicals are thought to cause degenerative change in the immune system, perhaps leading to cataract formation, atherosclerotic plaques, arthritis and Parkinson's disease. Studies have shown that elderly patients taking 200 mg of vitamin E daily had an enhanced immune responsiveness. Protection from DNA damage is believed to enhance the body's self defence mechanisms.

Substances in food such as phytochemicals may be as important as any single nutrient in supplemental form.

There is a decline in the relative mass of immune tissue over the life-cycle, beginning with the involution of adenoids in childhood and the thymus in young adults, and an associated decline in immune function. The immune system is influenced by dietary lipids that are precursors of eicosanoids, prostaglandins and leukotrienes; eicosanoid synthesis can be modified by dietary antioxidants such as vitamins E and C, selenium and copper. The decline with age in T-cell mediated immune function has been attributed to defective interleukin II production and responsiveness. Healthy elderly subjects supplemented with 800 IU of vitamin E for 30 days had a significantly greater production of interleukin II than those consuming a placebo. Vitamin B_6 depletion in healthy elderly subjects caused significant reduction in interleukin II production, which returned to normal following vitamin B_6 repletion.

Eating an antioxidant-rich diet may help keep cognitive skills strong during old age, according to a recent animal study.

Cosmic Rays
Some scientists believe that antioxidants may help defend astronauts from brain-damaging cosmic rays on future manned mission to mars.

Cataract

Human eye lens consists of high-density crystalline proteins which help in its transparency. Cataract is the impairment in the vision caused due to the loss of transparency in lens.

Accumulation of large amounts of insoluble proteins derived from the otherwise soluble protein is the major biochemical change in cataract. As a result of age and chronic exposure to near UV light, the crystallins undergo chemical modification and oxidative damage over a period of time. The changes observed in lens enzymes and crystallins by UV radiation could thus atleast in part be due to oxidative damage.

Studies conducted at National Institute of Nutrition, Hyderabad, indicated that cataract patients have lower levels of certain micronutrients such as riboflavin, copper, zinc in the blood compared to normal subjects. Strikingly, a high incidence (80%) of riboflavin deficiency was observed in cataract patients.

Antioxidant status is low in people with cataract. Antioxidant status can be assessed by measuring the levels of enzymes like catalase, superoxide dismutase and glutathione peroxidase. Cataract patients have lower intake of antioxidants such as β-carotene, riboflavin, ascorbic acid and minerals such as copper, zinc and manganese.

Cancer

Table 19.6 shows the beneficial effects of antioxidant nutrients in preventing cancer.

Table 19.6: Beneficial effects of some antioxidants

Nutrient	Beneficial effect
β-carotene	Reduced risk of various cancers especially lung cancer and also stomach, cervix, oesophageal and throat cancers, reduced risk of cardiovascular disease especially in smokers.
Vitamin C	Reduced risk of upper gastrointestinal tract, cervix cancer, cardiovascular disease.
Vitamin E	Significant decrease in the risk of oral and pharyngeal cancer, cardiovascular disease.
Selenium	Reduced risk of oesophageal and stomach cancers.

Source: Mathur Pulkit, *Natural Antioxidants in Our Diet*, Nutrition 31,4,1997.

Dietary deficiencies of selected antioxidant micro-nutrients and their association with known risk factors in the pathogenesis and potential prevention of various cancers. Concurrent correction of suboptimal plasma antioxidant levels may be important part of optimal nutrition that help to prevent early stages of cancer.

PEM

Odema is a typical clinical feature of kwashiorkor. Various theories like hypoalbuminemia, disturbances in renin-angiotensin system, increased blood cortisol and ferritin levels have been proposed to explain the occurrence of oedema in kwashiorkor. Increased free radical generation has also been suggested since levels of antioxidant nutrients in protein energy malnutrition have been reported to be low.

Copper as a constituent of the body, play an important role in the aetiology of oedema in kwashiorkor. Plasma copper and its carrier protein ceruloplasmin and RBC superoxide dismutase are significantly decreased in marasmic-kwashiorkor children compared to normal and marasmic children. These results suggest that oedema formation in kwashiorkor could be due to lowered levels of copper and its metallo enzyme superoxide dismutase. Recurrent infections and diarrhoeal episodes as well as inadequate dietary intake could have contributed to diminished copper nutritional status.

Neurological Conditions

The tight microglial cellular junctions that form the blood-brain-barrier protect the CNS from large molecules. Disease such as Alzheimer's disease and stress can make the blood-brain-barrier more permeable. Proper inclusion of specific nutrients such as antioxidants may play a role in maintaining this barrier.

α-tocopherol has been found to be useful in slowing the progression of moderately severe Alzheimer's. Antioxidants in foods have been shown to be effective in maintaining memory; folate, vitamin C, and β-carotene seem to be the best protective agents that are present in fruits and vegetables. Cognitive ability is also supported by adequate intakes of vitamins B_6 and B_{12} in addition to folate.

Cardiovascular Disease

Two dietary components that affect the oxidation potential of LDL cholesterol are the level of linoleic acid in the particle and the availability of antioxidants. Vitamin C, E and β-carotene at physiologic levels have antioxidant roles in the body. At supplement levels, they can be either pro-oxidant or antioxidant, depending on concentrations of other metal ions.

The French have relatively low rates of CHD, but a saturated fat intake and plasma cholesterol levels which do not differ appreciably from countries with much higher rates of CHD. Consumption of antioxidant nutrients may mitigate the detrimental effects.

Vitamin E is the most concentrated antioxidant carried on LDL, the amount being 20 to 300 times greater than any other antioxidant. A major function of vitamin E is to prevent oxidation of PUFA in the cell membrane.

American Heart Association recommends that vitamin E be obtained from a diet low in saturated fat. Evidence shows that vitamin E is more effective against CVD than β-carotene or vitamin C. Carotenoid studies suggest that these nutrients play a role later, rather than early in the atherosclerotic process by preventing arterial plaque formation. Higher intakes of flavonoids have been associated with reduced risk of cardiovascular disease.

Exercise

Endurance exercise can increase oxygen utilization from 10 to 20 times over the resting state. This greatly increases the generation of free radicals, prompting concern about enhanced damage to muscles and other tissues. Regular physical exercise enhances the antioxidant defence system and protects against exercise induced free radical damage. On the other hand, intense exercise in untrained individual overwhelms defences, resulting in increased free radical damage.

Most of the data suggest that increased intake of vitamin E is protective against exercise induced oxidative damage. Balanced training programme should be followed that emphasises regular exercise and eating 5 servings of fruit or vegetables per day. Athletes who exercise a lot produce free radicals that can be tackled by anthocyanidins.

SOURCES

Dietary components identified as antioxidants are vitamins C and E, niacin, riboflavin, sulphur containing amino acids (they provide the reducing thiol groups for proteins and GSH and have positive antioxidants properties). Phytochemicals like flavonoids and polyphenols also contribute to antioxidants.

Selenium a trace element, plays an important role in cellular function as it forms the intergral part of an important antioxidant enzyme, glutathione peroxidase (Se – GSH – Px) which protects the body against the oxidative tissue damage.

Table 19.7: Sources of nutrient antioxidants

Nutrient	Sources
β-Carotene	Green leafy vegetables, ripe yellow fruits and vegetables like papaya, musk melon, mango, pumpkin, carrots.
Vitamin C	Citrus fruits: orange, lemon, sweet lime, guava, goose berry sprouted pulses.
Vitamin E	Cereals, cereal products, oil seeds, nuts.
Selenium, Zinc	Meats, sea foods and cereals.
Copper	Oysters, liver, mushroom, nuts, chocolate.
Iron	Meat, liver, green leafy vegetables, cereals, millets, pulses.

Whole grains

Selenium is present as selenomethionine in cereals and millets. Its bioavailability is 85–100% through dietary source as compared to inorganic selenium.

Among cereals, selenium content is more in jowar and bajra. Rice is not rich in selenium compared to other cereals.

Table 19.8: Selenium content of cereals

Cereal	Selenium ng/g
Jowar	213
Bajra	179
Wheat	173
Rice	83

Whole grains contain phenolic compounds such as ferulic, caffeic acid and phytic acid.

It was found that the process of baking bread produces a novel type of antioxidant, called pronyl – lysine that is eight times more abundant in the crust than in the crumb. Pronyl – lysine is formed by the reaction of protein bound amino acid L-lysine and starch as well as reducing sugars in the presence of heat. Maillard reaction produces not only flavour compounds but also other types of antioxidants.

According to studies conducted at NIN (2000–2001) domestic processing of wheat like boiling, deep frying, sprouting and malting significantly increases phenolic content.

Pulses

Of 25 g of soya protein that is recommended in our daily diet, 45 mg are isoflavones. These are compounds that act as antioxidants and as protective agents against cancer and heart disease.

Phytoestrogen found in soyabean is a polyphenolic compound and has anticarcinogenic effect on the breast tissue and positive effects on the lipoprotein profile and bone density. In the whole grams – green gram, black gram and bengal gram – boiling and pressure cooking significantly increases the total phenolic content. Sprouting increases total phenolic content in green gram.

Pulses like red gram (203 ng/g) and bengal gram (180 ng/g) are rich source of selenium. Green gram contains only 98 ng/g of selenium.

Red wine

Crushing the grapes and allowing the skins, seeds and even the grape stems to ferment together with the pulp and juice, a process that creates a mixture rich in antioxidant compounds. Grape seeds in particular contain large amounts of flavonoid substances known as proanthocyanidins. In red wine, flavonols form part of a wider group of antioxidant chemicals called polyphenols. Grape seeds and grape skins used in wineries showed a significant decrease in total cholesterol as well as in LDL in subjects having high cholesterol.

Tea and Coffee

Polyphenols like chlorogenic acid present in coffee beans and tea leaves are antioxidants. Flavanoids like catachins and quercetin are found to have antioxidant properties. Tea derived from the plant camellia sinensis contains polyphenols in the form of flavonoids and its sub group flavonols, which give the tea its antioxidant properties. Polyphenols can stop the damage that free radicals do to cells, neutralise enzymes essential for tumour growth and deactivate cancer promoters.

NIN studies indicated that flavonoids in green and black tea have stronger antioxidant activity than standard antioxidant vitamins.

A cup of tea supplies around 200 mg of flavonoids. The antioxidant potency in a cup of tea is 400 per cent greater than a cup of orange juice. Black tea contains other polyphenols such as thearubigins and theaflavins which are very powerful.

Tea has been shown to contain several polyphenolic compounds and their derivatives which are reported to possess antioxidant activity. These can be divided into four groups-flavonols, flavondiols, flavonoids and phenolic acids. Studies have shown that colon cancer appears to show a negative association with tea consumption.

Higher the flavonoid intake lower is the risk of death from coronary heart disease. Men who drink more than four cups of tea a day (about 500 ml) are benefited most.

Figure 19a gives antioxidant activity of fruits.

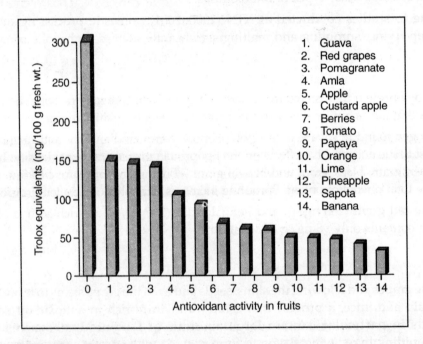

Figure 19a. Antioxidant activity in fruits.

Antioxidant activity of the methanolic extract of fruits were analysed and the results are expressed in mg of trolox equivalents (TE/100g fresh weight of edible portion of the fruits)

Source: Annual report 1998-99, National Institute of Nutrition, Hyderabad 500 007.

Fruits and Vegetables

Plants produce vitamins, vitamin C, β-carotene and tocopherols. These chemicals are known as high value, low volume chemicals. The secondary plant metabolites other than vitamins are referred to as nutraceuticals. Most of these compounds are flavonoids, polyphenols which are also known to inhibit free radicals generated in the cellular system when they are obtained through the diet.

Guava and amla, due to their vitamin C content, are rich in antioxidants. Red grapes and pomegranates contribute to antioxidants due to the presence of anthocyanins. Apples contain polyphenols. Banana is poor in antioxidants.

Green leafy vegetables are exceptionally rich source of β-carotene, the nature's most potent antioxidant that can inhibit atherosclerosis and prevent heart disease. They also contain bioactive agents — phyto chemicals.

Brinjal, spinach and onion are rich in phenolics and processing increases them. In brinjals and french beans the phenolic content increases during domestic methods of processing. Method of processing has no effect in spinach and other vegetables and onion. In amaranth, boiling and pressure cooking significantly decreases the phenolic content. Polyphenols are believed to prevent conversion of substances into carcinogens and inhibit mutations.

Cooked tomatoes are associated with greater health benefits, compared to uncooked, because the heating process makes lycopene more easily absorbed by the body. It has been associated with a reduced risk of many cancers and protection against heart attacks. Water melon, tomatoes, red peppers and pink grapes are rich in lycopene.

Some extracts from plants like lencos, cessampetos showed very high levels of tannins, flavonoids and vitamin C which have antioxidant performance. Some varieties of lettuce, small tomatoes and red onions are rich in flavonols. An apple a day (110 g/day) prevents heart attack by providing flavonoids.

Strawberries, rasberries, black berries contain polyphenols.

Lutein carotenoid is found in green leafy vegetables. Evidence suggests that eating foods high in lutein may prevent/slow macular degeration, a leading cause of blindness in the elderly. As an antioxidant, it may also prevent formation of cataracts, reduce the risk of heart disease and protect against breast cancer.

Glucosinolates such as glucobrassicin are metabolised to produce two other phytochemicals, isothiocyanates and indoles, which trigger production of enzymes that block cell damage due to carcinogens. Food sources include cruciferous vegetables such as broccoli, cabbage and brussels sprouts. Sulforaphane in broccoli has cancer preventive properties. Beet juice boosts man's immune building function.

Flavonoids are found in a wide variety of fruits and vegetables. They act as antioxidants. Resveratrol, anthocyanins, quercetin, hesperidin, tangerin, myricetin kaempferol and apigenin are some flavonoids. They act as anticarcinogen, anti allergen, anti-inflammatory and reduce the risk of heart diseases, cancer and urinary tract infection. They are found in apples, pears, cherries, grapes, citrus fruits, onion, kale, broccoli and lettuce.

Terpenes are found in citrus fruits, carrots, parsley, broccoli, cabbage, cucumber and mint.

Spices

Saffron and annoto contain carotenoids which are effective antioxidants.

Observations in animal studies show that ginger has the ability to stimulate protective enzymes involved in xenobiotic metabolism. Stimulation of the quinone reductase activity suggests that ginger can counteract the oxidative damage in tissues of liver and lungs.

Curcumin a diferuloyl methane, present in turmeric reduces the mutagenicity in smokers and promote mechanisms for detoxification and production of GSH. It is also antiinflammatory. The antioxidant properties of curcumin are attributed to its ability to inhibit lipid peroxidation and scavenging capacity of superoxide anion and hydroxyl radicals. The amount of turmeric required appears to be well within cultural norms and safety limits.

Eugenol, 4–allyl–2–methoxyphenol, active principle of clove oil has antioxidant properties.

The selenium content of coriander seeds (136 ng/g) and mustard (128 ng/g) contributes to their antioxidant activity.

Oils

Rice bran oil contains a high amount of unsaponifiable components such as tocotrienols and oryzanol. These possess antioxidant activity. Palmoil is a rich source of tocopherols and tocotrienols. The remarkable stability of sesame oil is attributed to its inherent lignans (sesamol, sesamin and sesamolin) present in its non-glyceride fraction. Sesame lignans have antioxidant properties.

Whey Proteins

Whey proteins have been shown to stimulate cell mediated and humoral immunity to improve the body's nutritional status in stressed individuals. Whey proteins have an antioxidant role by increasing tissue glutathione and inhibiting the growth of several types of tumours. Water soluble antioxidant components are present in a low molecular weight ultrafiltration permeate obtained from milk or whey.

The natural antioxidants are easily absorbable in human system. To meet the antioxidant requirement and to prevent degenerative diseases, the diet should include foods rich in antioxidants particularly a minimum of five servings of fruits and vegetables.

Nuts

Nuts are sources of phytosterols and other phytochemical compounds with potential serum cholesterol modulating effects. The phytochemicals in nuts include ellagic acid, flavonoids, phenolic compounds, luteolin (a major antioxidant) and tocopherols.

QUESTIONS

1. Define "Antioxidant".
2. Explain the need of antioxidants.
3. Give the list of nutrient and non-nutrient antioxidants.
4. Explain the role of antioxidants in combating free radicals and Reactive Oxygen Species.
5. Discuss the role of antioxidants in preventing degenerative disease.

6. Explain the beneficial effects of antioxidants in relation of cancer.

7. Differentiate between exogenous and endogenous antioxidants.

8. Discuss antioxidant activity in fruits.

9. Describe the sources of antioxidants.

10. Explain the effect of cooking on antioxidants.

SUGGESTED READINGS

• Raghunath Rao D. Antioxidants in Human Health. Nutrition 36, 2002 .
• Information on fruits and vegetables : www.dcpc.nci.nih.gov/5aday

CHAPTER 20

WATER AND ELECTROLYTE BALANCE

DISTRIBUTION OF WATER AND ELECTROLYTES

In human adults, total body water accounts for about 70 per cent of the lean body mass. Variations observed are mainly due to differences in fat contents. In obese males, water constitutes a lower percentage of body weight (45–60 per cent) than in lean individuals (55–70 per cent). Adult lean females have a low water content (45–60 per cent) and the value in infants can be in the range 65–75 per cent. A loss of 10 per cent of water in the body is serious; a loss of 20 per cent is fatal.

In an adult male of 70 kg body weight, 70 per cent of water, 30 litres, is found in intracellular fluids. Of this about 4 litres are found in bones which does not readily participate in fluid exchange. Nearly, 30 per cent of water, about 12 litres, is found in extracellular fluid. 3 litres of plasma, 8.5 litres of interstitial fluid and one litre of transcellular fluid come under extracellular fluid. Transcellular fluid are collections formed by the 'transport' or 'secretory activity' of cells, e.g., fluids secreted from salivary gland, pancreas etc. Aqueous humour and cerebrospinal fluid are also transcellular fluids.

Figure 20a illustrates body fluid compartments.

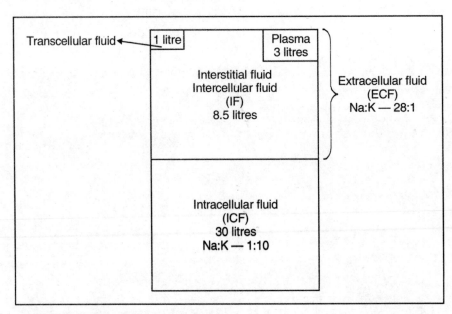

Figure 20a. Body fluid compartments.

Source: Pike Ruth Land Myrtle L. Brown, 1975, Nutrition an integrated approach, John Wiley & Sons Inc. New York.

Table 20.1: Chemical composition of extracellular and intracellular fluids

Chemical substance		ECF	ICF
Na$^+$	mEq/L	142	10
K$^+$	mEq/L	4	140
Ca^{++}	mEq/L	2.4	0.0001
Mg^{++}	mEq/L	1.2	58
Cl$^-$	mEq/L	103	4
HCO$_3$	mEq/L	28	10
Phosphates	mEq/L	4	75
SO$_4$	mEq/L	1	2
Glucose	mg/dl	90	0.20
Proteins	g/dl	2	16

Source: Guyton, A.C., 1991, Textbook of Medical physiology, Prism Books (Pvt.) Ltd., Bangalore.

Note that the extracellular fluid contains large quantities of sodium but only small quantities of potassium. Intracellular fluid contain more potassium than sodium. The extra cellular fluid contains large quantities of chloride but the concentrations of phosphates and protein in the intracellular fluid are considerably greater than in the extracellular fluid.

Sodium

The human body contains about 1.8 g Na/kg fat free body weight, most of which is present in extracellular fluids. The content in serum normally is about 140 mEq/litre (300–355 mg/100ml). Since sodium is the chief cation of the extracellular fluid, the control of body fluid osmolarity and therefore body fluid volume is largely dependent on sodium ions and the ratio of sodium to other ions.

Sodium is capable of permeating the cell membrane. Muscle contraction and nerve transmission involve a temporary exchange of extra cellular sodium and intracellular potassium. The subsequent transfer of sodium out of the cell is by means of an active mechanism of pump. A very small amount of sodium occurs intracellularly.

In bone, sodium is bound for the most part on the surface of bone crystals. The amount present in bone is by no means small and accounts for 30 to 45 percent of total body sodium. This reservoir apparently is part of the active labile sodium pool in the body.

Potassium

Potassium is the cation of the ICF and is also an important constituent of the ECF. It is this fraction that influences muscle activity. It is essential for growth and for building up of cells. This is indicated by a fairly high retention of potassium during infancy, childhood and pregnancy. During muscular contraction, potassium from the muscle cells are lost into the ECF and after muscle contraction they are returned to the muscle cells.

Any variation in the concentration of potassium causes abnormalities in the conduction and activity of cardiac muscle. Hypokalemia, low serum potassium is associated with extreme weakness of muscles and sometimes paralysis.

Potassium levels decrease in the blood when the rate of protein synthesis or glycogen deposition within the cell increases and in alkolosis, which indicates that potassium is leaving the blood and entering the cell.

Potassium levels increase in blood when there is a break down of body tissue (catabolism) and also in acidosis which occurs with diarrhoea and indicates that potassium is leaving the cell to help establish a normal acid-base balance.

Most of 250g of potassium is within the cells. Therefore blood potassium is a poor indicator of potassium status.

If the level of potassium in the blood and hence in the extracellular fluids increases above 7mEq per litre, muscular coordination is disturbed and in severe cases cardiac arrest occurs. This is the result of failure of the kidney to excrete potassium.

Seven per cent of potassium is lost in urine. Presence of chlorine aids in the conservation of potassium.

Within the cell, potassium acts as a catalyst in many biological reactions – release of energy and in glycogen and protein synthesis. If the sodium level increases in the intracellular material, it may counteract the catalytic effect of potassium and may interfere with cellular metabolism, specially protein synthesis.

Potassium is a major factor in maintaining the osmotic pressure of the cell. It helps in maintaining acid-base balance though not as effective as sodium.

Factors Influencing Distribution of Body Fluid

The principal factors controlling, the location and the amount of fluid in the various compartments are, the osmotic forces which are maintained by the solutes, that is, the substances dissolved in the body water. The solutes are:

- organic compounds having small molecular size e.g., glucose and urea. They do not exert much effect on the distribution of water because they diffuse freely across the cell membranes.
- organic compounds having large molecular size e.g., proteins. They help in the exchange of fluid between the circulating blood and the interstitial fluid. The plasma proteins are responsible for about 25mm of total osmotic pressure of the plasma.
- the inorganic electrolytes like various cations and anions of the body fluids. The main cations are Na^+ and K^+ ions. Ca^{++} and Mg^{++} are present in smaller amounts. The main anions are Cl^- and HCO_3^-. The inorganic electrolytes are important factors in directing the movement of the fluid in the various compartments and in determining their quantity.

FUNCTIONS

Water performs its functions within the body by acting as the following:

Part of structure

Water is a part of all tissues and is essential for growth. Glucogen is two-thirds water. Fat tissue is one-fifth water and muscle is close to three-fourths water.

Turgor

The cell water and its contents in solution provide a normal turgor or fullness to the tissues, a distension or degree of rigidity of the cells resulting from the fluid pressure of the cell contents on the cell membranes. Without this normal tissue turgor that cell water makes possible, the body form would not exist.

Solvent

Water is the solvent of life. In the presence of water as a solvent, many metabolic reactions of life are able to proceed and the remaining chemicals can react together to generate the integrated chemical complexity of a living body. By being dissolved in or otherwise exposed to intracellular and extracellular water, the chemistry of life gains the fluidity and flexibility that makes life possible.

When food enters the body, it is soon exposed to the watery secretions of saliva and the watery solutions in the stomach and intestine that allow the food to mix with and react with the compounds responsible for digestion. The digested nutrients are then absorbed into the blood, which contains an average of about 3 litres of water. It is this intravascular water that actually makes blood a fluid and allows absorbed nutrients to dissolve in blood and so be transported to every tissue of the body. The water of blood also acts as a solvent transporting many internally generated substances such as hormones and antibodies from their sites of manufacture in the body to the sites where they perform their function. Waste products of metabolism, such as carbon dioxide and urea also dissolve in the intravascular water to be transported to the lungs or kidneys for excretion.

The 12 litres or so of intercellular fluid found in the spaces between cells, carry nutrients from the blood capillaries to the outer membranes of the body's cells, allowing them to be transported across the membranes and into the watery intracellular fluid within the cells. Within cells the intracellular water serves as a suitable medium for nutrients to be transformed into the compounds needed to build and maintain cells.

Water is a solvent for electrolytes. It helps to regulate the electrolyte balance of the body and maintains a healthy equilibrium of osmotic pressure exerted by the solutes dissolved in water.

Some of the compounds of the body are not dissolved in water, such as the lipid-based cell membranes, but water plays an important role in allowing such structures to form and maintain their structural integrity.

Reactant

Water is a reactant that participates directly in a variety of different reactions within the body. During these reactions the water molecules often split up, to donate hydrogen atoms (H), hydrogen ions (H^+), oxygen atoms (O), oxide ions (O^{2-}), hydroxyl groups (OH) or hydroxide ions (OH⁻) to other reactants of the reactions concerned. Common examples of such reactants are polysaccharides, fats and proteins which are split into smaller molecules by reaction with water. During hydrolysis reactions a hydrogen atom derived from a water molecule ends up attached to one of the smaller products of the reaction, while a hydroxyl group containing the remaining atoms of the original water molecule is attached to the other product of the reaction. Water is also formed as a product of many chemical reactions within the cell, such as the reversal of hydrolysis, known as condensation.

Lubricant

Water-based fluids act as lubricants in various parts of the body, most notably within joints, where synovial fluid makes movement easier and minimises wear and tear on cartilage and bone. The water in saliva and mucus acts as lubricant in the mouth and oesophagus.

Temperature Regulator

Water plays an important role in the distribution of heat throughout the body and the regulation of body temperature. Heat in the body is generated by the metabolism of the energy yielding nutrients. All of the energy released by the oxidation of these nutrients is eventually released as heat, apart from any stored within the compounds involved in net growth. Some of this heat, is required to maintain the body's normal temperature of 98.6°C. The excess heat must be released to the surroundings because any significant rise in temperature to above normal levels causes illness and eventually death. Some heat is lost by radiation and simple conduction between the body and the air. The most effective route of heat loss from the body, however, is via the evaporation of the water as perspiration from the surface of the skin. The evaporation of 1 litre of perspiration from the skin is accompanied by the loss of 600 kcal of heat energy from the body.

Water Provides Dietary Minerals

Water contains significant amounts of minerals such as calcium, magnesium, sodium, zinc, copper and fluoride. The actual amounts depend on the source of the water.

Because water is an effective solvent for many minerals and other chemicals it may also carry significant quantities of toxic elements such as lead or cadmium, pesticides, herbicides and industrial waste products.

REQUIREMENTS

The requirement of water depends on a person's age, weight and life style and the climate in which he is living. When the body is too hot, the blood vessels just beneath the skin expand (dilate), increasing blood flow and accelerating heat loss. When the body is too cold, these blood vessels become narrow (constrict) reducing heat loss. In hot weather obese people feel more discomfort than do nonobese people as they have thicker insulating layer of subcutaneous fat and the blood vessels tend to be farther from the surface from the surface of the skin.

Adults should consume 1 litre of water for every 1000 kcal in their diet, infants should consume 1.5 litre/1000 kcal.

Table 20.2: Fluid requirement per kilogram of body weight

Group	Fluid ml/kg
Infants	110
10 year old children	40
Young adults	40
Older adults	30
Elderly adults (>65 years)	25
Adults (by environmental temperature)	
22.2°C	22
37.8°C	38

Source: Guthrie Helen, A. and Mary Frances Picciano, 1999, Human Nutrition, WCB McGraw-Hill Boston.

SOURCES

Most of the requirement of water is met by drinking as such. Part of the requirement is met by the foods consumed and water used in cooking and the beverages consumed. Metabolic water also contributes to the source of water. Water, in addition to carbondioxide and energy is an end product of combustion of carbohydrate, fat and protein. Oxidation of 100 g each of fat, carbohydrate and protein yields 107, 55 and 41 g of water, respectively. This is called metabolic water. Table 20.3 gives water content of solid foods.

Table 20.3: Water content of foods

Name of the foodstuff	Amount g/100g
Ash gourd	96.5
Water melon	95.8
Tomato	94.0
Spinach	92.1
Papaya	90.8
Sweetlime	88.4
Milk, cow's	87.5
Amaranth tender	85.7
Apple	84.6
Banana	70.1

WATER BALANCE

In a normal individual the maintenance of water balance is achieved by adjusting the input versus the output. The input of water as well as its loss can be highly variable due to individual habits and environmental factors. Inspite of this the total body water needs to be maintained constant to achieve normal osmolality for physiological functions.

Table 20.4: Daily water intake and output (or loss) from the human body in litres

Intake/Output	Temperate climate		Tropical climate	
Intake				
As liquids	1.5	⎫	2–5	⎫
In foods	1.0	⎬ 2.8	1–2	⎬ 3.3–7.3
Oxidation of foods	0.3	⎭	0.3	⎭
Output (or loss)				
Urine	1.5	⎫	1.0–1.5	⎫
Faeces	0.1	⎬ 2.8	0.1–0.2	⎬ 3.3–7.3
Evaporation through skin	0.8		1.8–5.2	
Evaporation through lung	0.4	⎭	0.4	⎭

Source: Jain, J.L. *et. al.*, 2005, Fundamentals of Biochemistry, S. Chand & Company Ltd., Ram Nagar, New Delhi – 110055.

Water balance is achieved in two ways – regulation of fluid intake through changes in thirst sensations and regulation of fluid loss through the kidneys.

Thirst Mechanism (Neural Mechanism)

The intake of fluid is regulated by the mechanism of thirst. A deficient intake of water with continuing 'obligatory' losses leads to concentration of body fluids with respect to solutes and a rise in osmotic pressure. This tends to draw water from ICF, the dehydration of the cells seems to be the main stimulus for their mechanisms through osmoreceptors as well as sensory nerves of mouth and phyrynx, which respond to dryness of the mouth and pharynx.

Kidneys

'Internal circulation of salts' is a process where the principal ECF ions enter the lumen of GI tract and renal tubules and their near complete reabsorption regulates electrolyte levels.

This process constantly occurring in the kidneys, is at a much faster rate than that observed in the GI tract. In the kidneys, a volume of plasma equal to ECF (12 to 15 litres) is filtered and reabsorbed every 2 hours and about 25,000 mEq of Na^+ are filtered and reabsorbed every day.

ELECTROLYTE BALANCE

Electrolytes namely sodium, potassium are present in intracellular and extracellular fluids. The concentration of electrolytes is affected by water balance, sodium chloride intake and intake of other minerals present in the diet. The body has several mechanisms by which it can keep the electrolyte balance in the intracellular and extracellular fluids at a constant level.

Gastrointestinal tract constantly regulates electrolyte levels. About 8 litres of fluid of different electrolytes enter GI tract every day and are reabsorbed almost completely with fluid loss approximately 100–150 ml and electrolyte loss of Na^+ approximately 10–30 mEq and of K^+ approximately 10 mEq.

When too much fluid is lost, the concentration of electrolytes, particularly sodium, in the extracellular fluid increases. This increase will cause water to be absorbed from the saliva, leaving a dry sensation in the mouth that stimulates thirst and then fluid intake. In addition, the hypothalamus in the brain responds to the higher sodium content of the blood in two ways; it stimulates the thirst sensation and it also signals the pituitary gland to release the antidiuretic hormone (ADH – also known as vasopressin as it elevates blood pressure) which influences the kidneys to reabsorb more water, restoring blood volume to a normal level. As water is reabsorbed, the volume of the urine decreases. Conversely, when the level of sodium in the fluid being filtered through the kidneys is low, the kidneys release a substance that triggers another hormone, aldosterone. This hormone causes the kidneys to retain more sodium. Stimulation of thirst secretion of ADH is triggered by changes in sodium concentration of as little as 1 per cent.

In diabetes insipidus, due to the failure of ADH secretion, there is excessive excretion of urine.

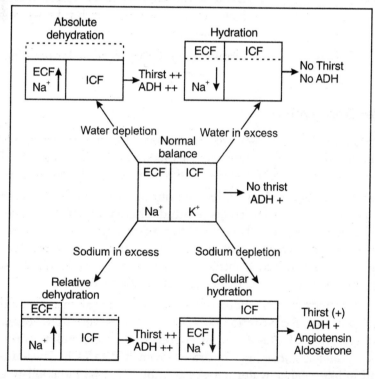

Figure 20b. Changes in body fluid distribution and composition during negative and positive water and salt balances. ECF, extra cellular fluid compartment; ICF, intracellular fluid compartment; ADH, antidiuretic hormone, vasopressin.

Source: Pike Ruth L and Myrtle L. Brown,1975, Nutrition, an integrated approach, John Wiley & Sons, Inc. New York.

WATER DEPLETION

Water can be depleted in the body due to reduced intake or increased losses. The possible reasons for these are given below:

Reduced intake

Water unavailable	:	After a calamity like shipwreck, earthquake or floods.
Inability to obtain water	:	Infants, elderly and debilitated patients, unconscious patients.
Inability to swallow		Diseases of mouth and esophagus.

Increased losses

From the skin	:	Hot environment, excessive exercise, fever, hyperthyroidism.
From the lungs	:	Hyperventilation, fever, high altitudes.
From the alimentary tract	:	Prolonged vomiting, diarrhoea.
In the urine	:	Osmotic diuresis in diabetes mellitus, too concentrated food e.g., with tube feeding and infant milk powders.
		Drinking sea water, various kidney disorders, diabetes insipidus.

Effect of Water Deprivation

Evidence of dehydration is sunken features, particularly the eyes which recede into the orbit. The skin and tongue are dry. The skin becomes loose and lacks elasticity. On pinching, it stands away from the subcutaneous tissues. The patient is usually but not always thirsty.

Water deprivation causes a reduction in the volume of the extracellular fluid (ECF) and intracellular fluid (ICF). The urine output is reduced. There is a rapid decrease in body weight and a state of dehydration of the cells occur. After a few days, a decrease in plasma volume (and also in blood volume) occurs which will reduce cardiac output and lead to circulatory failure. An adult who has lost 5 to 10 litres of water from the body will be seriously ill and death will occur when the water loss from the body is about 15 litres.

Dehydration of the body comes about when water is not taken in adequate amounts to make up for the water loss. Dehydration occurs rapidly in severe diarrhoea and vomiting in infants and children. The ECF is reduced in volume and its electrolyte content and osmotic pressure increase. Water is consequently drawn from ICF to ECF. The initial water loss is from the ECF but in later stages water is lost from the ICF. The metabolism of the shrunken cells is disturbed, leading to breakdown of protein and loss of K^+. The volume of urine excreted is diminished to the minimum by increased secretion of ADH to minimise water loss. The excretion of electrolytes is also increased.

In simple water deprivation, there is not only water loss but also losses of both K and Na for reasons given above. As the plasma volume decreases, the venous and capillary pressures fall while the osmotic pressure of the plasma proteins increases. These two factors tend to maintain plasma volume at the expense of ICF. Plasma electrolytes and NPN are significant, the clinical state is serious. The subject should be given water, electrolytes and glucose intravenously.

WATER EXCESS (WATER INTOXICATION)

Overhydration with a reduced plasma (Na⁺) and plasma osmolality may occur with an excessive intake. This may happen if large quantities of water are drunk to quench thirst in a hot climate when at the same time there are additional sodium losses in sweat. Overhydration may also arise in conditions where water excretion by the kidneys is impaired e.g., in nephrotic syndrome.

Overhydration leads to an increase in intracellular water and is a potentially dangerous and even lethal condition. There is difficulty in concentrating, drowsiness and giddiness sometimes associated with headache and nausea. In severe cases there may be confusion, behavioural disturbances, convulsions and coma.

Hyponatremia is commonly caused by either retention of water or loss of sodium. Loss of potassium may cause hyponatremia as sodium shifts into the cell in exchange for potassium.

OEDEMA

When NaCl is taken in excess in the form of solution, the plasma crystalloid osmotic pressure rises. Water moves from the interstitial spaces into the plasma, initially increasing the plasma volume and hence the blood volume; but at the same time, NaCl diffuses into the interstitial fluid. The outflow of salt also causes flow of water from plasma to interstitial fluid. The net result is a uniform increase in the salt concentration of the extracellular fluid. The raised osmotic pressure of ECF leads to a flow of water from the cells into ECF. This results in an increase in the volume of ECF and decrease in the volume of ICF.

Requirement of salt

According to WHO, the upper limit of sodium chloride from mixed food sources per day is 6 g. The lower limit is not defined.

This is usually associated with excess water giving rise to oedema. Pure sodium excess may arise from infusion of too much hypertonic solutions of sodium salts. It also arises in infants whose mothers have repeatedly made up their milk powder with insufficient water. The full capacity to excrete Na⁺ only develops some weeks after birth. With a high plasma Na⁺ there is irritability, overbreathing and often fever. Lowering plasma Na⁺ should proceed slowly and take 2 to 3 days.

Oedema, an increase in extracellular fluid is common in many conditions. Generalised oedema occurs in starvation and in liver disease, associated with diminished formation of plasma albumin. Generalised oedema is also associated with some kidney diseases, especially the nephrotic syndrome, when large losses of protein in the urine lead to a low plasma albumin.

Diuretics inhibit the action of carbonic anhydrase in the renal tubules and so prevent reabsorption of sodium and increase its urinary output. With their use a low sodium diet is seldom necessary but it is sensible not to overload the body with sodium by taking a high sodium diet.

World water day is observed on 22nd March.

QUESTIONS

1. Discuss the importance of water in the body?
2. What are the sources of water for the body?
3. What is water balance of the body? How does body maintain water balance?
4. What is oedema?
5. Explain the factors influencing distribution of body fluid.
6. Explain how the body maintains electrolyte balance.
7. Explain the role of hormones in maintaining normal water and electrolyte balance.
8. What is water intoxication?
9. Give the fluid requirement for different age groups.
10. Give the effect of electrolyte deficiency.
11. What is hyponatraemia?
12. What is hypokalaemia?

SUGGESTED READINGS

- Sodium in foods : www.fda.gov/fdac/foodlabel/sodium.html
- Importance of water : www.ificinfo.health.org/insight/waterref.htm

CHAPTER 21

ASSESSMENT OF NUTRITIONAL STATUS

Assessment of nutritional status of community is one of the first steps in the formulation of any public health strategy to combat malnutrition. The principle aim of such an assessment is to determine the type, magnitude and distribution of malnutrition in different geographic areas, to identify 'at risk' groups and to determine the contributory factors. In addition, factual evidence of the exact magnitude of malnutrition is essential to sensitise administrators and politicians to obtain allocation of material and human resources and to plan appropriately.

Nutritional status can be assessed by the following methods:

Direct methods	Indirect methods
Anthropometry	Dietary assessment
Clinical examination	Vital health statistics
Biophysical or radiological examination	
Functional assessment	
Laboratory and Biochemical estimation	

ANTHROPOMETRIC ASSESSMENT

Anthropometric measurements of human body reflect changes in morphological variation due to inappropriate food intake or malnutrition. A variety of anthropometric measurements can be made either covering the whole body or parts of the body.

Anthropometric measurements can be taken for cross sectional and longitudinal studies. In anthropometric measurements, there is no permanent standards as there is no uniformity of growth in subsequent generation. Local standards need to be developed of various ethnic groups.

Figure 21a shows dietary, biochemical, functional, clinical and anthropometry measurements which assess the nutritional status at different levels.

Body Weight

Body weight is the most widely used and the sensitive and simplest reproducible anthropometric measurement for the evaluation of nutritional status of young children. It indicates the body mass and is a composite of all body constituents like water, mineral, fat, protein and bone. It reflects more recent nutrition than does height.

Serial measurements of weight, as in growth monitoring are more sensitive indicators of changes in nutritional status than a single measurement at a point of time. Rapid loss of body weight in children should be considered as an indicator of potential malnutrition.

For measuring body weight, beam or lever actuated scales, with an accuracy of 50–100g are preferred. Bathroom scales may give errors upto 1.5 kg. Beam balances are extensively used in Integrated Child Development Services projects. Periodically scales need to be calibrated for accuracy using known weights. Weights should be taken with the individual under basal conditions with minimum clothing and without shoes. The zero error of the weighing scale should be checked before taking the weight and corrected as and when required.

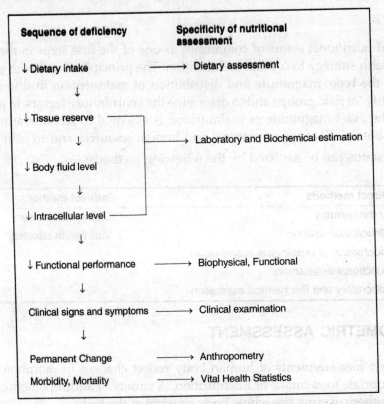

Sequence of deficiency	Specificity of nutritional assessment
↓ Dietary intake	→ Dietary assessment
↓	
↓ Tissue reserve	
↓	→ Laboratory and Biochemical estimation
↓ Body fluid level	
↓	
↓ Intracellular level	
↓	
↓ Functional performance	→ Biophysical, Functional
↓	
Clinical signs and symptoms	→ Clinical examination
↓	
Permanent Change	→ Anthropometry
Morbidity, Mortality	→ Vital Health Statistics

Figure 21a. Sequence of nutritional deficiency and specificity of assessment of nutritional status.

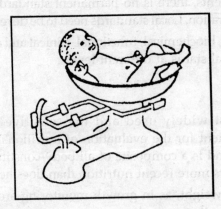

Figure 21b. Different type of scales are used for different age groups.

Height

The height of an individual is influenced both by genetic and environmental factors. The maximum growth potential of an individual is decided by hereditary factors, while the environmental factors, the most important being nutrition and morbidity, determine the extent of exploitation of that genetic potential. Height is affected only by long-term nutritional deprivation, it is considered an index of chronic or long duration malnutrition.

In children below the age of two years who cannot stand properly, recumbent length (crown-heel length) should be measured with infantometer (Figure 21c). The legs need to be held straight and firm with the feet touching the sliding board.

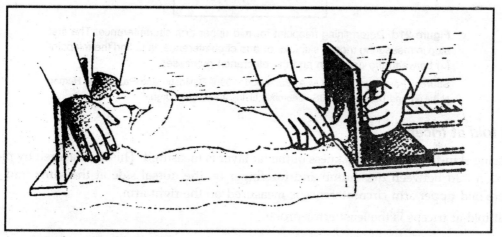

Figure 21c. Infantometer.
Source: Mahan Kathleen L. and Sylvia Escott. Stump (ed.), 2000, Krause's Food, nutrition and diet therapy, W.B. Saunders Company, Philadelphia (with permission).

In the older children and adults, heights are measured with a vertical measuring rod using anthropometer or stadiometer. The subject should stand erect looking straight on a levelled surface with heels together and toes apart, without shoes. The moving head piece of the anthropometer should be lowered to rest flat on the top of the head and the reading should be taken. Height should be read to the nearest 1/4" or 0.5 cm. An average of three measurements is taken as the final measurement.

Mid-Upper Arm Circumference (MUAC)

Mid-Upper Arm Circumference is recognised to indicate the status of muscle development. It is useful not only in identifying malnutrition but also in determining the mortality risk in children. It correlates well with weight, weight for height and clinical signs.

On the left hand, the mid-point between the tip of the acromion of scapula and tip of the olecranon of the fore-arm bone, ulna is located with the arm flexed at the elbow and marked with a marker pen. Fibre glass tape is used and the reading is taken to the nearest millimeter.

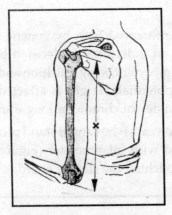

Figure 21d. Determining midpoint for mid upper arm circumference. The first step in measuring triceps skinfold, or arm circumference, is to find the midpoint (x) between the acromion and the olecranon processes.

Source: Passmore R. and M.A. Eastwood, 1990, Davidson and Passmore, Human Nutrition and Dietetics, ELBS, Churchill, Livingstone, Edinburgh.

Fat fold at triceps

By using skin-fold calipers thickness of the fat layer is measured. This is measured by picking the skin fold between the thumb and forefinger on the dorsal side at the same mid point where mid upper arm circumference is measured on the right arm.

Fat fold at triceps is the least error-prone.

Fat Fold at Sub-scapula

The fat fold is measured just below and lateral to the angle of the left scapula by picking it up with the thumb and forefinger in a line running approximately 45° to the spine, in the natural line of skin cleavage. The calipers used should have a standard contact surface (pinch area) of 20-40 mm and an accuracy of 0.1 mm.

Some of the standard calipers used are Harpender, Lange and Best. Una caliper is used in India.

Head and chest circumference

Head size relates mainly to the size of brain which increases quite rapidly during infancy. The chest in a normally nourished child grows faster than head during the second and third year of life. As a result, the chest circumference overtakes head circumference by about one year age. In protein energy malnutrition due to poor growth of chest, the head circumference may remain to be higher than the chest even at the age of 2½ to 3 years. Flexible fibre glass tape is used. The chest circumference is taken at the nipple level preferably in mid inspiration. The head circumference is measured passing the tape round the head over the supra-orbital ridges of the frontal bone in front and the most protruding point of the occiput on the back of the head (Figure 21e).

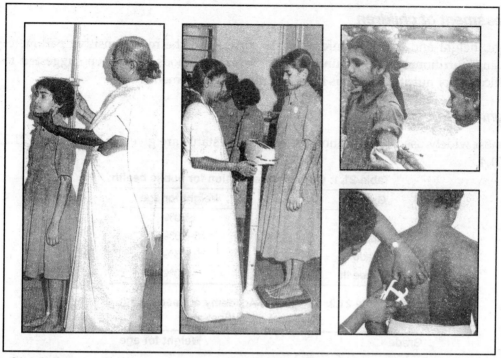

Figure 21e: Anthropometric measurements – Height, Weight, mid upper arm circumference, subscapular skin fold thickness.

Source: Proceedings of symposium on Micronutrient supplementation in health and disease. NIN, Hyderabad and Centre for Research on Nutrition support systems, New Delhi 2002.

Figure 21f shows the sites and types of anthropometric measurements used to assess body composition.

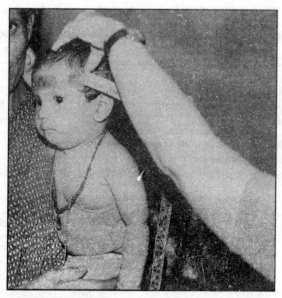

Figure 21f. The author measuring the head circumference.

Assessment of children

Weight, height and arm circumference are considered the most sensitive parameters for assessing nutritional status of under fives. Several methods have been suggested for the classification of nutritional status based on these measurements.

Weight for age

The most widely used classifications of nutritional status are given in Tables 21.1, 21.2, 21.3 and 21.4.

Table 21.1: Gomez classification for public health

Grade	Weight for age
Normal	>90%
Grade I	75–90%
Grade II	60–75%
Grade III	<60%

Table 21.2: IAP (Indian Academy of Paediatrics) National classification

Grade	Weight for age
Normal	> 80%
Grade I	70–80%
Grade II	60–70
Grade III	50–60%
Grade IV	> 50%

Table 21.3: Waterlow malnutrition classification

Type/degree of malnutrition	Cut of level as % of NCHS median Indicat or	
	% Wt/age	%Wt/Ht
Normal	>90	>80
Short duration malnutrition	>90	<80 wasted
Long duration malnutrition (Nutritional dwarf)	<90	<80 stunted
Current and long duration malnutrition	<90	<80 stunted and wasted

This classification identifies type and duration of malnutrition.
*National Center for Health Statistics.
Children with oedema are classified according to Welcome as given in TAble 21.4

Table 21.4: Welcome clinical classification

Type	% of wt for age	Oedema
Normal	>80%	–
Undernutrition	60-80%	–
Kwashiorkor	60-80%	+
Marasmus	< 60%	–
Marasmic kwashiorkor	< 60%	+

Most often accurate assessment of age may not be possible. Weight for height is age independent.

Mid-upper Arm Circumference for Age

Mid arm circumference varies little between the age of one and four years. It correlates well with weight and weight for height. Use of tricolour tape (Shakir Tape), QUAC stick (arm circumference and height) and arm circumference/head circumference ratio have been suggested for assessment of nutritional status.

Assessment of PEM Children

Assessment can be made by using anthropometric measurements. Table 21.5 gives anthropometric measurements of normal and PEM children.

Table 21.5: Anthropometric Measurements of normal and PEM children

Measurement	Normal	PEM
• Rao index $\dfrac{wt \text{ in kg}}{(ht \text{ in cm})^2} \times 100$	> 0.15	< 0.15
• Wt/age	Normal	80–60% kwashiorkor oedema <60% Marasmus without oedema.
• Skin fold thickness	>10 mm	< 6 mm
• Bangle test – 4.0 cm diameter	Does not pass	Passes above the elbow
• Mid arm cirumference	16 cm	Mild — 13.5 cm Moderate — 12.5 cm Severe < 12.5 cm
• Kanawati index $\dfrac{\text{Mid arm circumference}}{\text{Head circumference}}$	> 0.32	Mild — 0.28–0.32 Moderate — 0.25–0.28 Severe < 0.25
• $\dfrac{\text{Chest circumference}}{\text{Head circumference}}$	> 1.0	< 1.0

Composite Classification

Table 21.6 gives composite classification of Kanawati and Mcharen's index of thriving.

Table 21.6: Kanawati and Mcharen's Index of thriving

Sl. No.		Measurement	% range	Score
I.	1.	Weight	>100	0
	2.	Mid arm circumference	90-100	1
			80-90	2
			70-80	3
			60-70	4
			<60	5
II.	1.	Height	>100%	0
	2.	Head circumference	90-100	1
			85-90	2
			80-85	3
			<80	4

Final score is calculated by adding individual scores for weight, mid arm circumference, height and head circumference.

Normal children – Index = 0-1

Failure to Thrive – Index = >9.

Prediction of Birth Weight of the Newborns

Maternal height and weight for height (%) are useful in predicting the birth weight of the newborn. Women with height of more than 145 cm and weight of 45 kg or more are found to have good birth weights and good weight gain during pregnancy. Prematurity rates are very low with better stature, better body weight and better weight/height[2].

Assessment of Adults

Body Mass Index

After the cessation of linear growth around 21 years, weight for height indicates muscle fat mass in the adult body. The ratio of Weight in kg/Height[2] m is referred to as Body Mass Index.

BMI has good correlation with fatness. It may also be used as an indicator of health risk.

Table 21.7: BMI in relation to energy status

Presumptive diagnosis	BMI
Chronic energy deficiency-grade III severe	< 16.0
Chronic energy deficiency-grade II moderate	16.0–17.0
Chronic energy deficiency-grade I mild	17–18.5
Low weight-normal	18.5–20.0
Normal	20.0–25.0
Obese grade I	25.0–30.0
Obese grade II	> 30

For similar BMI, Indians have a grater proportion of body fat which renders them susceptible to morbidity.

Broka's Index

Broka's index = Ht in cms –100 = ideal weight in kg.

Broka's index is simple and easy to use index for assessment of nutritional status of adults. Broka's index correlates with BMI and wt/ht.

Determination of arm muscle circumference and arm muscle area: Waist and Hip Circumference Ratio

To calculate muscle circumference and area, lay a ruler between the appropriate values for arm circumference and muscle area from the middle line. Waist hip ratio gives distribution of fat in the human body. A waist hip ratio greater than 1.0 in men 0.8 in women is indicative of android obesity and increases the risk of atherosclerosis.

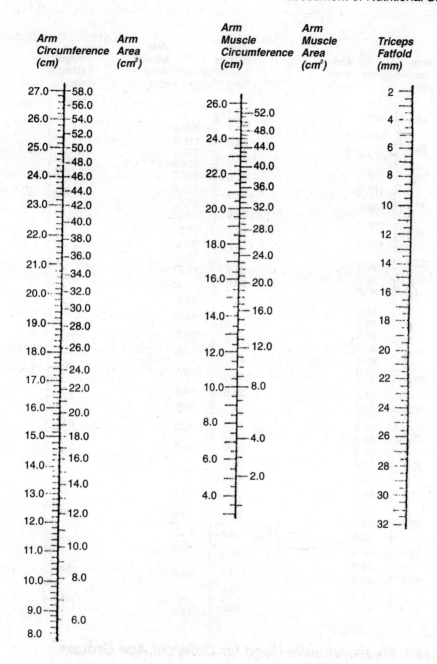

Figure 21.g. Nomogram for determination of arm muscle circumference and arm muscle area

Source: Gurnery J Jelliffe D. 1973, Arm anthropometry in nutritional assessment nomogram for rapid calculation of muscle circumference and cross-sectional muscle and fat areas. Am. J. Clin. Nutr 26: 912.

Contd....

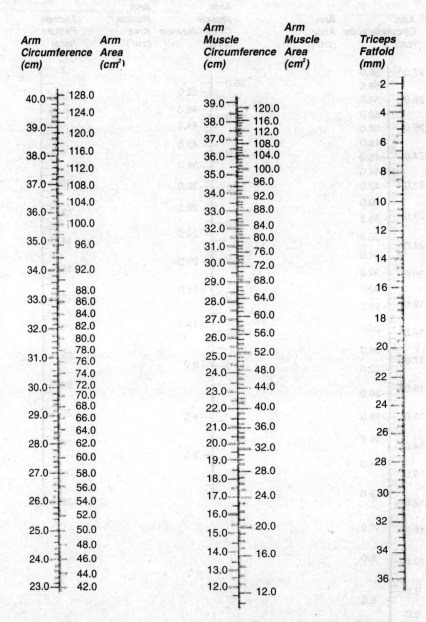

Anthropometric Measurements Used for Different Age Groups

The best combinations of measurements found useful for the assessment of the growth status of infants, pre-school and school age children and adolescents are given in Table 21.8.

Table 21.8: Best set of measurements/indices found useful for nutritional status

Details	Measurement/indices
Newborns	Weight, height, weight for height (%) or weight/height^2
Infants	Weight, height, weight for height (%) or weight/height^2 head cir, chest cir.
Preschool children	Weight, height, weight for height (%) or weight/height^2 arm cir, calf cir.
School age children And adolescents	Weight, height, weight for height (%) or weight/ height^2
Adults	Weight for height (%) weight/height^2, weight/height, weight/height^3 or Broka's index

Source: Visweswara Rao, K. 1999, Biostatistics, Jaypee Brothers, Medical Publishers (P) Ltd., New Delhi.

For screening short-term malnutrition at a high level of specificity, weight for height is superior to weight for age. For monitoring malnutrition for long-term periods, with the usual random errors in age data, weight for age is better. For those interested in assessing the type and duration of malnutrition, Waterlow's classification is recommended.

Anthropometric measurement can easily be carried out without much technical knowledge. The results can be used immediately. This is the most inexpensive method. It is faster and not time consuming and a large community can be covered in a short time. This method can be done in a remote village where no facilities are available. It has no side effects. It is noninvasive and better cooperation can be achieved from community.

Limitations: The results may not be accurate if the instruments used are not calibrated properly. This may not be the conclusive method and another method may be needed to support. Standards need to be revised constantly. Sometimes it may be difficult to find the age of the child.

One cannot use the same percentiles for height and weight and skin folds for early maturers, late maturers and those of intermediate maturing timing. This limitation is inherent in existing standards.

CLINICAL EXAMINATION

Clinical examination assess levels of health of individuals or of population groups in relation to the food they consume. It is the simplest and practical method. When two or more clinical signs characteristic of a deficiency disease are present simultaneously, their diagnostic significance is greatly enhanced.

Table 21.9 shows clinical signs and symptoms of nutritional inadequacy in adults for different nutrients.

Table 21.9: Clinical signs and symptoms of nutritional inadequacy.

Site	Sign	Deficiency
General appearance	Loss of subcutaneous fat Sunken or hollow cheeks	Calories Calories, fluid
Hair	Easily plucked hair, alopecia Dry, brittle hair Corkscrew hairs	Protein Protein, biotin Vitamin C

Contd...

Site	Sign	Deficiency
Nails	Spooning	Iron
	Transverse depigmentation	Protein
Skin	Dry and scaly flaky paint	Vitamin A, zinc
	Nasolabial seborrhea	Essential fatty acid, riboflavin
	Psoriasiform rash	Vitamin A, zinc
	Pallor	Iron, vitamin B_{12}, folate
	Follicular hyperkeratosis	Vitamin A, essential fatty acid
	Perifollicular hemorrhage	Vitamin C
	Easy bruising	Vitamin K or C
	Hyperpigmentation	Niacin
Eyes	Night blindness	Vitamin A, zinc
	Photophobia, xerosis	Vitamin A
	Conjunctival inflammation	Riboflavin, vitamin A
	Retinal field defect	Vitamin E
Mouth	Glossitis	Riboflavin, pyridoxine, niacin, folic acid, vitamin B_{12}, iron
	Bleeding gums	Vitamin C, riboflavin
	Angular stomatitis	Riboflavin, pyridoxine, niacin
	Cheilosis	Riboflavin, pyridoxine, niacin
	Decreased taste or smell	Zinc
	Tongue fissuring	Niacin
	Tongue atrophy	Riboflavin, niacin, iron
	Loss of tooth enamel	Calcium
Neck	Goitre	Iodine
	Parotid enlargement	Protein
Heart	High output failure	Thiamin
Chest	Respiratory muscle weakness	Protein, phosphorus
Abdomen	Ascites	Protein
	Hepatomegaly	Protein, fat
Extremities	Edema	Protein
	Bone tenderness	Vitamin D
	Bone/joint pain	Vitamin A or C
	Muscle pain	Thiamin
	Joint swelling	Vitamin C
Muscles	Atrophic muscles	Protein
	Decreased grip strength	Protein
Neurological	Dementia	Thiamin, vitamin B_{12}, folate, niacin
	Acute disorientation	Phosphorus, niacin
	Nystagmus	Thiamin
	Ophthalmoplegia	Thiamin
	Wide-based gait	Thiamin
	Peripheral neuropathy	Thiamin, pyridoxine, vitamin E
	Loss of vibratory sense	Vitamin B_{12}
	Loss of position sense	Vitamin B_{12}
	Tetany	Calcium, magnesium
	Paresthesias	Thiamin, vitamin B_{12}
	Wrist or foot drop	Thiamin
	Diminished reflexes	Iodine

Source: Shils Maurice E. *et. al.* (Editors), 1998, Modern nutrition in health and disease, Lippincott Williams & Wilkins, Philadelphia.

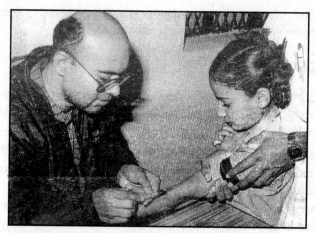

Figure 21h: Drawing blood for biochemical assessment.

Source: Proceedings of symposium on 'Micronutrient supplementation in health and disease, NIN, Hyderabad and Centre for Research on Nutrition support systems, New Delhi, 2002.

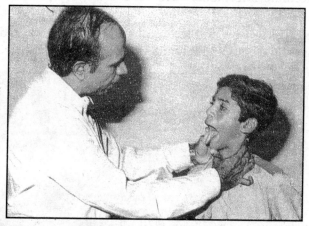

Figure 21i: Clinical examination

Source: Proceedings of symposium on 'Micronutrient supplementation in health and disease, NIN, Hyderabad and Centre for Research on Nutrition support systems, New Delhi, 2002.

For clinical examination cooperation of the subject can be achieved easily because the procedure is noninvasive and the symptoms are observed externally. This method is reliable and easy to organise. Age of the subject need not be ascertained. Symptoms are specific to a particular nutrient. This method is not very expensive. It does not require elaborate apparatus and reagents.

However it requires an experienced investigator to assess the symptoms.

Early clinical symptoms and signs of malnutrition are rather vague and often include weakness, lethargy, irritability and light headedness. Many of the symptoms and signs are nonspecific for a single nutrient deficit and may be caused by insufficiency of one or several nutrients e.g., flaking dermatitis may be due to protein, riboflavin or linoleic acid deficiency. Some symptoms like angular stomatitis may be due to several deficiencies.

Changes in the conjunctiva, lips and skin can be caused by non-nutritional factors like cold, dryness, irritation and injection. In a well nourished community, signs of malnutrition are infrequent and so more easily overlooked or misinterpreted.

BIOPHYSICAL OR RADIOLOGICAL MEASUREMENT

These tests are used in specific studies where additional information regarding change in the bone or muscular performance is required. Radiological methods have been used in studying the change of bones in rickets, osteomalacia, osteoporosis and scurvy.

When clinical examination suggests following radiographic examination is done:

- In rickets, there is healed concave line of increased density at distal ends of long bones usually the radius and ulna.
- In infantile scurvy there is ground glass appearance of long bones with loss of density.
- In beriberi there is increased cardiac size as visible through X-rays.
- Changes in bone also occur in advanced fluorosis.
- Endocardiograph, a tool for graphing heart sounds and a means for measuring nutritional status.

These give more accurate information. The results can be used as a supporting data for other methods.

Equipment required is expensive and technical knowledge is required in interpreting data. It is difficult to transport the equipment to interior parts of any village.

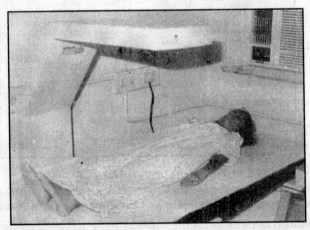

Figure 21j: Biophysical assessment—Measuring bone parameters using Dhel Energy X-Ray Absorptiometry.

Source: Proceedings of symposium on 'Micronutrient supplementation in health and disease, NIN, Hyderabad and Centre for Research on Nutrition support systems, New Delhi, 2002.

FUNCTIONAL ASSESSMENT

Functional indicators of nutritional status are diagnostic tests to determine the sufficiency of host nutriture to permit cells, tissues, organs, anatomical systems or the host him/herself to perform optimally the intended nutrient dependent biological function.

Functional indices of nutritional status include cognitive ability, disease response, reproductive competence, physical activity, work performance and social and behavioural performance.

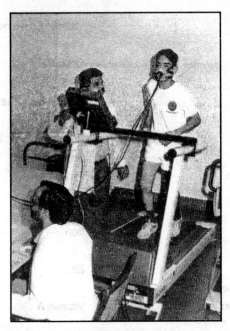

Figure 21k: Functional assessment—Tread Mill test.

Source: Proceedings of symposium on 'Micronutrient supplementation in health and disease, NIN, Hyderabad and Centre for Research on Nutrition support systems, New Delhi, 2002.

Submaximal test using tread mill might be useful as an adjunct to biochemical and anthropometric measures in the assessment of nutritional status. Since it involves only counting of heart rates, it could be applied in field conditions suitable for stepping test. Increased severity of malnutrition was associated with an increased heart rate response to the same submaximal work rate. The heart rates and O_2 intakes are obtained during maximal O_2 consumption test by using treadmill.

Lactation performance may be yet another functional index of individual nutriture. Milk volume is reduced in malnourished women as is fat and total energy content of the milk.

Growth velocity represents a more sensitive and at the same time a functional index. Growth rates are suboptimal in PEM, zinc deficiency and iodine deficiency. The use of this index requires serial, accurate anthropometric measurements. Severe deficiencies of several nutrients will delay the onset of menarche. Chronic malnutrition will influence sexual maturation.

Fertility and birth weight reflect nutritional status at the population level. Nutritional supplements can reduce the duration of postpartum amenorrhoea. A number of studies have demonstrated a dose - response relationship between maternal energy consumption during pregnancy and the birth weight of the infant.

Social performance, the ability of an individual to interact with his or her peers and environment, is an index for functional nutritional status. Prenatally undernourished infants show several behavioural impairments that could negatively affect the development of social competence including reduced activity and less interaction with caretakers.

Table 21.10: System classification of functional indices of nutritional status

System	Nutrients involved
Structural Integrity	
Erythrocyte fragility	– Vitamin E, selenium
Capillary fragility	Vitamin C
Tensile strength of skin	– Copper
Experimental wound healing	– Zinc
Lipoprotein peroxidation	– Vitamin E, sodium
Host defence	
Leucocyte phagocytic activity	– Protein, energy, iron
Leucocyte metabolism	– Protein, energy
White cell interferon production	– Protein, energy
Transport	
1. Intestinal absorption	
Iron absorption	– Iron
Cobalt absorption	
2. Plasma tissue transport	– Zn
Zinc uptake by erythrocyte	
Retinol relative dose response	– Vitamin A
Haemostasis	
Prothrombin time	Vitamin K
Platelet aggregation	Vitamin E, zinc
Reproduction	
Sperm count	– Energy, zinc
Nerve Function	
Dark adaptation	Vitamin A, zinc
Olfactory acuity	Vitamin A, B_{12} and zinc
Taste acuity	Vitamin A, zinc
Nerve Conduction	Protein, energy, vitamin B_1 and B_{12}
Work capacity Haemodynamics	
Task performance endurance	– Protein, energy, vitamin, B_1, B_2, B_6 and iron
Heart rate (cumulative)	– Protein, energy and iron

Source: Solomons Noel and Lindsay H. Allen. The functional assessment of nutritional status: Principles, Practice and Potential, Nutrition Reviews, 41,2,1983.

The direct relevance of functional impairment and its improvement with supplementation are more likely to convince healthcare administrators and the community of the appropriateness of expenses involved in an intervention.

Functional indices have several potential advantages over static indices with respect to the validity of the information about nutritional status. A defective function may be uncovered despite an apparently "adequate" circulating or tissue level of a nutrient. Conversely, functional competence may be preserved even though the static index has fallen below the level of adequacy. Moreover, functional performance can to some extent be normalised on an individual basis rather than on a population standard, especially where performance can be assessed serially and a maximum output after nutritional supplement defined.

LABORATORY AND BIOCHEMICAL ASSESSMENT

a. Laboratory Tests

Haemoglobin estimation: It is a useful index of the overall state of nutrition irrespective of its significance in anaemia. RBC count and a haematocrit determination are also valuable.

Stools and urine: Stools should be examined for intestinal parasites. History of parasitic infestation, chronic dysentery and diarrhoea provides useful background information about the nutritional status of persons. Urine should be examined for albumin and sugar.

b. Biochemical Tests

In the development of any deficiency disease, biochemical changes can be expected to occur prior to clinical manifestation. Therefore, biochemical tests which can be conducted on easily accessible body fluids such as blood and urine, can help to diagnose disease at the subclinical stage. These tests confirm clinical diagnosis if symptoms are nonspecific.

Biochemical tests are precise and measure individual nutrient concentration in body fluids (serum retinol, serum iron) or detection of abnormal amounts of metabolites in urine (urinary iodine) frequently after a loading dose or measurement of enzymes in which the vitamin is a known co-factor (riboflavin deficiency) to help establish malnutrition in its preclinical stages.

Modern analytical instruments (e.g., high performance liquid chromatography) techniques (e.g., radio or enzyme immunoassay) and computerisation have greatly increased the capability of nutritional bio-chemical testing.

Table 21.11 shows normal and deficiency indices for assessing nutritional status with regard to vitamins and minerals.

Table 21.11: Biochemical methods for assessing nutritional status

Nutrient	Principle Method	Normal	Deficiency
Vitamin A	S. vitamin A	30 µg/dl	< 20 µg/dl
	Relative Dose Response test (450–1000µg retinol) 100 µg/kg dehydroretinol;	–	> 20% RDR
	Dehydroretinol : vitamin A	–	> 0.06
Vitamin D	S.25-hydroxy cholecalciferol	>10 ng/ml	< 5 ng/ml
Vitamin E	S.vitamin E/total lipid ratio	> 0.8	–
Vitamin K	Protein induced by vitamin K absence PIVKAS	Absent	Accumulate

Contd....

Nutrient	Principle Method	Normal	Deficiency
Thiamin	Urinary thiamin	100 μg/24 hr 65 μg/g of creatinine	–
	Erythrocyte Transketolase Test (ETK-AC) Activated coefficient	< 1.15	> 1.25
Riboflavin	Erythrocyte glutathione reductase (EGR-AC)	< 1.2	> 1.4
Niacin	N-methy 1-2 pyridone-5 carboxylamide (2-pyridone) and N1- methyl nicotinamide ratio	1–4	< 1.0
Vitamin B₆	Urinary excretion B₆		< 20 μg/g creatinine
	Erythrocyte asparatate amino transferase (EAspAT - AC)	< 1.7–2.0	–
Folic acid	Serum folate	> 6.0 ng/ml	< 3.0 ng/ml
	RBC folate	> 160 ng /ml	< 140 ng/ml
	Formimino glutamic acid FIGLU	< 20 mg FIGLU in 8 hours after histidine load of 0.26 g/kg body weight	> 100 mg
Vitamin B₁₂	Serum B₁₂	200–900 pg/ml	80 pg/ml
Ascorbic acid	P. ascorbic acid levels	> 0.3 mg/dl	< 0.2 mg/dl
	Leucocyte ascorbic acid	> 15 mg/dl	< 8 mg/dl
Iron	Serum ferritin levels	–	12μg/l
	Serum iron	–	< 40 μg/dl
	Serum transferrin	–	< 0.16
	Haemoglobin	>13 g/dl (Men)	–
		> 12 g/dl (Women)	
Iodine	Urinary excretion of iodine	> 50 mg/g creatinine	–
Zinc	P. zinc	84–104 μg/dl	–
Copper	S. copper	75–125 μg/dl	–

Source: Bamji Mehtab.S., Biochemical tests for the assessment of nutrition status from (ed.) Bamji Mehtab. S et. al., text book of Human Nutrition, 1998 Oxford and IBH Publishing Co. Pvt. Ltd., New Delhi.

TESTS FOR PROTEIN ENERGY MALNUTRITION

Serum Proteins

The first indication of malnutrition is the lowering of serum total proteins and serum albumin. The normal albumin levels are 3.5–5.5 g/dl. During PEM the levels may slow down to 2.0–2.5 g/dl. α-globulin and γ-globulin fractions show a small rise but the albumin globulin ratio shows a tendency to decrease.

Serum Amino Acid Ratio

This ratio of non-essential/essential amino acids is very sensitive at an early stage of PEM as also for kwashiorkor. This test is not sensitive to marasmus.

$$\frac{\text{Glycine} + \text{Serine} + \text{Glutamine} + \text{Taurine}}{\text{Leucine} + \text{Isoleucine} + \text{Valine} + \text{Methionine}}$$

Normal mean value	– 1.5
Subclinical malnutrition	– 2 to 4
Frank kwashiorkor mean value	– 5

Urinary Hydroxyproline Index

$$\text{Hydroxyproline Index} = \frac{\mu\,\text{moles hydroxyproline/ml}}{\mu\,\text{moles creatinine/ml/kg body weight}}$$

In normal children the index is 4.7. The index declines in kwashiorkor and marasmus. In growth retardation the index is –2.

Urinary Creatinine Height Index

$$= \frac{\text{mg creatinine / 24 hour excreted by the malnourished child}}{\text{mg creatinine / 24 hour excreted by a normal child of the same height}} \times 100$$

Normal and recovery from PEM	– 1
Kwashiorkor	– 0.24 to 0.75
Marasmus	– 0.33 to 0.85

The measurement provides an approximate idea of the musculature of the child and it is of value in assessing the recovery of malnourished children as well as, in the detection of marginal nutrition.

Fasting Urinary Urea Nitrogen and Creatinine Nitrogen Ratio

$$\text{Urea - creatinine ratio} = \frac{\text{mg urea nitrogen / ml}}{\text{mg creatinine nitrogen / ml}}$$

Children eating diets low in protein show low ratios of urinary urea to creatinine.

The establishment of normal nutrient values in body fluids or tissues for each sex varies from laboratory to laboratory. Optimally, a low biochemical nutrient value in body fluids or tissue should be coupled with a specific functional abnormality before making the diagnosis of a nutrient deficiency. For some nutrients like vitamin A, children have a different normal range than adults.

Biochemical tests are time consuming and expensive. They cannot be applied on a large scale as, for example, in the nutritional assessment of a whole community. They are often carried out on a subsample of the population. Most biochemical tests reveal only current nutritional status. They are useful to quantify mild deficiencies.

DIETARY ASSESSMENT

A diet survey provides information about dietary intake patterns of specific foods consumed and estimated nutrient intakes. It indicates relative dietary inadequacies, which is helpful in planning health education activities and changes needed in the agriculture and food production industries. Most of the time, the surveys are carried out for 7–10 days. If needed in different seasons surveys can be repeated.

Food Balance Sheet Method

This method is employed when information regarding the availability of food is needed at macro level — region or country.

$$\text{Per capita availability per day (g)} = \frac{\left(\begin{array}{c}\text{Stocks at the beginning}\\\text{of the year + total food}\\\text{produced + imports}\end{array}\right) - \left(\begin{array}{c}\text{Stocks at the end of the year}\\\text{+ exports + seeds}\\\text{+ cattle / poultry feeds}\end{array}\right)}{\text{Mid year population} \times 365 \text{ days}}$$

Food balance sheets are most useful for administrators and planners to monitor food position in the country and to take appropriate decisions.

This method is of little use to health/nutrition workers since the actual dietary consumption will not be known from balance sheet.

Inventory Method

This method is often employed in institutions like hostels, army barracks, orphanages and homes for the aged, where homogenous groups of people take their meals from a common kitchen. In this method, the amounts of food stuffs issued to kitchen as per the records maintained by the warden are taken into consideration. No direct measurement or weighing is done. A reference period of one week is desirable.

This method can also be used for assessing food consumption at household level provided the respondent maintains a regular record.

$$\text{Average intake per person per day} = \frac{\begin{array}{c}\text{Stocks at the beginning of the week}\\\text{- Stocks at the end of the week}\end{array}}{\begin{array}{c}\text{Total no. of inmates partaking the meal}\\\text{and no. of days of survey}\end{array}}$$

Though a large sample can be covered in a relatively short time, active cooperation of the respondent is very necessary. This method is possible only when the community is fairly educated and subsists on cash economy where food is usually purchased from the market.

Weighment Method

In this method, food either raw or cooked is actually weighed using an accurate balance. It is ideal to conduct the survey for 7 consecutive days to know the true picture of diet.

Every day food is weighed in the morning and evening before actual cooking is begun by the housewife. Only edible portion of raw food is weighed. All family members who consume their food, the age, sex, physiological status should be noted down. Consumption of food by guests and additional food consumed by the family members like those brought in a cooked form, sweets and foods accepted from the friends and relatives should be noted with the details. Survey should not be done on fast and festival days.

Foods are converted to nutrients by referring to food composition tables. The nutrient intakes thus can be expressed per consumption unit or per capita. Though weighment method is relatively more accurate as it involves direct weighing of foods, it is time consuming and needs cooperation of the housewives. The coefficient for computing caloric requirement cannot be calculated for other nutrients.

Housewives may not cooperate. They may exaggerate or underestimate the food consumption. All the cooked food may not be eaten on the same day. The investigator has to stay in the village or the place where the survey is being conducted. This method does not give the actual intake of the individual in the family.

Expenditure Pattern Method

In this method, money spent on food as well as non-food items is assessed by administering a specially designed questionnaire. The reference period could be either a previous month or week.

This method, apparently is less cumbersome as it avoids actual weighing of foods. The reference period too is usually longer. In trained hands, both the methods, weighment and expenditure pattern method have yielded comparable results.

Diet History

This method is useful for obtaining qualitative details of diet and studying patterns of food consumption household level or industrial level. The procedure includes assessment of the frequency or consumption of different foods daily or number of times in a week or fortnight or occasionally. This method has been used to study meal pattern, dietary habits, peoples food preferences and avoidances during physiopathological conditions like pregnancy, lactation, sickness etc. Infant weaning and breast feeding practices and the associated cultural constraints which are often prevalent in the community can also be studied by this method. At times, information on approximate quantities of foods, consumed by the households like 30 kg of rice per month or half a litre of milk per day can also be collected.

Oral Questionnaire (24 hour recall)

In this recall method of oral questionnaire diet survey, a set of standardised cups suited to local conditions are used. Information on the total cooked amount of each preparation is noted in terms of standardised cups. The intake of each food item by the specific individual in the family such as the preschool child, adolescent girl or pregnant or lactating woman is assessed by using the cups. The cups are used mainly to aid the respondent recall the quantities prepared and fed to the individual members.

Chemical Analysis

In this method, the individual is required to save a duplicate sample of each type of food eaten by him during the day. These samples are then collected and sent to the laboratory for chemical analysis. It is the most accurate method but is costly and needs a good laboratory support.

Dietary Score

This method is useful where one is trying to assess the dietary intake of specific nutrient e.g., iron content of diet. Depending on the content of iron, a food item is given a score. The frequency of intake of those foods is noted by questionnaire method. The frequency of consumption of foods, the total score and percentages are then calculated. The value of this qualitative assessment method is enhanced when it is combined with quantitative method of survey and nutritional status assessment.

Recording Method

It involves maintenance of dietary records of weighed quantities of foods consumed by an individual/family according to number of days of survey. If this method is followed well with proper instructions, a large sample can be covered in a short time, sometimes through mailed questionnaire, provided the population is educated.

Even the best of diet surveys, give only an approximate estimate of foods and nutrients consumed, but not the amount absorbed or utilised. Twenty four hour recall method together with diet history (food frequency) would yield reasonably accurate estimates of the prevalent dietary situation. A combination of dietary, clinical and biochemical assessment is desirable for assessment of nutrition status of individuals or communities.

The errors which occur generally in diet surveys are :

- memory lapses.
- long reporting period may give rise to a lot of errors.
- prestige and other considerations influencing the responses.
- non-response due to non-cooperation.
- conversion factors for the various crude local measures (inventory method).
- inaccurate weighing of food stuffs (weighment method).
- housewife deviating from the normal pattern of food consumption during the survey period (response errors).
- seasonal variations and improper selection of the reporting period.
- problems in the use of tables on nutritive value of foods.

VITAL HEALTH STATISTICS

The term vital statistics signifies the data and analytical methods for describing the vital events occurring in communities. The raw data of vital statistics are generally obtained through the sources of population census, sample surveys and vital statistics registers.

For public health and nutrition the vital statistics are most useful. Vital statistics include the counts of births, deaths, illnesses, movements and the various rates and ratios that may be computed from them and utilised.

Some types of malnutrition have a particularly high incidence at certain ages so that the mortality rates at these specific age periods have been suggested as indicators of the incidence of certain type of malnutrition. Malnutrition can be either the direct cause or indirect cause. There are measures of fertility, measures of mortality and measures of morbidity under vital health statistics.

Measures of Mortality

Infant mortality rate: This is the number of babies dying in the first year of life per 1000 live births. The rates are falling as there is improvement in infant feeding. In most prosperous countries the rate lies between 10 and 20. In India the rate is 80 per 1000 live births. It has come down from 129 per 1000 live births in 1971.

$$\text{Infant mortality rate (IMR)} = \frac{\text{Number of deaths under one year of age in a year}}{\text{Number of live births in a year}} \times 1000$$

Perinatal mortality rate: This is the number of deaths of infants under 1 month and stillbirths per 1000 total births. This rate gives an index of maternal nutrition through many other factors like genetic make up of mother and child, the degree of exposure to infections and the standard of medical care available.

$$\text{PNMR} = \frac{\left(\begin{array}{c}\text{Late foetal deaths after}\\ \text{28 weeks or more gestation}\end{array}\right) + \left(\begin{array}{c}\text{Deaths under}\\ \text{one week}\end{array}\right)}{\text{Mid year population of the same age group in the same year}} \times 1000$$

The Perinatal, Neonatal and Infant Mortality Rates in India are given in Figure 23h.

Toddler mortality rate: This is the number of deaths between 1 to 4 years per 1000 toddlers born. The manifestations and effects of malnutrition are well known to be severe in toddlers. Although death certificates may record gastroenteritis or respiratory infections, malnutrition contributes to many of the deaths.

In addition, disease specific mortality rate, maternal mortality rate, family size and fertility rate are also an indication of nutritional status of the community.

If in any community the perinatal, infant and toddler mortality rates are all falling, then it can be inferred that the general level of nutrition of the people is improving.

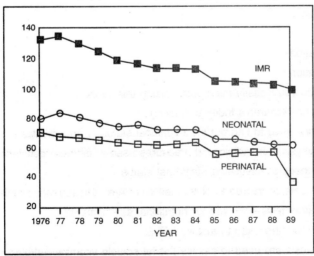

Figure 21I. IMR Neonatal and perinatal mortality rates from 1976–1989.

Source: Reddy Vinodini et al., 1993, Nutrition trends in India, National Institute of Nutrition, Hyderabad.

Measures of Morbidity

Morbidity relates to types and varieties of diseases one faces or experiences affecting the day-to-day activity.

Rates which are utilized are

$$\text{Incidence rate} = \frac{\text{Total number of new cases of a specific deisease during year}}{\text{Mid year population}} \times k$$

$$\text{Prevalence rate} = \frac{\text{Total number of cases new or old existing at a point of time}}{\text{Total population at that point of time}} \times k$$

k can be 100 or 1000, 10,000 or 1,00,000.

Case fatality ratio and immunity ratio are also measures of morbidity.

Morbidity hospital data or data from community health and morbidity surveys, particularly in relation to protein energy malnutrition, anemia, xerophthalmia and other vitamin deficiencies, endemic goitre, diarrhoea, measles and parasitic infestations can be of value in providing additional information contributing to the nutritional status of the community.

QUESTIONS

1. List the methods used to assess the nutritional status of a community.
2. Explain the sequence of nutritional deficiency and specificity of assessment of nutritional status.
3. Which anthropometric measurements are used to assess nutritional status of a community?
4. Explain the anthropometric methods needed to assess PEM.
5. Explain the following and bring out the differences among them.
    Gomez classification
    IAP classification
    Waterlow classification
    Welcome classification
6. What is BMI, how do you classify malnutrition using this index?
7. What is Kanawati and Mcharen's Index of thriving?
8. Give the clinical signs used to find out the nutritional status of an individual.
9. Give the list of biophysical or radiological measures used in different deficiency diseases.
10. Explain indirect methods of assessing nutritional status.
11. How are functional tests compared to other methods? Are they superior or inferior? Why?
12. What kind of laboratory tests are used for nutritional assessment?
13. Which biochemical tests are used to assess PEM?
14. Which biochemical tests are used to assess the fat soluble vitamins nutrition status?
15. What is food balance sheet method? When is it used?
16. Compare diet surveys with other methods of nutritional assessment.

17. "Diet surveys may not give the accurate value in knowing the nutritional status", Give reasons.
18. What are the different dietary methods used to know the nutritional status of a community?
19. Define the following:

    Infant Mortality Rate

    Perinatal Mortality Rate

    Toddler Mortality Rate
20. How will you assess the iron nutritional status of an adolescent community?
21. How will assess the vitamin A nutritional status of pre-school children?

SUGGESTED READINGS

- Feasibility of Broka's index for assessing nutritional status of adults in rural population. National Institute of Nutrition, Annual Report, 2000-2001.

- Chheda K. Mayoor, 2000, Practical aspects of paediatrics, Balam Book Depot, Mumbai 400 014.

CHAPTER 22

NATIONAL NUTRITION POLICY AND PROGRAMMES OF TENTH FIVE YEAR PLAN

NATIONAL NUTRITION POLICY

One of the most significant achievements on the nutrition scene in the country has been the adoption of the National Nutrition Policy by the Government in 1993. It advocates a comprehensive, integrated and inter sectoral strategy for alleviating the multi-faceted problem of malnutrition and achieving the optimal state of nutrition for the people.

Nutrition affects development as much as development affects nutrition. It is therefore, important to tackle the problem of malnutrition both by direct nutrition intervention for specially vulnerable groups as well as through various development policy instruments which will create conditions for improved nutrition.

A. DIRECT INTERVENTION : SHORT TERM

Nutrition Intervention for Vulnerable Groups

The universal Immunisation Programme, Oral Rehydration Therapy and the Integrated Child Development Services have had a considerable impact on child survival and extreme forms of malnutrition. The position, however, is that the silent form of hunger and malnutrition continues with over 43.8 per cent (1988–90) children suffering from moderate malnutrition and about 37.6 per cent from mild malnutrition. Therefore, more children are surviving today, though an overwhelmingly large number of them are destined to remain much below their genetic potential. An immediate imperative is to substantially expand the nutrition intervention net through ICDS so as to cover all vulnerable children in the age group 0–6 years.

Improving growth monitoring between the age group 0 to 3 years in particular, with closer involvement of the mothers is a key intervention. Getting involved in the growth monitoring of her child will give her a feeling of control over the child's nutrition process. This combined with adequate nutrition and health education will empower her to manage the nutrition needs of her children effectively.

The Government's recent initiative of including the adolescent girl within the ambit of ICDS should be intensified so that they are made ready for a safe motherhood, their nutritional status is improved. They are given some skill upgradation training in home-based skills and covered by non formal education, particularly nutrition and health education.

In order to reduce the incidence of low birth weight coverage should include supplementary nutrition right from 1st trimester and should continue during the major period of lactation at least for the first one year after pregnancy.

Fortification of Essential Foods

Essential food items shall be fortified with appropriate nutrients like salt with iodine and/ or iron. Research in iron fortification of rice and other cereals should be intensified. The distribution of iodised salt should cover all the population in endemic areas of the country to reduce the iodine deficiency to below endemic levels.

Popularisation of Low Cost Nutritious Food

Efforts to produce and popularise low cost nutritious foods from indigenous and locally available raw material shall be intensified. It is necessary to involve women particularly in this activity.

Control of Micronutrient Deficiencies amongst Vulnerable Groups

Deficiencies of vitamin A, iron and folic acid and iodine among children, pregnant women and nursing mothers shall be controlled through intensified programmes. Iron supplementation to adolescent girls shall be introduced. The programme shall be expanded to cover all eligible members of the community. The prophylaxis programme of vitamin A covers only 30 out of about 80 million.

B. INDIRECT POLICY INSTRUMENTS: LONG TERM INSTITUTIONAL AND STRUCTURAL CHANGES

Food Security

In order to ensure aggregate food security, a per capita availability of 215 kg/person/year of food grains needs to be attained. This requires production of 230 millions of food grains per year taking into account the possibility of improved availability of non-cereal food items.

Improvement of production

The production of pulses, oil seeds and other food crops will be increased with a view to attaining self sufficiency and building surplus and buffer stocks. Preference shall be given to growing foods such as millets, legumes; vegetables and fruits, like green leafy vegetables, guava, papaya, amla and carrots. The prices of pulses, which were below cereal prices before the Green Revolution are now almost double the price of cereals. Our food policy should be consistent with our national nutritional needs and this calls for the introduction of appropriate incentives, pricing and taxation policies.

Policies for effecting income transfers

Improving the purchasing power: Poverty alleviation programmes, like the Integrated Rural Development Programme and employment generation schemes like Jawahar Rozgar Yojana and Nehru Rozgar Yojana are to be reoriented and restructured to make a forceful dent on the purchasing power of the lowest economic segments of the population. It is necessary to improve the purchasing power of the landless and the rural and urban poor by implementing employment generation programmes so that additional employment of at least 100 days is created for each rural landless family and employment opportunities are created in urban areas for slum dwellers and the urban poor.

Public Distribution System: The public distribution system shall ensure availability of essential food articles, such as coarse grains, pulses and jaggery, besides rice, wheat, sugar and oil. They should be available at reasonable prices to the public particularly to those living below the poverty line not only in urban areas but throughout the country.

Land Reforms

Implementing land reform measures so that the vulnerability of the landless and the landed poor could be reduced. This will include both tenurial reforms as well as implementation of ceiling laws.

Health and Family Welfare

Though "Health for all by 2000 A.D." programme increased health and immunisation facilities shall be provided to all. Improved prenatal and postnatal care to ensure safe motherhood shall be made accessible to all women. The population in the reproductive age group shall be empowered through education, to be responsible for their own family size. Small family norm and adequate spacing shall be encouraged so that the food available to the family is sufficient for proper nutrition of the members.

Basic Health and Nutrition Knowledge

Basic health and nutrition knowledge, with special focus on wholesome infant feeding practices, shall be imparted to the people extensively and effectively. Nutrition and health education are very important in the context of the problems of overnutrition also.

Prevention of Food Adulteration

This should be strengthened by gearing up the enforcement machinery.

Nutrition Surveillance

The NNMB/NIN of ICMR need to be strengthened so that periodical monitoring of the nutritional status of children, adolescent girls and pregnant and lactating mothers below the poverty line takes place through representative samples and results are transmitted to all agencies concerned. The NNMB should also serve as an early warning system for initiating prompt action.

Monitoring of nutrition programmes

Monitoring of nutrition programmes like ICDS and of nutrition education and demonstration by the Food and Nutrition board should be continued.

Research

Research must accurately identify those who are suffering from various degrees of malnutrition. Research should enable selection of new varieties of food with high nutritive value which can be within the purchasing power of the poor.

Equal Remuneration

The wages of women shall be at par with that of men in order to improve women's economic status. This requires a stricter enforcement of the Equal Remuneration Act. Special emphasis have to be given for expanding employment opportunities for women.

Communication

Communication through established media is one of the most important strategies to be adopted for the effective implementation of the Nutrition Policy. While using the communication tools, both mass communication as well as group or inter-personal communication should be used. Not only the electronic media but also folk and print media should be used extensively.

Minimum wage administration

The minimum wage should be linked with the price rise through a suitable nutrition formula. A special legislation should be introduced for providing agricultural women labourers the minimum support and atleast 60 days leave by the employer in the last trimester of pregnancy. Excessive loss of energy during the working seasons has serious nutritional implications. The legislation should take care of this problem also.

Community Participation

Generating awareness among the community regarding the National Nutrition Policy and encouraging the participation, particularly women in all programmes is vital for improving nutritional status of families.

Education and literacy

It has been shown that education and literacy particularly that of women, is a key determinant for better nutritional status. For instance, Kerala State has the highest literacy level, and also has the best nutrition status.

Improvement of the status of women

The most effective way to implement nutrition with mainstream activities in agriculture, health, education and rural development is to focus on improving the status of women, particularly the economic status. There is evidence that women's employment does benefit household nutrition, both through increase in household income as well as through an increase in women's status, autonomy and decision making power, particularly those relating to nutrition and feeding practices.

Nutritional anaemia prophylaxis programme

Government of India launched this programme in 1970. Under the programme, the expectant and nursing mothers as well as women acceptors of family planning are given one tablet containing 60 mg elemental iron (180mg ferrous sulphate) and 0.5 mg of folic acid and children in the age group 1–5 years are given one tablet containing 20 mg elemental iron (60 mg of ferrous sulphate) and 0.1 mg folic acid daily for a period of 100 days. This programme covered children and pregnant women with haemoglobin level less than 8 g per cent and 10 g per cent respectively. Fortification of salt with iron has been identified as a measure to control anaemia.

Prophylaxis programme against vitamin A deficiency

Initiated by the Government in 1970, the children in age group 1–5 years are given an oral dose of 0.2 million I.U. of vitamin A in oil every 6 months. During 1980, the Department of Food introduced a scheme of fortification of milk with vitamin A to prevent nutritional blindness. Presently the milk supplied by Tamilnadu Government is fortified with vitamin A.

IDD Control Programme

This programme was initiated by the Government of India in 1962 to identify goitre endemic regions and to assess the impact of goitre control measures.

There is an increasing awareness about the broad spectrum of Iodine Deficiency Disorder (IDD) in the country. The Government of India has started a scheme with effect from 1986 envisaging, "Universal Iodisation of Edible Salt" in a phased manner to cover the whole country. The States/UTs have been requested to arrange for distribution of iodised salt through their public distribution system.

National Diarrhoeal Diseases Control Programme

The programme was launched in 1981 to reduce the mortality due to diarrhoeal diseases in children below five years, through introduction of Oral Rehydration Therapy (ORT). The Anganwadi centres of the ICDS scheme have served as nucleus for the propagation of Oral Rehydration Therapy.

Functions of Food and Nutrition Board

The FNB advises Government, co-ordinates and reviews the activities with regard to food and nutrition, extension/education; development, production and popularisation of nutritious food and beverages; measures required to combat deficiency diseases and conservation and efficient utilisation as well as augmentation of food resources by way of food preservation and processing.

OBJECTIVES OF TENTH FIVE YEAR PLAN—2002-2007

During the Tenth Plan, there will be focussed and comprehensive interventions aimed at improving the nutritional and health status of the individuals.

There will be a paradigm shift from

- household food security and freedom from hunger to nutrition security for the family and the individual.
- untargeted food supplementation to vulnerable groups to screening of all the persons from these groups, identification of those with various grades of undernutrition and appropriate management.
- lack of focussed interventions on prevention of over-nutrition to promotion of appropriate life styles and dietary intakes for prevention and management of over-nutrition and obesity.

Interventions will be initiated to achieve the following :

Adequate availability of food shifts: This is to be achieved by ensuring production of cereals, pulses and vegetables to meet the nutritional needs. Also making them available at affordable cost throughout the year to urban and rural population through reduction in post harvest losses and appropriate processing.

More cost effective and efficient targeting of PDS to address macro and micro nutrient deficiencies such as providing coarse grains, pulses and iodised/double fortified salt to below poverty line families through the Targeted PDS (TPDS) is another measure for adequate availability of food stuffs. People's purchasing power is to be improved through appropriate programmes including food for work schemes.

Prevention of under nutrition through nutrition education: This is aimed at ensuring appropriate infant feeding practices (universal colostrum feeding, exclusive breast feeding up to six months, introduction of semisolids at six months). Appropriate intra-family distribution of food based on requirements is to be promoted. Dietary diversification is to be encouraged to meet the nutritional needs of the family.

Screening of vulnerable groups: All pregnant women, infants, preschool and school children are to be screened for under nutrition.

Nutrition interventions: Undernutrition is to be managed through targeted food supplementation and health care and effective monitoring of these individuals and their families. Panchayati Raj institutions are to be utilised effectively for intersectorial coordination and convergence of services. Community participation is to be improved in planning and monitoring of the ongoing interventions.

Prevention of micronutrient deficiencies: Nutrition education is to be promoted through dietary diversification to achieve balanced intake of all nutrients. There should be universal access to iodised/double fortified salt. Screening of all children with severe under nutrition, pregnant women and school children for early detection of micronutrient deficiencies. Timely treatment would be given for micronutrient deficiencies.

Management of obesity: Appropriate dietary intake and life style are promoted to prevent and manage obesity and diet related chronic diseases.

Nutrition monitoring and surveillance: This is done to enable the country to track changes in the nutritional and health status of the population. Existing opportunities for improving nutritional status are ensured for full utilisation. Also emerging problems are identified early and corrected expeditiously.

Research efforts: This will be directed to review the recommended dietary intake of Indians. Epidemiological data is built on relationship between birth weight, survival, growth and development in childhood and adolescence. Body mass index norms of Indians and health consequences of deviation from these norms are to be stressed.

In view of the massive inter-state variations in the access to nutrition related services and nutritional status, state specific goals to be achieved by 2007 have been worked out. National goals have been drawn taking into account the state specific goals.

GOALS SET FOR THE TENTH PLAN

The major goals to be achieved by 2007 are

- intensify nutrition and health education to improve infant and child feeding and caring practices so as to
  * bring down the prevalence of underweight children under three years from the current level of 47 per cent to 40 per cent.
  * reduce prevalence of severe undernutrition in children in the 0–6 years age group by 50 per cent.
- reduce prevalence of anaemia by 25 per cent and that of moderate/severe anaemia by 50 per cent.
- eliminate vitamin A deficiency as a public health problem and
- reduce prevalence of IDD in the country to less than 10 per cent by 2010.

QUESTIONS

1. What are the salient features of National Nutrition Policy?
2. Explain NNP's short term objectives and long term objectives.
3. What are the steps taken under NNP regarding iodine deficiency and vitamin A deficiency?
4. Describe the objectives of Tenth Five Year Plan.
5. Explain the goals set for the Tenth Plan.

SUGGESTED READINGS

- Vijayaraghavan, K, National Nutrition programmes-current status, Proceedings of Nutrition Society of India, NIN, Hyderabad.
- Tenth Five Year Plan (2002–2007). Vol. II, Sectorial Policies and Programmes Nutrition, Planning Commission, Govt. of India, New Delhi.

CHAPTER 23

ROLE OF INTERNATIONAL AND NATIONAL AGENCIES IN COMBATING MALNUTRITION

INTERNATIONAL AGENCIES

WORLD HEALTH ORGANISATION

The World Health Organization is an agency of the United Nations. The headquarters is in Geneva. The organization came into function on 7th April 1948, which is celebrated as World Health Day. On this day, for each year a theme is chosen on a certain aspect of public health and all attention is focussed on it.

The most important objective that the WHO seeks is the attainment of the most optimum level of health of the people which would enable them to lead a socially, economically and mentally productive life.

The WHO seeks to :

- act as directing and co-ordinating authority on international health activities.
- collaborate the member states and other agencies in planning and carrying out health programmes.
- give technological assistance in emergencies or upon the request of the government.
- promote medical research and improve the underdeveloped countries.
- bring the health status to international level.
- keep communicable diseases under constant surveillance, to give knowledge about health.
- set certain standards for the quality control of drugs, vaccines and other detrimental substances to the well being.
- widen the spectrum of maternal and foetal health and to live harmoniously.

The WHO consists of 3 principal organisations:

World health assembly: This is the supreme growing body of the WHO, which meets the assembly composed of delegates representing the member states.

Executive board: This has 32 members technically qualified in the field of health. The main work of the board is to give effective decision and policies to the assembly.

Secretariat : It is the organisation staff consisting 5000 people mainly physicians, medical scientists, health administrators. The main function is to give technical and managerial support for the national health development programmes.

In order to meet the special health needs of the different nations WHO has established regional headquarters.

Region	Headquarters
South East Asia	New Delhi
Africa	Brazzaville
America	Washington DC
Europe	Copenhagen
East Mediterranean	Gilekandia (Egypt)
Western Pacific	Manila

Functions

Feeding special food: WHO has recently increased its nutrition work to develop low cost foods for babies and infants, which are rich in protein. It educates the people and also encourages the governments to educate people about the importance of correct foods - basically the mothers, because they are involved in selection, preparation and handling of food.

Research work: It conducts medical research programme, which includes human reproduction, drug evaluation, pollution and to improve sanitary conditions. The WHO is studying the different types of medical disorders and their treatment. The main function of WHO is to sponsor the training and research for the medical practitioners of different countries.

Other functions: WHO continuously stresses on the importance of National Health Planning, and the need for each country to make best utilisation of the social resources. The WHO is always ready to serve in case of major natural calamities like floods, famines or quakes. WHO now directs its resources in underdeveloped countries to accelerate the growth of primary healthcare in rural areas. WHO provided vaccination for cholera and eradicated in Nigeria.

WHO is collaborating with Indian Government in the programme of medical research in areas of epidemics like cholera, typhoid, occupational health, medical technology, pathology etc. WHO gives support to the Cholera Research Centre, Kolkata and the National Institute of Occupational Health, Ahamedabad.

Almost all communicable diseases have been the subject of WHO. The global emancipation from small pox is an example of this. WHO is currently and directly involved in the global battle against AIDS. Immunisation against common diseases during childhood is given the utmost priority in WHO programmes. WHO provides vaccinations for measles, polio and tablets for deworming.

WHO is working closely with health authorities in the SARS (Severe Acute Respiratory Syndrome) affected countries to provide clinical, epidemiological and logistical support to eradicate it.

WHO acts as a source of information regarding various health problems. A wide variety of morbidity and mortality statistics relating to health problems are published by WHO in the weekly epidemiological records and quarterly world health statistics. The technical reports of WHO publication compiles hundreds of topics on a wide variety of health issues. The WHO also has a public information service booth at the headquarters and at each of the regional offices.

There has been a regional advisory committee on health research and a global advisory committee which is in collaboration with policy of global health.

WHO is involved in nutrition programmes by promoting general awareness of the prevalence of deficiencies and supporting the development and application of improved methods of prevention, detection and control of diseases. It also provides technical and other support to countries for strengthening their capabilities for preventing and managing nutritional problems.

FOOD AND AGRICULTURE ORGANISATION

The Food and Agricultural Organization came into existence in October 1945 with a mandate to raise levels of nutrition and standards of living, to improve agricultural productivity, and to better the condition of rural populations. Today, FAO is the largest autonomous agency within the United Nations system.

The motto of FAO is "FIAT PANIS" (let there be bread) and leads international efforts to defeat hunger.

Functions

- The organization shall collect, analyse, interpret and disseminate information relating to nutrition, food and agriculture. In this constitution the term "agriculture" and its derivatives include fisheries, marine products and forestry products. FAO publishes hundreds of newsletters, reports and books and creates CD-ROMs. Millions visit FAO Internet for technical consultation.
- The organisation shall promote and where appropriate, shall recommend national and international action with respect to :
  - a. scientific, technological, social and economic research relating to nutrition, food and agriculture.
  - b. the improvement of education and administration relating to nutrition, food and agriculture and the spread of public knowledge of nutritional and agricultural license and practice.
  - c. the conservation of natural resources and the adoption of improved methods of agricultural products.
  - d. the improvement of the processing, marketing and distribution of food and agricultural products.
  - e. the adoption of policies to the provision of adequate agricultural credit - national and international.
  - f. the adoption of international policies with reference to agricultural commodity arrangement.
- It shall furnish the technical assistance as Governments may request. Since its inception, FAO has worked to alleviate poverty and hunger by promoting agricultural development, improved nutrition and the pursuit of food security— the access of all people at all times to the food they need for an active and healthy life. The organization offers direct

development assistance, collects, analyses and disseminates international forum for debate on food and agricultural issues.

FAO is active in land and water development, plant and animal products, forestry, fisheries, economic and social policy, investment, nutrition, food standards and commodities and trade. It also plays a major role in dealing with food and agricultural emergencies.

A specific priority of the organization is encouraging sustainable agriculture and rural development, a long-term strategy for the conservation and management of natural resources. It aims to meet the needs of both present and future generations through programmes that do not degrade the environment and are technically appropriate, economically viable and socially acceptable.

FAO under "Farmer Field Schools" gives training to farmers of Asian countries in using biopesticides.

In crisis situations, FAO works with World Food Programme to help people rebuild their lives.

The Challenges of the Future

- To reduce the number and proportion of the world's people affected by hunger and malnutrition.
- To speed up the development of food production in low income food deficit countries.
- To conserve and protect natural resources.
- To achieve a higher degree of rural equity.
- To strengthen the position of the developing countries in world trade.

UNITED NATIONS CHILDREN'S FUND

United Nations International Children's Fund was created at the end of World War II in 1946 to relieve the suffering of children in war torn Europe. It continues today to respond rapidly in crisis helping to recreate a sense of stability and normalcy, in children when war, flood and other disruptions occur. It is now known as UN Children's Fund.

For more than 55 years UNICEF has been helping governments, communities and families to make the world a better place for children. Part of the United Nations systems, UNICEF has an enviable mandate and mission, to advocate for children's rights and help to meet their needs.

UNICEF now works in 161 countries, areas and territories on solutions to the problems plaguing poor children and their families and on ways to realize their rights. UNICEF's regional office for South Central Asia is in New Delhi. Its activities are as varied as the challenges it faces.

UNICEF Nutritional priorities include:

Infant and child feeding: UNICEF works to promote, protect and support exclusive breastfeeding and to educate families about care and feeding practices. The end goal: to empower all women to breastfeed their children exclusively for the first six months and to continue breastfeeding, with complementary food, well into the second year. UNICEF has two active ongoing programmes; the Baby-Friendly Hospital Initiative (BFHI) and International Code of Marketing of Breastmilk Substitutes.

Delivering vital micronutrients: Micronutrients enhance the nutritional value of food and have a profound impact on a child's development and a mother's health. UNICEF works with governments to deliver key minerals and vitamins – iodine, iron, vitamin A and folate – through supplementation, fortification and promotion of micronutrient-rich diets. To achieve the goals of virtual elimination of vitamin A and iodine deficiencies, UNICEF collaborates with a diverse group of public and private organizations, forming alliances such as the Vitamin A Global Initiative.

Promoting maternal nutrition/preventing low birth weight: Improving the nutritional status of pregnant women is essential to reduce maternal deaths, miscarriage, stillbirth and low birth weight. UNICEF focusses on the need to improve the status of women and to provide adequate nutrition, care and rest during pregnancy and breastfeeding. UNICEF is also working to prevent low birth weight in infants through the Low Birth Weight Prevention Initiative. This programme provides multi-micronutrient supplements for pregnant women and is being piloted in 11 countries.

Monitoring infant growth rates: Poor physical growth is linked closely to overall health and development, and affects a third of the world's children. UNICEF works with governments and non-governmental organizations on a range of issues from growth monitoring to prevention and management of childhood illness. At this time, UNICEF supports growth monitoring in health facilities and communities in more than 40 countries, generating information that is used by the immediate care takers and local health workers to assess child growth, analyse the causes of any problems that exist, and determine necessary action.

Providing nutrition in emergencies: Young children and pregnant and lactating mothers are extremely vulnerable in emergencies. UNICEF's foremost priority is to prevent death from starvation and disease and to reduce malnutrition by supporting therapeutic and supplementary feeding, providing essential micronutrients and feeding orphans. The long-term goal is always to work with communities to address the underlying problems that create these dire situations to prevent a future occurrence or to devise better coping strategies.

Nutrition and HIV: With HIV/AIDS, UNICEF's focus is two fold: reducing mother-to-child transmission of the virus during breastfeeding and meeting the nutritional needs of those who are HIV positive or affected by HIV/AIDS, such as orphans and children living in households where family members have HIV. Strategies include providing voluntary, confidential testing and infant feeding counselling for pregnant women, helping governments develop infant and young child feeding policies with HIV guidelines, encouraging and supporting breastfeeding, and promoting optimal infant feeding in hospitals.

Supporting community-based programmes: Families and communities are the key players in the battle against childhood malnutrition and must work together to assess, analyse and take action to solve any problems. UNICEF's strategy is to empower community members to become their own agents of change. UNICEF's role is to work with governments to support participatory, community-based programmes focussing on children's survival, growth and development.

The Tamil Nadu Integrated Nutrition programme in South India and the Iringa Programme in Tanzania are among the largest and most well known community-based child survival, growth and development programmes. Thailand, Cambodia, Indonesia, Sri Lanka, Bangladesh, Uganda, Kenya, Madagascar, Ghana, Niger, Oman, Brazil and others are working on similar programmes.

Related programming: UNICEF's programmes in the area of child and maternal health, basic education, water and sanitation, and improved child protection contribute to the reduction of child malnutrition.

The development of a milk supply within a country has also received UNICEF support. More than 200 milk processing plants in 41 countries, have been set up in cooperation with FAO. Fish farming, poultry raising, gardening, digging of wells, testing of protein mixtures and iodisation of salt in areas of endemic goitre prevailing are some of the programmes supported by UNICEF.

UNICEF depends entirely on voluntary contribution. Nearly three-fourth of its income comes from various governments. The rest comes from organisations and from individuals through the sale of greeting cards and other fund raising campaigns.

NATIONAL AGENCIES

INDIAN COUNCIL OF AGRICULTURAL RESEARCH

The ICAR is an autonomous apex national organisation. It was set up in 1929. The head office is at Krishi Bhavan, New Delhi. It operates through 46 Central Research Institutes, 4 National Bureaus, 10 Project Directorates, 27 National Research Centres, 90 All India Coordinated Research Projects, 261 Krishi Vigyan Kendras and 8 Training Centres.

From the past 74 years the Indian council of Agricultural Research has been striving for the development of agriculture at the national level through planning, promoting, conducting and coordinating research and education in agriculture. This is ensured by optimal utilisation of land, water and plant and animal genetic resource.

Salient Achievements

National Agricultural Technology Project (NATP): A World Bank aided project has made significant progress in agro-ecosystem research, innovation in technology, dissemination and organisation and management system. Two quality protein maize hybrids, Shaktiman–1 (for U.P and Bihar) and Shaktiman–2 (for Bihar) have been released. This will be a boon for removing protein malnutrition of people subsisting on maize.

Natural Resource Management: The addition of organic manure and zinc sulphate and growing of crops like green gram and groundnut reduced arsenic uptake in west Bengal.

Crop Science: The ICAR participated in the Yellow Revolution brought out through increased production of oil seeds. National Gene Bank of the NBPGR, Delhi, now holds more than 0.22 million accessions of plants. A total of 738 varieties in 15 crops have been finger-printed using recent molecular marker techniques. A super fine rice hybrid Pusa RH-10 and two scented varieties have been released. Technology for baby corn production in hills has been standardised.

Horticulture: India is the 2nd largest producer of fruits and vegetables after Brazil and China respectively in the world. India holds number one position in banana, mango and coconut production in the world. The technology for fruit based carbonated drinks on pilot plant scale has been developed. Various new promising varieties/hybrids in horticultural crop have been released. Medicinal mushroom, *Ganoderena lucldum* was successfully cultivated for the first time on saw dust and wheat straw substrates.

Animal Science: Technologies of instant kheer mix, probiotic cheese, cheddar cheese flavour base, mango – whey beverage and Jaljeera - whey beverage were developed. A test for detecting adulteration in cow's milk with buffalo milk was developed and is being used in various dairies and milk collection units.

Fisheries: Easy and effective polymerase chain reaction (PCR) technique for detection of white spot syndrome virus for all stages of shrimps has been developed. The rainbow trout, a fish of coldwater aquatic system, has been cultured successfully in the warmer agro-climatic condition of Uttaranchal. The break through has been achieved in the seed production and larvae rearing of sea cucumber-*Holothuria spinifera* for the first time in hatchery.

Agricultural Engineering: Tractor mounted till planter was developed which performs two operations simultaneously i.e., tilling and sowing. Rural soya milk enterprises was initiated at 4 places under NATP activity on Household food and Nutritional security, in which, the village women produced soyamilk and distributed sweetened milk to rural children. A soyamilk preparation facility was set up in village Gunga of district Bhopal.

Education : ICAR prepared 15 university level Text books with Indian data in agriculture and allied fields. ICAR brought uniformity of standards across 29 agricultural universities. It conducts summer and winter school, short courses and training, which benefits faculty members/scientists and provides senior research fellowship and National talent scholarships. A World Bank assisted project on the Agricultural Human Resource Development (AHRD) has been launched to improve the educational system in agriculture and meet its future challenges. M.Sc degree course in plant genetic resource has been introduced.

Agricultural Extension: The front line extension programmes implemented by ICAR include a network of Krishi Vigyan Kendras and establishment of Agricultural Technology Information Centre.

International Linkages : Work plan (2002) was signed between ICAR and International Water Management Institute, Colombo.

Publication: ICAR brings out a number of periodicals, news letters, bulletins and project reports.

INDIAN COUNCIL OF MEDICAL RESEARCH (ICMR)

The Indian Council of Medical Research, ICMR, New Delhi is the apex body in India for the formulation, coordination and promotion of biomedical research.

In 1911, the Government of India had set up Indian Research Fund Association (IRFA) for medical research. It was redesignated in 1949 as the Indian Council of Medical Research with expanded scope of functions. The ICMR is funded by the Government of India through the Ministry of Health and Family Welfare.

The Governing Body of the Council is presided over by the Union Health Minister. It is assisted in scientific and technical matters by a Scientific Advisory Board comprising eminent experts in different biomedical disciplines. The Board in its turn is assisted by a series of scientific advisory groups, expert groups, task forces and steering committees which evaluate and monitor different research activities of the Council.

The Council promotes biomedical research in the country through intramural as well as extramural research.

Intramural research is carried out currently through the Council's 21 permanent research institutes. They do research on specific areas such as tuberculosis, leprosy, cholera and diarrhoeal diseases, viral diseases including AIDs. They also do research on malaria, kala-azar, nutrition, food and drug toxicology, reproduction, immunohaematology, oncology and medical statistics.

Intramural research is also carried out through 6 Regional Medical Research Centres which concentrate on regional health problems.

Extramural research is promoted by ICMR through setting up advanced research centres in non-ICMR Research Institutes and Universities and Medical Colleges.

In addition to research activities, the ICMR encourages human resource development in biomedical research through research fellowships, short-term visiting fellowships, short-term research studentships. ICMR also conducts various training programmes and workshops. For retired medical scientists and teachers, the Council offers the position of Emeritus Scientist. At present, the Council offers 38 awards of which 11 are meant exclusively for young scientists.

In recent years, ICMR is also intensifying research in non-communicable diseases such as cardiovascular diseases, metabolic disorders, mental health problems, neurological disorders, blindness, liver diseases and cancer. Research on Traditional Medicine is also revived. Medical information is strengthened to meet the growing demands and needs of the biomedical community.

NATIONAL INSTITUTE OF NUTRITION

The National Institute of Nutrition, located at Hyderabad is one of the permanent research Institutes of the Indian Council of Medical Research under the ministry of Health and Family Welfare, Government of India. It was founded in 1918 as part of Coonoor Pasteur Institute.

The objectives of National Institute of Nutrition are:

- to identify various dietary and nutrition problems prevalent among different segments of the population and continuously monitor diet and nutrition situation of the country.
- to evolve suitable methods of prevention and control of nutrition problems through research, keeping the existing economic, social and administrative set up in view.
- to conduct operational research, to pave the way for planning and implementation of national nutrition programmes.

- to investigate nutritional deficiencies, nutrient interactions and food toxicities at basic level for understanding the biochemical mechanism involved.
- to provide training and orientation in nutrition to key health professionals.
- to disseminate authentic health and nutrition information through appropriate extension activities.
- to integrate the institute's research programmes with other health, agricultural and economic programmes as envisaged by the government.
- to advise governments and other organisations on problems of nutrition.

The institute's activities can be broadly categorised under four major heads.

Clinical studies

The clinical aspects of the Institute's work are carried out mostly in the three major teaching hospitals in the twin cities of Hyderabad and Secunderabad.

Presently, studies are being conducted on the role of intrauterine infections and vitamin nutritional status on the pregnancy outcome. Field studies are being conducted on the impact of women's work load on health and on survival of the under fives.

The paediatric unit is carrying out research on the interactions of nutrition immunity and infectious diseases of childhood. Efficacy of immunisation programmes in relation to the widely prevalent nutritional disorders like protein energy malnutrition and vitamin A deficiency have also been investigated.

Clinical studies in adults include nutritional disorders like pellagra and degenerative diseases like diabetes, cancer and cardiovascular diseases. This unit has also been engaged in studies on absorption, metabolism and toxicity of commonly used drugs in various deficiency states in both experimental animals and human beings.

Laboratory Studies

The Institute has excellent facilities for undertaking some of the most sophisticated laboratory investigations covering a wide range of specialities like biochemistry, food chemistry, pathology, immunology, hematology, microbiology, endocrinology, physiology and toxicology. Excellent facilities exist for laboratory animal breeding and experimentation.

Community Studies

A range of investigations in community nutrition and operational research are carried out in rural areas not only in Andhra Pradesh but in many other states as well. The Institute collaborates with the State and Central Governments and international agencies in planning and conducting diet and nutrition surveys, evaluating ongoing nutrition programmes and conducting studies on socio-cultural aspects of nutrition.

Recent studies include:

- relationship between vitamin A deficiency and child mortality.
- impact of community feeding programmes on the incidence of low birth weight infants.

- operational research on the off take of iron fortified salt through the fair price shops and its effect on prevalence of anaemia in the community.
- energy requirements of different groups have received special attention in view of their importance in planning national food strategy.
- body composition studies have also been initiated using a Whole Body Monitor.

Teaching Programmes

Though primarily a research oriented institution, teaching and training activities are also given priority. The Institute has been recognised as a centre for research leading to Ph.D and M.D. degrees by many Indian Universities. The Institute has been recognised by WHO as a centre for advanced training in health and nutrition.

At present the following courses are offered every year.

- Master of science.
- Certificate course in nutrition.
- Orientation course for Middle level personnel from Primary Health Care and Nutrition Programmes (sponsored by WHO/ICMR).
- Certificate course in Endocrinological techniques and their application.
- Advanced programme leading to Ph.D. biochemistry.

A number of ad hoc orientation programmes of short duration are also arranged for medical and public health administrators at the request of sponsoring authorities.

Publications are brought out on specific nutrition themes of importance to major target groups like auxiliary health workers, teachers, women and children. Publications such as "Nutritive value of Indian foods" "Nutrition for mother and child" "Your Health and Nutrition" "and "A manual of Nutrition" belong to this category.

NUTRITION FOUNDATION OF INDIA

Nutrition Foundation of India (NFI) was founded by Dr. C. Gopalan in 1980 with the active cooperation and support of a large body of scientists and leading citizens. NFI is a non-governmental, nonprofit, voluntary institution dedicated to the cause of eradication of undernutrition in the country. It is recognized officially by the Government of India as a "Scientific Research Body".

The foundation derives financial support for its activities from enlightened private donors and from national and international agencies interested in the improvement of nutritional status of populations. The Government of India's continued support and goodwill facilitated the growth of the foundation.

The objectives of NFI are as follows:

- Highlight and focus public and government attention on national problems related to malnutrition; assess their causation, magnitude and implications; and offer short term as well as long term action plans for their control.

- Initiate, conduct and support action oriented studies and research on these problems through existing institutes, university centres and other suitable bodies in order to evolve appropriate solutions capable of application in the current context.
- Investigate means to offset existing deficiencies in the pattern of production and distribution of foods and to ensure wholesomeness and nutritive value of foods sold for public consumption.
- Disseminate information on diet and nutrition, promote nutrition education in schools and through mass media, publish periodically a Bulletin in order to disseminate information on important facts of nutrition.
- Interact with the planning commission and governmental agencies to facilitate the formation, implementation and evaluation of nutrition programmes.

Some of the research projects undertaken by NFI are as follows:

- Investigation of current prevalence, nature and etiology of obesity in urban Delhi.
- Nutritional status and cognitive function in 3–10 year olds in Delhi slums.
- Low-cost technology for promotion of consumption of carotene rich foods.
- Control of anaemia in adolescent girls of poor communities.

The foundation has always recognised the fact that the growing knowledge regarding diet and nutrition should be widely disseminated to the public and play an important role in extension education.

Foundation has also set up a separate body which will deal with dietary and nutritional management of nutrition related chronic degenerative disease.

The publications of NFI are the Bulletin of the NFI, proceedings of the conferences and symposia being organised by the foundation, study circle meetings and the Director General's special lectures. NFI maintains an up-to-date library.

FOOD AND NUTRITION BOARD

The Food and Nutrition Board is under the Department of Women and Child Development. The FNB has a technical wing at the centre, 4 regional offices at Delhi, Mumbai, Kolkata and Chennai. It is engaged in its conventional activities as well as in new initiatives undertaken as a followup of National Nutrition Policy. Some of the important areas of FNB activities are as under.

Nutrition education and orientation: Nutrition education of the people in rural, urban and tribal areas is one of the primary activities of the infrastructure of FNB. Nutrition Demonstration programmes in rural, urban and tribal areas are organised by each of the 43 Community Food and Nutrition Extension Units (CFNEUS) in different states, 12,000 programmes benefiting about 5 lakh persons are organised annually.

Training in Home scale Preservation of fruits and vegetables: The CFNEUS impart education and training in home-scale preservation of fruits and vegetables to housewives and adolescent girls with a view to promote preservation and consumption of fruits and vegetables which could be useful for income generation purposes.

Monitoring of supplementary feeding under ICDS: The CFNEUS monitor the supplementary feeding component of ICDS in areas of their location, 6900 anganwadis are inspected by CFNEUS annually.

Development and distribution of educational/training material: Development, production and distribution of educational and training material on nutrition for use by grass root level functionaries and others agents of the Government is done by FNB. Efforts are made to promote nutrition facts about infants, pregnant and lactating women.

Mass awareness campaigns: FNB celebrates National events like World Breast Feeding week (1–7 August), National Nutrition week (1–7 September), World Food Day (16th October), Global Iodine Deficiency Disorders Day (21st October), Universal Children's day (14th November) in collaboration with concerned agencies by organising special programmes for creating nutritional awareness.

Mass Media Communication: Video spots and radio spots on infant nutrition have been developed. Newspaper supplements are given on topics like green leafy vegetables, malnutrition in 0–2 years and supplementary feedings. A radio sponsored programme on "Poshan our Swasthya" with 30 episodes on various aspects of nutrition has been prepared and is being launched shortly.

Advocacy and sensitization of policy makers and programme managers: Advocacy and sensitization of policy makers for integrating nutritional concerns in developmental programmes is a key issue for promoting nutrition of the people in the country. Regional workshops are planned for this.

Follow up action on National Nutrition Policy: A number of initiatives have been taken up since the National Nutrition Policy was adopted by Government of India in 1993. A National plan of Action on Nutrition was formulated and approved by the Inter Ministerial Coordination Committee and released in 1995. A task force on micronutrient deficiency like vitamin A and iron was constituted and details are worked to eradicate them.

The National Nutrition Mission aims at eradicating malnutrition in a time bound fashion. The three important areas for action are vigorous awareness campaign in malnutrition and its prevention, direct interventions for preventing malnutrition, nutrition monitoring, mapping and surveillance to be established in the country for reducing high levels of malnutrition.

CENTRAL FOOD TECHNOLOGICAL RESEARCH INSTITUTE

Central Food Technological Research Institute (CFTRI), Mysore, is a constituent laboratory of the Council of Scientific and the Industrial Research, New Delhi. This institute popularly known as CFTRI was on 21st October 1950. Through its Research and Development programmes it seeks to promote and aid the conservation of food resources and maximise the utilization and value addition for the economic growth and thereby contribute to ultimate food security through science and technology.

While the main campus and headquarters of CFTRI is located at Mysore, the region specific Research and Development problems are investigated and solutions offered at the CFTRI Regional Centres located at Bombay, Hyderabad, Lucknow, Ludhiana, Mangalore and Nagpur.

The 15 Research and Development departments at CFTRI have been created to be the centres of excellence in every discipline of food science and technology. The Research and Development is ably supported by specific departments of Technical Assistance, Technology Transfer, Analytical and Advisory Assistance and Certification of Quality, Information and Database. Manpower Training is given special attention as a part of industrial services.

Technology Transfer

CFTRI transfers classified technologies against a prescribed fee for each process. Apart from this, it also offers services, namely, answering of technical enquiries, advise and counselling at the Institute and its Regional Centres through preparation of technical reports, techno-economic feasibility reports; project engineering reports; evaluation/appraisal of project/feasibility reports; consumer acceptability studies; resource and techno-economic surveys; research and development project evaluation of packaging materials, analysis and quality control guidance; sponsored research and development projects; general technical consultancy; advisory consultancy and engineering consultancy for food industry; sensory evaluation and consumer acceptance of food products; and selected turnkey projects.

Human Resource Development

A 2 year M.Sc. (Food Tech.) programme is conducted by the Institute, affiliated to the University of Mysore. Students trained by the qualified and trained food technologists will cater to the needs of industry in India and other developing countries. Numerous national and international short-term refresher courses are organized for technical personnel from the industry in order to update the skills of candidates already working in industry as well as to create new entrepreneurship.

A 10– month course in Milling Technology trains personnel from India and other developing countries in flour milling technologies. Doctoral programmes in food science and technology are offered to the institute staff, Research fellows and Faculty members of University. M.Sc. Food Science by Research for employees of CFTRI and other Research and Development organizations is being conducted to improve the knowledge and expertise and career prospects in R & D are also included in HRD programmes.

Some Important Industrial Services

These include, Project identification and evaluation; Preparation of industrial feasibility and project reports for processes and products; Technoeconomic and pre-investment surveys; Resource inventories; Project engineering and design; Identification of post-harvest problems of regional food materials; Market research related to Processed foods; Assistance in process control; Quality assurance; Packaging; Product diversification as well as machinery selection and installation, commissioning and operation of plants and operational research in food industries. These services are undertaken on a prescribed fee.

CFTRI publishes books, monographs, directories and annotated bibliographies and publishes 3 periodicals; Food Technology (Monthly), Food Digest (Quarterly) and Food Patents (Quarterly).

CFTRI offers a variety of technologies in post-harvest handling, storage and processing of food. Over 300 processes have been developed in Food Science and Technology and allied fields.

NATIONAL NUTRITION MONITORING BUREAU

NNMB was set up by ICMR in the year 1972 in 10 states with the Central References Laboratory (CRL) at NIN, Hyderabad.

The objectives of NNMB are :

- To collect data on dietary intakes and nutritional status of the population on a continuous basis.
- To evaluate the ongoing national nutrition programmes. In addition to coordinating the activities of the state units, CRL is also responsible for sampling, training, supervision and analysis of the data. Linkages with the National sample survey organisation have also been forged. At present there are 10 units of NNMB in different states.

The NNMB has evaluated the following nutrition programmes and published the findings as special reports.

- Vitamin A prophylaxis programme, 1977-78.
- Applied Nutrition Programme, 1977-78.
- Indian Population Project, Karnataka, 1979.
- Special Nutrition Programme, 1979-80.
- World food-assisted feeding Programme, 1981-82.
- National Anaemia Prophylaxis Programme, 1986-87.

The evaluation reports published by NNMB have helped in identifying the corrective steps which need to be taken with respect to the vitamin A prophylaxis Programme, the Special Nutrition Pogramme and the world food-assisted feeding programme. It also identified the basic weakness in the Applied Nutrition Programme-the ineffective education component.

CHILD SURVIVAL AND STATE MOTHERHOOD PROGRAMME (CSSM)

In 1992, Child Survival and State Motherhood Programme was implemented with financial assistance from World Bank and UNICEF. It has the following objectives:

- Sustaining and strengthening the ongoing Universal Immunisation Programme; continuing ORT Programme for Children below the age of 5 years; introducing and expanding the programme for control of acute respiratory infection for children below 5 years of age.
- Universalising the existing prophylaxis scheme for control of blindness due to deficiency of vitamin A for children up to the age of three years and prophylaxis scheme against nutritional anaemia among pregnant and lactating women as well as children upto 5 years of age through administration of iron and folic acid tablets.
- Improving new born care and maternal care at the community level.

In addition to continuing supply of vaccines, cold chain equipment, needles and syringes, ORS packets are supplied to control diarrhoea induced dehydration. The programme includes training of peripheral level health worker on recognition of pneumonia and treatment with cotrimoxazole. The drug is being supplied to the health worker through CSSM drug kit.

The CSSM programme has given priority to anaemia control measure and massive vitamin A doses programme. The CSSM Programme accords high priority to speeding up the training of traditional birth attendants.

CENTRAL SOCIAL WELFARE BOARD

The Central Social Welfare Board was set up by the Government of India in 1953. CSWB is an autonomous organisation under the Ministry of Education. It is the first organisation in post independent era to achieve people participation for implementing welfare programmes for women and children. Its motto is to implement welfare programmes for women and children through voluntary organisation.

Activities

Condense Courses of Education and Vocational Training: Under CCE, a two year course is conducted for women aged above 15 to pass secondary, middle and primary level examination. Under VT deserving women are given training in vocations such as draft designing, computer courses, type setting, batik, handloom, weaving, nursery teacher training and stenography.

Awareness: An awareness of various social issues is created so that they can realise their potential in the family and society.

Socio Economic Programmes: Under SEP, voluntary organisations are given financial assistance to take variety of income generating activities like industrial components ancillary units, handicrafts, sericulture and vegetable and fish vending.

Voluntary Action Bureau and Family Counselling Centres: They provide preventive and rehabilitation services to women and children who are victims of family maladjustments and atrocities.

Mahila Mandal Programmes: It is a decentralised programme of the board and it is run by state board. In those areas where there is no voluntary organisation to take up welfare service for women and children, they help in promoting and setting up social welfare organisation on voluntary basis.

Balwadi's Nutritional Programme: Under this scheme, supplementary foods, health education and recreation facilities are provided to children of 3–5 years belonging to low income families.

Innovative schemes: Special group of women and children like mentally retarded children, children of prostitutes and widows are helped.

Supportive service: They provide day care centres to the children of mothers from low income group families who are working or ailing. The Board gives assistance to voluntary organisation for running working women's hostel.

CSWB monitors and evaluates the schemes being implemented in the state. They also organise play centres for children.

CSWB brings out two publications in Hindi 'Samaj Kalyan' and in English 'Social Welfare'.

NUTRITION SOCIETY OF INDIA

The Nutrition Society of India (NSI) is an organization dedicated to keep abreast of the latest developments in the basic and applied aspects of Science of Nutrition. Established in 1965 at the National Institute of Nutrition, Hyderabad, the Society continues to analyse issues related to the diverse aspects of nutrition. The Society activities involve scientists, programmers and policy makers throughout the country and abroad who are working in the field. Through its

Annual Conference, the Society provides a forum for new ideas, encourages innovations, recognizes important research findings, increases awareness of the latest survey data and promotes action programmes.

COSTED — IDA Information Centre

The Indian Dietetic Association has approached COSTED (Committee on Science and Technology in Developing Countries) which has facilities to store information and retrieve the same, for collaboration to run an information centre. COSTED has agreed to collaborate and allow the centre to be established in COSTED Office.

The Centre will :

- Collect information on Dietetics from different chapters and Dietetic associations abroad and store in the computer.
- Publish Dietetics Newsletter.
- Run refresher course for dietitians every year.
- Prepare booklets for different courses for Registration Board Examination.
- Maintain question bank for Registration Board Examination and supply question papers when required.

QUESTIONS

1. Explain the functions of WHO.
2. Discuss the achievements of UNICEF in relation to nutrition.
3. What is FAO? How is it helping in preventing malnutrition?
4. Explain the role of ICMR in alleviating malnutrition.
5. Explain the contributions of NIN.
6. Who founded NFI? Explain its objectives and projects it has under taken.
7. Under which department does FNB come? What is the contribution of FNB?
8. Explain CFTRI under the following:

   Related industrial services

   Technology transfer

   Human Resource Development.
9. How does ICAR help in combating malnutrition in India?
10. Explain the role of following agencies in combating malnutrition.

    CSSM, NNMB, CSWB.

SUGGESTED READINGS

- Food and Agriculture Organisation : www.fao.org
- World Health Organisation : www.who.org/nut
- UN World Food Programme : www.wfp.org
- World Bank : www.worldbank.org

CHAPTER 24

COMPUTERS IN MANAGEMENT OF NUTRITION PRACTICE

Computer applications have multiplied so rapidly that the heart of its technology — tiny miracle chips—now touch almost all aspects of our lives. Computer literacy is becoming increasingly essential not only in personal lives but also in professional practice. In healthcare and nutritional care in particular, management information systems require both the development of the components to meet our needs and our ability to use them with skill and wisdom.

GENERAL INFORMATION

Data input

The computer can store large amounts of data, depending on its capacity. These data then are in the computer's memory for use according to need. These pieces of information may be in the form of numbers or words, as well as directors for use of these units.

Data output

Whether called up to be viewed upon a screen or printed out as hard copy, the computer output is made up of pieces of data that it gives back to the user. Stored data may be retrieved for use or data analysis results from a task performed by the computer or the initial data stored may be returned.

Data Analysis

The computer can perform a number of functions on data it has received from the user. It can sort, file, tabulate, calculate, edit, rewrite, reformat, compare, contrast, project cost and plan according to "what if" scenarios provided.

Data Communication

Anyone with a personal computer can send messages via "electronic mail" to another person with a computer by use of a MODEM (telephone hook up) and dialling one of the several nation wide "electronic mail box" networks. Also a local network of personal computers at various work stations may be set up in almost any environment, thus sharing data and equipment with gains in productivity and economy. Connections may also be made between computers and a large main frame computer within an organisation, thus unlocking the larger power of the mainframe computer for wider use.

By and large, the type of tasks required to be done by a computer in providing nutritional services may include the following:

Business Management: Whether the activity is food service or patient care, business management principles must underlie its operation. These include fiscal responsibility, such as accounting, forecasting, budgets and cost control and working activities including both material and human resources.

Primary client / patient care: Business management principles again are involved in handling cost-effectiveness studies, program planning and evaluation.

Education: Computer assisted instruction finds use in both patient education and professional / staff education as well as employee training.

Research: Activities concerning clinical problems and the most cost effective methods of providing services are necessary working activities.

Writing: Word-processing capabilities of the computer provide support for a variety of writing tasks including records and reports, communications, articles or educational materials and books.

Historically, the earliest and most extensive applications of computer managed services in nutrition and dietetics have been in the area of food service systems. However, many other areas of application in clinical nutrition practice, community nutrition, nutrition education and research are currently developing.

CLINICAL CARE

A first basic area of computer application in nutrition practice is in clinical care in the hospital setting. The clinician is constantly involved in the basic aspects of patient care assessment, analysis, intervention, implementation and evaluation. The patient care team uses computer management system in constantly coordinating communications. This is essential in planning all aspects of patient care, including nutritional assessment and support services, nutritional analysis and nutritional therapy.

Communication in Patient Care

Computer system has applications in various aspects of patient care
- storage and retrieval of clinical and statistical data
- a base of educational materials that may be consulted in patient care problems.
- guidance for patient care planning
- patient care audits to ensure quality standards and
- clinical research

In addition to the dietary order entry module, additional applications modules in the system support patient care; clinic scheduling / patient registration, census, financial management, clinical laboratory, electrocardiogram, medical record abstracting etc.

Nutritional assessment and support services: A broad range of anthropometric, biochemical, clinical and historical data is gathered in the process of the required comprehensive nutritional assessment involved. The computer can quickly analyse these data so that the nutrition support team can screen and identify patients at risk, institute therapy and monitor individual patients closely.

Nutrition analysis: Nutrition analysis of diets is an important basis of comprehensive nutritional assessment. Computerised nutrient analysis enables primary care clinical dietitian to obtain the necessary detailed individual patients nutrient information with speed and relative accuracy and generate reports via data processing.

Such rapid practical data processing through the computer system allows the nutrition practitioner to spend more professional time with other nutritional assessment work as well as personal interaction with the patient.

Nutritional Therapy

In the hospital setting, computerised medical records provide a basis for the nutrition staff to analyse comparative therapy for various conditions in the light of implications for nutritional status of patients and contribution to healing. The widespread hospital malnutrition of past years has been well documented.

In the special units of critical care within the hospital setting such as burn units, clinicians use continuous computer graphic programmes to monitor the nutritional status of critically ill patients. The nutrition - support team can quickly evaluate continuous nutritional needs and plan effective patient care. These bedside graphs also motivate patients and their families to work closely with the clinical dietitians to facilitate progression from a negative nutritional balance to a positive balance in early catabolic periods following massive injury.

COMMUNITY NUTRITION

This work involves surveys, special projects, nutritional counselling, and programme planning.

Nutrition Surveys

Various population surveys provide data for identifying nutrition needs and planning programmes to help meet these needs. Such surveys are conducted at both national and local levels. With the recent development of an optical scanning process, survey data may be read rapidly by the Optical Character Reader. It is now used by public health departments for health surveillance of population groups.

Programme-planning: Using the data from community population surveys, public health nutritionists are able to assess particular community needs and base programme planning on these identical needs. Computers are used in such analysis of data.

Nutrition Counselling: To meet special nutritional therapy needs in client - centered counselling, computer assisted programmes are developed for special clinical problems such as diabetes or hyperlipidemia. In addition to dietary analysis and calculation of individual nutrition prescription, computer-planned menus for these clients can be generated and ongoing care can be monitored.

Special nutrient data bases are constructed for such specific nutritional therapy purposes. For example, a data base used with hyperlipidemia, clients would not only list values for kilocalories, protein and carbohydrate but also give specific ratios of the total fat in terms of saturated, monounsaturated and polyunsaturated fatty acids and cholesterol. Using such a computerised nutrient data storage with an interactive retrieval programme, clinical nutritionists are able to diagnose various eating problems of their clients and plan and implement their specific food plan. The practitioner may use such an interactive retrieval system directly while interviewing clients or for followup computing of nutrient values in individual food records, family menus and recipes.

This learning process takes place in both formal school settings and in general healthcare agencies.

Impact of educational technology: Over the next few decades, society will increasingly rely on the computer to collect, distribute and control massive amounts of information economically.

An electronic classroom: All questions, answers, homework and project reports as well as student team messages are sent through the computer and "posted" on the electronic bulletin board for all to read. The student papers are critically evaluated by the professor on a word processor with comments written into the paper itself. Multiple copies of all instructional documents are sent to all students electronically. Students log on daily to read the bulletin board and to get any specific messages. Many messages are transmitted back and forth including notes for the bulletin board, problem statements, queries of the system staff, short assignments, team projects, messages to other faculty and others.

The computer bulletin board serves as a central information point, and its data are always available, which is especially important to students who lost assignments or who missed class. The professor is able to answer questions immediately so that students with difficulties can continue their projects without delay and assignments could be submitted in return from several locations at any hour. Through these techniques, a strong group sense is created and individualised instruction is made available according to student need.

Professional Nutrition Education

Computers combined with other audiovisual instruction techniques are used for self paced courses in nutrition offered to dietetic, nutrition, nursing and premedical students. Computer simulated clinical encounters have been used in clinical nutrition courses and found to be effective in comparison with hospital based clinical experiences. Such simulation includes a medical record with nursing care cardex for a patient, an interview with the patient, a formulatory and a nutrient catalogue. The instructor gets a printout reporting the student's knowledge, responses to inquiries concerning the patient and organisation of the clinical encounter thus enabling the instructor to meet individual student needs.

The potential use of computers in nutrition-related education is found to encompass four areas:

- Instruction — drill, practice and dialogues
- Real-life simulations
- Hypothesis/idea testing - building process models
- Reduction of computational labour.

Investigators recommend that at the minimum, students should be exposed to courses dealing with computers and information processing, especially with use of microprocessors, for the wave of the future is in wide spread multi use computers.

Patient/client education: Computer assisted learning is used in a variety of ways in private practice, clinics and hospitals for patient/client education in healthcare. For example a computer and a programme can be used to develop a programme in diabetes education that does not require constant surveillance by the health professional. In addition to such specific programmes written by nutritionists to meet special learning needs, a number of general diet and exercise programmes are available for use in professional healthcare services.

Consumer education: In future computers may become a major tool for both food marketing and client nutrition education. Consumers can view the entire product lists of grocery stores on the monitor, compare prices and select the local store offering the lowest total cost of the day. Payment transaction can also be done through computer. Reductions of in-store advertising and resultant impulse buying would drastically affect food company marketing programmes. 'User friendly' ordering will offer the consumer the advantages of reduced shopping time and product costs. Opportunity for involvement of consumer nutrition education in such programmes is indeed vast.

NUTRITION RESEARCH

General research projects can be greatly assisted by computers. In metabolic clinical research, for example, the diets used must satisfy both the nutrient specifications of the research protocol and satisfy the individual subject's nutrient requirements and preferences. Computer based nutrition research involves selecting and using data bases, developing literature search strategies and writing resulting reports.

Use of Data base: More information is available through a computer terminal than in any library in the world. A number of computerised nutrient data banks are available for use in nutrient analysis, surveys and research projects. In addition, a large number of data bases exist for searching the scientific literature, on any desired topic such as EXCERPTA MEDICA and MEDLINE, CINAHC, AGRICOLA, BIOSIS, SCISEARCH etc. These files make available a variety of materials including scientific journal articles, monographs, proceedings of conferences and many other documents. Bibliographic and referral data bases can be searched via one or more of the three major, information service vendors. DIALOG, BRS etc. Proliferating traditional scientific journals have become increasingly specialised and expensive. Electronic journals give speedy scientific reports.

Report writing: Any writing of scientific reports or educational materials for professional students as well as the public is facilitated by use of word processing. Such programmes allow for initial drafts to be filed with the necessary follow-up work of revising, proof reading and editing accomplished much more quickly.

Computer communication can be grouped under two headings—stand-alone and on-line application.

STAND-ALONE APPLICATIONS

'Stand-alone' applications are computer programmes that run without connection to a network or modem. These applications have been designed to provide information and training in nutrition education for the public, the paraprofessional and the professional. The major types of programmes designed for both professionals and consumers include data collection, nutrition analysis, food service and recipe management. Those programmes which help in analysing nutrient intake are welcomed by researchers and dieticians who found that these programmes significantly reduced both the time and efforts of calculating intake.

Nutrient Analysis: The programme calculates the nutrient intake of individuals or groups of individuals and compares it to a nutrient standards. Computerised database for food consumption information are available from FAO on well as other international organisations. The International Network of Food Data Systems (INFOODS) has food composition databases organized for regions of the world.

Programmes that analyse nutrient intake are useful for researchers and hospital dietitians. They found computerised nutrient analysis significantly reduced both the time and effort of calculating intakes using calculators and food composition books.

The programmes have been used extensively for classroom assignments from elementary through medical school students and have been offered as a nutrition education service in shopping malls and health fairs, in science exhibits and by public health professionals, fitness trainers, food scientists and food service professionals. The programmes are used in physician offices as part of a medical assessment or nutrition counselling session. The popularity of these diet analysis programmes continues to grow as consumers become aware of the relationships between food intake and health and want to tailor their own dietary intake (e.g., to be lower/higher in calories or fat).

The effectiveness of these programmes in computing nutrient intake for research and education purposes, identifying nutrient excesses and deficiencies, and teaching food composition to varied audiences is well documented. The speed of calculation has allowed nutrient analysis is to be used more frequently in education and counselling settings.

Food Frequency Questionnaires: The FFQ is a short-cut method for collecting information about dietary intake. First, computerised software made it possible to easily estimate reliable nutrient intakes.

"Nutrition Discovery" is a CD-ROM available. It is based on the health habits and history questionnaire, dietary analysis system. Rather than selecting from a list of foods, the user identifies the foods eaten from 100 food items shown in colour on the screen. The user is asked the quantity and frequency of only those foods selected.

It is expected that multimedia programmes when compared with pencil and paper or partially automated questionnaires will result in more reliable data because serving sizes are represented better. The programme also allows collection of dietary data when the expert interviewer is unavailable or unaffordable.

Food Service and Recipe Management, Menu Planning: Basic software programmes used for nutrient analyses are used for these functions. Additional functions generate nutrient analyses, costing and quantity conversion of recipes, food production reports, inventory listing and purchasing.

One example of a consumer version of menu-planning multimedia software delivered on floppy disk is "Ready, set, Dinner". This software was developed for use in a communication programme designed to increase the consumption of fresh potatoes. Multimedia menu-planning software allows the users to easily search a library of 40 recipes, create menus and shopping lists, find nutrition information, use graphics, music and animation.

Nutritionists suggest that this type of programme may help individuals follow dietary guidelines. The programme demonstrates a benefit of computer application, that is, providing information when and where the public wants it.

Clinical Nutrition

Assessment tools: Applications that use computer capabilities in calculation and data management are widely available. Software for desk-top computers and programmes for hand–held computers are useful for many formulas used in nutrition assessment, including basal metabolic energy needs, Body Mass Index, desirable body weight, nitrogen and diabetic food exchanges. These tools are useful in hospital and community research and service settings. They allow the use of more precise calculations rather than "rule of thumb" calculations with fewer errors in making decisions about nutrition care. These tools can be less cumbersome than manuals.

Nutrient Drug interaction: This software is an example of a specialized data base for clinical nutrition. It allows the users to quickly assess any nutrients that may be compromised with a medication regimen. These aids make it more likely that interactions will be considered when prescribing medicines.

Patient education: Programmes to provide dietary information and education to patients are available for individuals with diabetes, hypertension heart disease and complex medication regimens. These programmes teach about causes of the disease, symptoms, complications, dietary management and menu-planning.

Computer-assisted instruction for health professionals: The nutrition programmes available generally include content such as the relationship of diet to a disease, components of nutritional assessment, diet history methods and patient case studies. Users have found text-on-screen applications valuable for the immediate feedback provided by drills and quizzes.

Text-on-Screen Examples: "Nutrition and the Practicing physician" (1994) is an example of a computer assisted instruction programme that addresses both the prevention and management of disease including obesity, hypertension, diabetes and lipid disorders. The programme provides nutrition information and counselling strategies known to foster a positive physician/patient relationship.

Multimedia Examples: One of the few nutrition interactive videodisc programmes produced is "cardio vascular health: Focus on Nutrition, Fitness and Smokings cessation" (Kolasa and Jobe, 1994). The technology is used for role modelling. Physicians are seen completing nutrition assessments and counselling their patients in ambulatory clinics. This is useful if subject matter experts are scarce.

Application to Distance Learning: Computer assisted instruction CAI is a distance learning approach. Computer based case studies teach the learner nutrition assessment practices, perform assessment tasks and interpret results. Here the lecturer becomes a guide.

Food and Nutrition Education Instructional Programmes and Games

For children delivered on floppy disk. For school going children an interactive programme "ship to shore" is devised. The programme, delivered on floppy disk, uses nutrition as the vehicle to integrate math, science, language arts and social studies for late elementary school age children. Students take the part of apprentices to Christopher Columbus and face a series of decisions about their food supply while sailing from Europe to the New World.

For children, delivered on CD-ROM. One of the most popular and widely distributed CD-ROM programmes is the "5-A-day-adventures" (Dole Food Co., 1994). It includes activities about nutrients in fruits and vegetabls, serving sizes, label reading, simple recipes and making salads.

"Dr. Health' n stein's Body Fun" (Cancer Research foundation of America, 1994) is a child's multimedia CD-ROM programme that is an adventure game and fantasy programme to encourage healthy choices and promote a life time of fitness and health.

For adults, delivered by interactive videodisc. "Stamp smart" is an effort to teach low fat, low cholesterol and high vegetable diets to women who receive food stamps.

"Health talk" is an example of a multimedia programme designed for low literacy populations (Strecher et al, 1993). It collects dietary information, processes it to create a computer personalised educational and behavioural change programme tailored to specific dietary and life style factors of the users.

Other kiosk applications. Several programmes described above either have been or could be delivered using a kiosk. Interactive kiosks that dispense information, coupons, recipes are increasing in popularity in the U.S. Kiosks are successful delivery systems, when requests for information are predictable.

Production Tools

Computer tailored messages: Word processing and desk-top publishing software enable nutrition educators without computer programming expertise to develop print materials personalised for their audiences. The programme eliminates extraneous material and presents only the information most relevant to the user.

Tailoring graphics for Nutrition Education: The American Dietetic Association prepared and distributed floppy disks with patient education handouts in files. Nutrition education programme developers could use this approach to design materials that would be tailored and printed at the delivery site.

Clip art and photo collections: Users can access professional art illustrations at low cost. These programmes can produce the graphics for print or slide or computer presentation.

Reading level evaluation: Nutrition educators use software programmes to evaluate reading grade. Electronic publishing improves access to information.

Presentation software: Presentation software allows nutrition educators with multimedia computers to enhance their presentations by incorporating visuals, sound, animation, texts and video. Nutrition instructors at many colleges and universities are beginning to use presentation programmes to enhance their lectures.

Nutrient Database

The U.S. Department of agriculture has just made it easier for people with palm pilots and other hand held personal digital assistants (PDAs) to maintain healthy diets while on the go. The National Nutrient Database of more than 6,000 food items can now be downloaded into PDAs, making nutrient information as easily accessible as the PDAs' calendars and calculators.

The database programme, which is categorized by food groups, allows users to scroll through an alphabetised list of foods and gives consumers information on approximately 30 nutrients in each food listed. It also includes a handy "portion modifier" feature that allows consumers to adjust the given portion size, either upwards or downwards, to the portion size that they would ordinarily eat.

Doctors can also use the database to recommend low-sodium foods to patients with heart conditions or to help their patients choose foods that are appropriate for their weight loss plan.

The database will also soon be available for down loading on to personal computers. Consumers who own hand-held personal digital assistants with the palm operating system can download the software in about 30 seconds from www.nal. usda.gov/fnic/foodcomp.

ON-LINE APPLICATION

On the web, one can be a seeker or a provider of information. Nutrition educators from different parts of the world are using e-mail to exchange ideas, projects and data easily, quickly and inexpensively. The Internet has become a very popular forum of communication, which allows researchers to carry out surveys. Discussion groups and chat rooms on specialised nutrition issues could be created to exchange ideas and seek solutions. The advantage is the informality that goes with it and all this happens in real time irrespective of distances. Using multimedia and web, nutritional brochures could be designed attractively and meaningfully and distributed instantaneously to a large group. Web offers not only freedom but also privacy. Information could be protected using passwords at will.

Nutrition on Web

Nutrition on web is a mind-boggling load of information that can be used to seek answers to almost any nutritional topic. Web can be a very useful tool to supplement the efforts of paranutritionists and to help remote healthcare centres. Though initial investment of establishing networks, at village, mandal, district and state levels, may seem discouraging in terms of finances and training, the investment could definitely pay off in forecasting and preventing nutrition related problems. Nutrition web would have to be run by professionals in the field of nutrition science. The site can develop programmes catering to school children, illiterate people, senior citizens, clinicians and paraprofessionals.

There are several computer based programmes on nutrition which are interactive, informative and interesting. 'Nutrition Discovery' for example is a CD-ROM based programme which evaluates an individual's nutritional intake and quality of diet in an engaging and interesting way. This programme presents food items as we see them in a super market and helps and reminds of all the food items consumed. Based on USDA's (United States Department of Agriculture) food guide pyramid and National Cancer Institute's Dietary Analysis system, this programme calculates individual's nutritional intake and suggests alternate foods.

There are many sites on nutrition accessible to us.

Web sites for Nutrition

1. General Resources

a.	Wadsworth Nutrition Resource Center	: www.wadsworth.com/nutrition
b.	The Tuffs University Nutrition Navigation	: www.navigator.tuffs.edu.
c.	US Government Healthfinder	: www.healthfinder.gov.
d.	American Dietetic Association	: www.eatright.org/
e.	Health Canada Nutrition	: www.hc-sc.gc.ca/hppb/nutrition/
f.	Thrive Online	: www.thriveonline.com/nutrition/index.html
g.	AMA Health Insight's Nutritional Basics	: www.ama-assn.org/insighVgen_hlth/
		: nutrinfo/nutrinfo.htm
h.	Personalised Counselling	: www.nutricise.com
i.	Healthy recipes, dictionary	: www.foodfit.com
j.	Health and Nutrition store	: www.thenutritionconnection.com
k.	Keeping fit	: www.naturalhub.com
l.	Dietary analysis	: www.nutrigenie.biz/products.html
m.	Nutrition Research	: www.nutrition.org

2. Nutrition Searches

a.	FDA Search	: www.fda.gov/search.html
b.	VSDA Search	: www.vsda.gov/searth/index.htm
c.	About.com: Nutrition	: Nutrition about.com
d.	The Blonz Guide	: www.blonz.com
e.	Arbor Nutrition	: arborcom.com
f.	Lifelines Nutrition and Fitness Links	: www.lifelines.com/ntnlnk.html

3. Nutrition Standards and Guidelines

a.	Food and Drug Administration	: www.fda.gov
b.	USDA Dietary Guidelines	: www.nal.usda.govlfnic/dga
c.	USDA Food Guide Pyramid	: www.nal.usda.gov/fnic/Fpyr/pyramid.html
d.	American Diabetes Association	: www.diabetes.org
e.	International Food Information Council	: ificinfo.health.org/infofsn.htm
f.	5 a Day for Better Health	: www.5aday.com
g.	Health Canada on line	: www hc-sc.gc.ca/english/food.htm + guide

4. The Nutrient

a.	American Diabetes Association	: www.diabetes.org
b.	International Food Information Council	: ificinfo-health-org/infofsn.htm
c.	FDA: Information about Dietary Supplements	: vm.cfsan.fda.gov/idms/supplmnt.html
d.	American Society for Nutritional Sciences Nutrient Information	: www.fascb.org/asns/intro.html
e.	NIH Osteoporosis and Related Bone Disorders National Resource Center	: www.osteo.org
f.	Iron Overload Diseases Association	: www.ironoverload.org
g.	Vitamin Update	: bookman.com.au/vitamins
h.	Vitamin and Mineral Guide	: www.thriveonline.com/eats/vitamins/ guide.index.html

5. Vegetarianism

a.	Vegetarian Resource Group	: www.vrg.org
b.	Vegetarian Pager	: www.veg.org/veg/

6. Diet and Health

a.	National Library of Medicine	: www.ncbi.nlm.nih.gov/PubMed
b.	Mayo Clinic Nutrition Center	: www.mayohealth.org/mayo/common/htm/ dietpage.htm
c.	Flax Council of Canada	: www.flax council.ca
d.	National Center for Complementary and Alternative Medicine	: nccam.nih.gov
e.	The Alternative Medicine Home Page	: www.pitt.edu/ncbw/altm.html
f.	Alternative Health News Online	: www.altmedicine.com/
g.	The International Food Information Council	: ificinfo.health.org/index.htm
h.	National Council Against Health Fraud	: www.ncahf.org
i.	Stephen Barrett's Ouackwatch	: www.quackwatch.com

7. Energy Balance and Weight Control

a.	Shape up America	: www.shapeup.org/sua
b.	American Anoreocia Bulimia Association	: www.aabainc.org
c.	Calories in Foods and Beverages	: www.nal.usda.gov/fnic/food comp
d.	Nutrition & Weight Maintenance	: www.niddk.nih.gov/health/nutrit/nutrit.htm
e.	Center for Drug Evaluation and Research (weight loss drugs)	: www.fda.gov/cder
f.	AMA Health Insight's Personal Nutritionist	: www.ama-assn.org/insightgen_hlth/pemutri/ permutri.htm

8. Nutrition and Physical Activity

a.	American College of Sports Medicine	: www.acsm.org
b.	Surgeon General's Report on Physical Activity	: www.cdc.gov/nccdphp/sgr/sgr.htm
c.	President's Council on Fitness & Sports	: www.whitehouse.gov/WH/PCPFS/html/ fitnet.html
d.	AMA Health Insight's Fitness Basics fitness/	: www.ama-assn.org/insightigen_hlth/ fitness.htm

| e. | Gatorade Sports Science Institute | : www.gssiweb.com |
| f. | Sports Science News | : www.sportsci.org |

9.   Nutrition and Disease Prevention

a.	CDC: National Center for Chronic Disease Prevention and Health Promoter	: www.cdc.gov/nccdphp
b.	National Institute of Health	: www.Nih.gov/od/oar
c.	American Heart Association	: www.americanheart.org
d.	Heart Information Network	: www.heartinfo.org
e.	National Heart, Lung and Blood Institute	: www.nh lbi.nih.gov/index.htm
f.	Heart & Stroke Foundation of Canada	: www.hsf.ca/
g.	National Stroke Association	: www.stroke.org
h.	American Cancer Society	: www.cancer.org
i.	American Institute for cancer Research	: www.aicr.org
j.	Dash Research Homepage	: dash.hwh.harvard.edu
k.	ANA Nutrition Fact Sheet: HIV/AIDS	: www.eatright.orglnfs42.html

10.   Life Cycle Nutrition

a.	La Leche League International	: www.lalecheleague.org
b.	USDA: Food and Nutrition Service	: www.fns.usda.gov/fns
c.	Mayo Health Clinic	: www.mayohealth.org
d.	American Health Association	: www.american heart.org
e.	March of Dimes	: www.modimes.org
f.	National Organization on Fetal Alcohol Syndrome	: www.nofas.org

Computer can do many jobs in handling a wealth of information in numbers and words to reshape our work, relieve us of tedious labour and provide greater opportunity to work directly with our patients and clients. What computers cannot do is supply the human factor. We need to learn how to use these revolutionary tools with skill and wisdom in providing sensitive, sound and humanistic healthcare.

QUESTIONS

1. Describe several different types of computer applications for management of clinical nutrition support services for hospitalized patients. What are the roles for the clinical nutritionist?

2. How would you use computer technology in doing a nutritional assessment for a hospitalized patient at risk for malnutrition?

3. What are nutrient data banks? How are they used?

4. Describe possible computer applications in nutrition education.

5. How would you use an interactive programme in nutrition counselling activities?

6. What are the computer resources available for nutrition research? How are they used?

7. What are Stand-alone application?

8. Explain on-line applications.

9. Computers are trendsetters of modern meal pattern. Justify.
10. Name five websites that can be used to get information on nutrients.

SUGGESTED READING

- Wang Samual J.A. Cost benefit analysis of Electronic Medical Records in Primary care, The American Journal of Medicine, 114, 2003.
- Clark. M. et al, Development and evaluation of computer based system for directory management of hyperilimedia, J Am Dict Assoc. 97, 1997.

APPENDICES

APPENDIX–1

Conversion Factors

I. Volume and weight conversions

1 Tbsp	= 3 tsp
2 Tbsp	= 1 fluid ounce
4 Tbsp	= ¼ cup
1 quart	= 2 pints
	= 4 cups
1 gallon	= 4 quarters
16 ounces	= 1 pound

II.
1 kilogram	= 2.2 lbs
1 litre	= 1.06 quarts
1 lb	= 454 g
1 cup	= 236 ml

III. Temperature conversions

$$°C = \frac{5}{9}(°F - 32)$$

$$°F = \left(\frac{9}{5} \times °C\right) + 32$$

IV. Biochemical conversions

1 milimole (mMol) = atomic weight in mg

mMol = mg ÷ atomic weight

mg = mMol × atomic weight

$$1 \text{ miliequivalent (mFq)} = \frac{\text{atomic weight in mg}}{\text{valency}}$$

$$mEq = \frac{mg \times valency}{atomic\ weight}$$

$$mg = \frac{mFq \times atomic\ weight}{valency}$$

APPENDIX–2

AVERAGE NUTRITIVE VALUE OF FOODSTUFFS (RAW) PER 100 g.

(Nutritive Value of Indian Foods, NIN, ICMR, 1982)

Sl. No.	Foodstuffs	Protein	Fat	Carbo-hydrates	Calories	Calcium	Phos-phorus	Iron	Carotene	Thiamin	Ribo-flavin	Niacin	Vitamin C
		g	g	g	kcal	mg	mg	mg	µg	mg	mg	mg	mg
1.	Cereals	9.9	2.3	71.0	344	79.8	277.3	5.6	56.7	0.34	0.17	2.42	0.00
2.	Bread	7.8	0.7	51.9	245	11.0	–	1.1	0.0	0.07	0.00	0.70	0.00
3.	Biscuit (salt)	6.6	32.4	54.6	534	–	–	–	–	–	–	–	–
4.	Biscuit (sweet)	6.4	15.2	71.9	450	–	–	–	–	–	–	–	–
5.	Dals	23.3	2.1	59.2	349	85.4	343.6	7.5	123.6	0.50	0.22	2.46	0.20
6.	Whole grams	21.9	1.9	57.6	335	156.7	331.7	7.0	68.6	0.44	0.20	2.24	1.00
7.	Green leafy vegetables	3.8	0.6	6.0	45	295.8	64.2	11.9	4390.3	0.09	0.22	1.30	63.87
8.	Roots and tubers	1.2	0.2	16.0	70	37.7	90.4	0.9	222.3	0.05	0.05	0.54	14.25
9.	Other vegetables	2.2	0.3	6.3	36	42.2	51.0	1.7	98.5	0.08	0.05	0.44	27.80
10.	Nuts & oilseeds	15.2	46.6	20.4	578	258.0	464.0	6.1	31.4	0.44	0.28	4.03	0.82
11.	Coconut milk	3.4	41.0	11.9	430	15.0	140.0	1.6	0.0	0.08	0.04	0.60	3.00
12.	Coconut water	1.4	0.1	4.4	24	24.0	10.0	0.1	0.0	0.10	0.00	0.10	2.00
13.	Condiments and spices	9.8	6.6	40.6	261	410.3	239.8	14.5	241.2	0.20	0.19	1.59	15.13
14.	Fruits	1.1	0.4	17.6	79	36.2	34.0	1.8	294.0	0.06	0.12	0.40	15.10

Contd....

Sl. No.	Foodstuffs	Protein g	Fat g	Carbohydrates g	Calories kcal	Calcium mg	Phosphorus mg	Iron mg	Carotene µg	Thiamin mg	Riboflavin mg	Niacin mg	Vitamin C mg
15.	Fish	19.6	2.6	3.0	112	344.8	308.9	2.6	0	0.03	0.11	1.63	14.50
16.	Meat[1]	20.4	4.9	0.4	127	41.0	179.0	1.8	9	0.29	0.09	5.33	2.00
17.	Chicken	25.9	0.6	0.0	109	25.0	245.0	0.0	0	0.00	0.14	0.00	0.00
18.	Egg[2]	13.3	13.3	0.0	173	60.0	220.0	2.1	600	0.10	0.40	0.10	0.00
19.	Milk[3]	3.6	5.8	4.7	85	166.7	113.3	0.2	53	9.04	0.34	0.16	1.33
20.	Curd[4]	3.1	4.0	3.0	60	149.0	93.0	0.2	34	0.05	0.16	0.10	1.00
21.	Butter[5]	0	81.0	0.0	729	0.0	0.0	0.0	1056	0.00	0.00	0.00	0.00
22.	Ghee[6]	0	100.0	0.0	900	0.0	0.0	0.0	479	0.00	0.00	0.00	0.00
23.	Oil	0	100.0	0.0	900	0.0	0.0	0.0	0	0.00	0.00	0.00	0.00
24.	Sugar	0.1	0.0	99.0	398	12.0	1.0	0.0	0	0.00	0.00	0.00	0.00
25.	Honey	0.3	0.0	79.5	319	6.0	16.0	0.9	0	0.00	0.00	0.00	0.00
26.	Jaggery	0.4	0.1	95.0	383	80.0	40.0	11.4	168	0.02	0.04	0.20	4.00
27.	Sago	0.2	0.2	87.1	351	10.0	10.0	1.3	0	0.01	0.04	0.50	0.00

Following foods contain vitamin A (retinol) also:

1. Meat—9 µg   2. Egg—420 µg   3. Milk—53 µg   4. Curd—34 µg   5. Butter—960 µg   6. Ghee—600 µg

Source: Pasricha Swaran, 1997, Count what you eat, National Institute of Nutrition, Hyderabad.

APPENDIX–3

Energy requirements of adult males and females aged 18–30 years with different body weights (kcal/24 hr)

Body Weight (Kg)	Male				Female			
		Activity				Activity		
	BMR	Sedentary	Moderate	Heavy	BMR	Sedentary	Moderate	Heavy
35					960	1536	1824	2400
40	1225	1960	2328	3063	1030	1648	1957	2575
45	1300	2080	2470	3250	1100	1760	2090	2750
50	1370	2192	2603	3425	1170	1872	2223	2925
55	1445	2312	2746	3612	1240	1984	2356	3100
60	1515	2424	2879	3788	1310	2096	2489	3275
65	1590	2544	3021	3975	1380	2208	2622	3450
70	1660	2656	3154	4150	1450	2320	2755	3625
75	1755	2806	3335	4388	–	–	–	–

Energy requirements at different ages of adult males and females with different body weights (kcal/24 hr)

Sex	Body Weight (Kg)	Age 30+ to 59+ years				Age 60+ years	
			Activity				Activity
		BMR	Sedentary	Moderate	Heavy	BMR	Sedentary
Males	45	1325	2120	2518	3313	1040	1664
	50	1380	2208	2622	3450	1105	1768
	55	1435	2296	2727	3588	1170	1768
	60	1485	2376	2822	3713	1235	1976
	65	1540	2464	2926	3850	1285	2072
	70	1595	2552	3031	3988	1360	2176
	75	1650	2640	3135	4125	1425	2280
Females	40	1120	1792	2128	2800	0965	1544
	45	1160	1856	2204	2900	1015	1624
	50	1200	1920	2280	3000	1065	1704
	55	1240	1984	2356	3100	1115	1784
	60	1285	2056	2442	3213	1165	1864
	65	1325	2120	2518	3313	1215	1944
	70	1365	2184	2594	3413	1265	2024

Source: Expert Group of the ICMR, 2000, Nutrient requirements and Recommended Dietary Allowances for Indians, ICMR, Hyderabad, 500 007.

APPENDIX–4

Expected Height and Weight Age

Age (Years)	Boys Height (cm)	Boys Weight (kg)	Girls Height (cm)	Girls Weight (kg)
0	50.5	3.3	49.9	3.2
3 months	61.1	6.0	60.2	5.4
6 months	67.8	7.8	66.6	7.2
9 months	72.3	9.2	71.1	8.6
1.0	76.1	10.2	74.3	9.5
1.5	82.4	11.5	80.9	10.8
2.0	85.6	12.3	84.5	11.8
2.5	90.4	13.5	89.5	13.0
3.0	99.1	15.7	93.9	14.1
3.5	99.1	15.7	97.9	15.1
4.0	102.9	16.7	101.6	16.0
4.5	106.6	17.7	105.1	16.8
5.0	109.9	18.7	108.4	17.7
5.5	113.1	19.7	111.6	18.6
6.0	116.1	20.7	114.6	19.5
6.5	119.0	21.7	117.6	20.6
7.0	121.7	22.9	120.6	21.8
7.5	124.4	24.0	123.5	23.3
8.0	127.0	25.3	126.4	24.8
8.5	129.6	26.7	129.3	26.6
9.0	132.3	28.1	132.2	28.5
9.5	134.8	29.7	135.2	30.5
10.0	137.5	31.4	138.3	32.5
10.5	140.3	33.3	141.5	34.7
11.0	143.3	35.3	144.8	37.0
11.5	146.4	37.5	148.2	39.2
12.0	149.7	39.8	151.5	41.5
12.5	153.0	42.3	154.6	43.8
13.0	156.5	45.0	157.1	46.1
13.5	159.9	47.8	159.0	48.3
14.0	163.1	50.8	160.4	50.3
14.5	166.2	53.8	161.2	52.1
15.0	169.0	56.7	161.8	53.7
15.5	171.5	59.5	162.1	55.0
16.0	173.5	62.1	162.4	55.9
16.5	175.2	64.4	162.7	56.4
17.0	176.2	66.3	163.1	56.7
17.5	176.7	67.8	163.4	56.7
18.0	176.8	68.9	163.7	56.6

National Centre for Health Statistics (NCHS). (USA). Standards.

Average or mean value (or) 50 percent of NCHS is taken as equivalent to 100 percent for (maximum) possible growth) Indian children.

APPENDIX–5

Coefficient for computing calorie requirements of different groups

Group	Cu-Units
Adult male (sedentary worker)	1.0
Adult male (moderate worker)	1.2
Adult male (heavy worker)	1.6
Adult female (sedentary worker)	0.8
Adult female (moderate worker)	0.9
Adult female (heavy worker)	1.2
Adolescents — 12 to 21 years	1.0
Children — 9 to 12 years	0.8
Children — 7 to 9 years	0.7
Children — 5 to 7 years	0.6
Children — 3 to 5 years	0.5
Children — 1 to 3 years	0.4

Source: Gopalan, C., B.V. Ramasastri and S.C. Balasubramanian, 1999, Nutritive value of Indian foods. National Institute of Nutrition, ICMR, Hyderabad.

APPENDIX–6

Energy expenditure of 60 kg person in activity zones

Activity zone	Example of activities and median energy cost	Kcal/min
1.	Sleeping, resting in bed, relaxing, lying still awake.	1.0
2.	Sitting, eating, listening, writing, sitting and light work.	1.5
3.	Standing, personal needs, sitting and doing respective tasks, standing and light work.	2.3
4.	Slow walk, standing and doing repetitive tasks, caring for children.	2.8
5.	Light manual work, house cleaning activities (Floor, doors, windows etc.), fast walk, caring for animals, gardening.	3.3
6.	Warm up activities in sports, light play of games, lifting light weights, carrying light weights.	4.8
7.	Manual work at moderate pace, mining, house building, loading, unloading, harvesting.	5.6
8.	Friendly matches with higher intensity, digging, swimming, speed cycling .	6.0
9.	Intense manual work, high intensity sports, activities or games, tournament matches, carrying heavy loads, running (9 km/hr), competitions, competitive swimming.	7.8

Source: Satyanarayana, K. "Exercise and physical fitness" Nutrition 23, **3**, 1989.

APPENDIX–7

Institutes offering post graduate diploma/degree in food science/nutrition/dietetics.

1. All India Institute of Hygiene and Public Health, Calcutta.
2. Avinashilingam Institute for Home Science and Higher Education for Women, Coimbatore.
3. Central Food Technological Research Institute, Mysore – 570013.
4. Christian Medical College and Hospital, Vellore.
5. College of Home Science, Acharya N.G. Ranga Agricultural University, Saifabad, Hyderabad.
6. College of Home Science, Agricultural University, Dharwar, Karnataka.
7. College of Home Science, HPKV, Palampur – 176 062.
8. College of Home Science, Punjab Agriculture University, Ludhiana.
9. Etheraj College, Egmora, Chennai.
10. Gandhigram Institute, Gandhigram, Ambathurai, Tamil Nadu.
11. IGNOU. SCS. Kothari Academy,Chennai– 600010
12. Institute of Home Economics, Delhi.
13. Institute of Hotel Management Catering Technology and Applied Nutrition, Bombay.
14. Kaveri College of Arts and Science, Trichy, Tamil Nadu.
15. Lady Irwin College, New Delhi.
16. M.S. University, Baroda – 390 002.
17. Madras Medical Mission, J.J. Nagar, Mogappair, Chennai – 600050.
18. Manasa Gangothri University, Mysore – 570005.
19. Mother Teresa Women's University Extension Centre, Saidapet, Chennai – 600 015.
20. Nirmala Niketan, 49 Marine Lines, Bombay – 400 020.
21. P.S.G. College of Arts and Science, Coimbatore – 641 914.
22. Prof. Dhanapalan College, Kelambakkam, Old Mahabalipuram Road, Chennai.
23. Queen Mary's College for Women, Chennai – 600 004.
24. S.V.T. College of Home Science, S.N.D.T. University, Juhu Campus, Santacruz West, Bombay – 400 049.
25. S.V.U. College, Thirupathi.
26. Sardar Patel University, Vallabh, Vidyanagar, Gujarat – 388120.
27. Smt. V.H.D. Central Institute of Home Science, Bangalore.
28. Sri Ramachandra Medical College and Research Institute, Porur, Chennai – 600116.
29. St. Teresa's College, Cochin, Kerala.
30. Tamil Nadu Agricultural University, Coimbatore – 641 003.
31. University College of Agriculture, Calcutta University, 35, Bailygunge Circular Road, Kolkata – 700 019.
32. Voluntary Health Services, Adayar, Chennai - 600 103.

33. Women's Christian College, College Road, Chennai – 600 006.
34. Women's Technical Education and Research Institute, Sitabuldi, Nagpur.

APPENDIX–8

To get information on nutrition these organisations can be contacted :

1. All India Institute of Medical Sciences, New Delhi.
2. CARE, 27, Hauz Khas village, New Delhi – 110 016.
3. Central Food Technological Research Institute, Mysore.
4. Council of Scientific and Industrial Research MS Complex, Tharamani, Chennai – 600 113.
5. Dairy Development Department, Madhavaram Milk Colony, Chennai – 600 051.
6. Food and Agriculture Organisation, 9, Chamier Road, Chennai – 600 018.
7. Food and Nutrition Board, Community Food and Nutrition Extension Unit, Rajaji Bhavan, Chennai – 600 090.
8. Food and Nutrition Board, Department of Women and Child Development, Ministry of Human Resources Development, Government of India, Shastri Bhavan, New Delhi – 110 001.
9. Foundation of Research in community health, Pune.
10. Indian Council of Medical Research, Ansari Nagar, Post Box No. 4911, New Delhi – 110 029.
11. Institute of Child Health and Hospital for Children, Halls Road, Chennai – 600 008.
12. King Institute of Preventive Medicine, Guindy, Chennai – 600 032.
13. M.S. Swaminathan Research Institute, Taramani, Chennai.
14. Madras Medical Mission, Mogappair, Chennai.
15. Ministry of Health and Family Welfare, ICMR Institute for Research in Medical Statistics, Spurtank Road, Chennai – 600 031.
16. National Institute of Nutrition, Indian Council of Medical Research, Jamai-Osmania, P.O. Hyderabad – 500 007.
17. Nutrition Foundation of India, C-13, Qutab Institutional Area, New Delhi – 110 016.
18. Nutrition Society of India, National Institute of Nutrition, Hyderabad – 500 007.
19. Swaminathan Research Foundation, Taramani, Chennai – 600 036.
20. The Indian Society for Parenteral and Enteral nutrition. Nutrition support service, Tamil Nadu, Hospital Cheran Nagar, Chennai – 601 302.
21. United Nations Center for Human, 8, Gandhi-Irwin Road, Chennai – 600 008.
22. United Nations Children's Fund, 20, Chittaranjan Road, Chennai – 600 018.

APPENDIX-9

Nutritive Value of Cereal Preparations (Per Serving)

Preparation	Wt. of cooked preparation g	One Serving Weight g	Measure/ No.	Calories kcal	Protein g	Carbohyd rates g	Fat g	Calcium mg	Iron mg
Rice	620	200	2k	222	4.4	50.0	0.3	6.5	2.0
Khicheri	520	200	2k	430	8.6	66.0	14.7	23.1	6.9
Pulao	915	300	2k	358	9.5	57.0	10.3	56.9	3.2
Paratha	293 (6)*	100	2	297	8.3	47.0	8.3	32.8	7.8
Phulka	280 (8)	70	2	170	6.0	35.0	0.9	24.0	5.7
Puri	298 (12)	75	3	240	6.1	35.0	8.4	24.2	5.8
Pathura	360 (10)	36	1	154	2.7	18.0	7.9	24.4	0.5
Potato paratha	520 (6)	90	1	213	4.8	35.0	6.9	31.5	4.5

* Figures in brackets indicate the number.

Contd....

Nutritive Value of Dal Preparations (Per Serving)

Preparation	Wt. of cooked preparation g	One Serving		Calories kcal	Protein g	Carbohydrates g	Fat g	Calcium mg	Iron mg
		Weight g	Measure/ No.						
Cooked dal									
Bengal gram dal	2470	123	1 k	124	5.6	16.0	4.1	17.5	2.5
Black gram dal	2365	145	1 k	161	9.0	21.0	4.5	60.9	4.9
Green gram dal	705	155	1 k	316	19.2	47.0	5.6	71.7	7.0
Lentil dal	1170	140	1 k	248	15.5	37.0	4.1	65.8	3.2
Lentil dal (Bengali)	780	130	1 k	79	4.2	12.0	1.8	13.2	1.0
Red gram dal	2760	135	1 k	109	6.0	17.0	2.0	27.1	1.6
Cuddy	2250	140	1 k	118	4.0	10.0	6.8	66.6	1.5
Kootu	2970	155	1 k	147	4.7	15.0	7.7	31.9	2.6
Spinach with dal	2750	140	1 k	113	5.6	12.0	4.6	77.9	10.4
Sambar	610	160	1 k	81	4.0	12.0	2.1	38.3	1.2

Contd....

* Figures in brackets indicate the number.

Nutritive Value of Preparations based on whole grams (Per Serving)

Preparation	Wt. of cooked preparation g	One Serving Weight g	Measure/ No.	Calories kcal	Protein g	Carbohydrates g	Fat g	Calcium mg	Iron mg
Chole	1665	160	1 k	119	6.8	8.0	6.6	85.9	3.8
Green gram (whole)	2800	145	1 k	113	6.4	15.0	3.3	33.7	2.5
Lentil (whole)	3220	130	1 k	95	5.3	13.0	2.5	20.8	1.5
Rajmah	2370	135	1 k	153	7.1	18.0	5.7	94.2	3.3
Rawan	2685	140	1 k	141	7.4	16.0	5.1	38.0	3.1

Nutritive Value of Vegetable Preparations (Per Serving)

Preparation	Wt. of cooked preparation g	One Serving Weight g	Measure/ No.	Calories kcal	Protein g	Carbohydrates g	Fat g	Calcium mg	Iron mg
Preparations with gravy									
Avial	3470	140	1 k	123	2.2	10.0	8.3	44.7	1.4
Baghara Baigan	2650	170	1 k	230	3.4	9.0	20.0	163.3	2.0
Chor-Chari	860	110	1 k	96	2.4	10.0	5.3	33.4	2.4
Mirchi Ka Salan	2200	95	1 k	89	1.5	9.0	7.7	56.7	0.7
Peas and Panir	1840	130	1 k	191	11.0	14.0	10.4	97.2	1.4
Peas and Potato curry	2850	135	1 k	132	3.2	13.0	6.4	23.6	1.5
Potato curry	285	110	¾ k	131	1.5	18.0	6.2	22.8	0.9
Potato stew	2425	160	1 k	130	1.8	21.0	4.9	10.4	0.8
Soup	2270	130	1 k	123	1.1	8.5	9.5	30.6	0.4
Veg Kotta curry	2060 (70)	145	1 k	217	3.9	20.0	13.7	139.7	2.2
Vegetable Khorma	2635	140	1 k	132	2.1	13.0	7.9	95.3	1.7

Contd....

* Figures in brackets indicate the number

Nutritive Value of Vegetable Preparations (Per Serving) (*Contd.*)

Preparation	Wt. of cooked preparation g	One Serving Weight g	Measure/ No.	Calories kcal	Protein g	Carbohydrates g	Fat g	Calcium mg	Iron mg
Dry Preparations									
Bean and Potato curry	910	70	1 k	94	1.7	3.0	6.1	41.9	1.5
Brinjal and Potato	2090	130	1 k	134	1.7	17.0	6.7	21.1	1.2
Capsicum-Potato	1995	125	1 k	116	1.9	16.0	5.1	24.3	1.3
Cauliflower and Carrot Bhaji	1250	95	1 k	100	1.9	10.0	6.0	59.2	1.7
Dondakaya	1545	110	1 k	78	1.6	6.0	5.5	51.2	1.6
Lady Fingers	775	140	1½ k	226	5.5	17.0	15.0	184.6	4.4
Pumpkin Curry	2050	165	1 k	110	2.6	11.0	6.3	33.1	1.4
Ridge Gourd Curry	1980	155	1 k	97	1.8	6.0	7.3	62.9	3.0
Bhurtha	1375	100	¾ k	115	2.3	8.0	8.2	47.4	2.3
Cabbage	1220	100	1 k	131	2.3	7.0	10.3	48.1	1.1
Stuffed Tomato	1140 (11)*	85	1	84	2.1	11.0	3.4	37.6	1.3
Vegetable Cutlets	900 (30)	60	2	132	1.9	10.0	9.4	70.4	0.4
Yams and Fenugreek Greek Leaves	1520	100	1 k	121	2.2	16.0	5.4	136.7	4.5

* Figures in brackets indicate the number

Contd...

Nutritive Value of Savoury Snacks (Per Serving)

Preparation	Wt. Of cooked preparation g	One Serving Weight g	Measure/ No.	Calories kcal	Protein g	Carbohydrates g	Fat g	Calcium mg	Iron mg
Awal (Pohe)	850	150	1½ k	298	3.7	41.0	13.1	33.2	7.7
Bajji or Pakora	550 (76)	58	8	280	3.8	17.0	22.0	15.7	1.7
Basen Ka Pura	607 (6)	100	1	222	7.2	22.0	11.7	50.4	3.2
Cashewnut-cutlets	920 (30)	60	2	198	3.8	22.0	10.5	65.8	0.8
Chat	2530 (60)	192	5	218	6.6	25.0	10.0	196.8	3.6
Cheese balls	1100 (80)	35	2	244	2.9	22.0	16.0	53.2	0.5
Dahi Vada	1415 (17)	166	2	343	11.3	31.0	19.2	286.4	2.6
Vada	340 (16)	43	2	138	6.1	15.0	5.9	40.1	2.3
Masala Vada	400 (20)	60	3	167	6.4	20.0	6.9	45.9	2.9
Dalia (salted)	665	140	1 k	166	5.1	21.0	6.8	16.5	1.9
Dosa	295 (7)	84	2	254	6.2	42.0	6.9	2.6	2.8
Masala Dosa	680 (7)	100	1	192	3.8	30.0	6.5	37.2	1.8
Onion Dosa	655 (9)	146	2	319	6.6	43.0	13.3	106.2	3.5
Idli	519 (9)	170	3	229	7.2	49.0	0.4	30.0	3.5
Kodai Shooter Kachori	365 (8)	90	2	383	6.2	33.0	25.1	20.2	1.5
Onion Pakori	215 (30)	60	8	242	6.6	25.0	12.8	82.0	3.0
Potato bonda	500 (12)	83	2	199	5.9	20.0	10.8	33.3	1.7
Sago Vada	865 (32)	60	2	214	1.8	22.0	13.1	9.6	0.6
Samosa	1045 (24)	65	1	207	2.5	21.0	12.6	5.8	0.7
Sandwiches	1000(30)	65	2	194	3.2	14.0	14.1	14.3	0.5
Savian Upma	650	80	1 k	130	2.9	21.0	4.0	25.5	0.7
Upma	505	160	1¼ k	260	6.4	33.0	11.3	35.7	1.3
Vegetable puff	1060 (19)	56	1	166	3.0	17.0	9.6	19.6	1.0

* Figures in brackets indicate the number.

Nutritive Value of Sweet Snacks (Per Serving)

Preparation	Wt. of cooked preparation g	One Serving Weight g	Measure/ No.	Calories kcal	Protein g	Carbohydrates g	Fat g	Calcium mg	Iron mg
Besan Ki Barfi	1195 (20)*	60	1 big piece	405	7.6	35.0	25.4	23.0	3.3
Chikki	900 (30)	60	2 pieces	290	8.0	37.0	12.0	23.1	0.9
Dalia (sweet)	1690	145	1 k	211	4.2	32.0	7.4	115.2	0.9
Fruit Cake	775	50	1 piece	273	3.3	31.0	15.1	13.9	0.9
Jam tart	590 (18)	35	1 piece	331	2.0	60.0	9.1	4.1	0.4
Lemon tart	1000 (18)	56	1 tart	204	2.8	28.0	9.2	22.6	0.6
Nut Biscuits	640 (32)	40	2 nos.	218	2.6	21.0	13.8	5.6	0.6
Rice Puttu	355	100	1 k	280	2.8	55.0	5.4	26.6	4.3
Sandesh	220 (10)	44	2 pieces	140	5.5	9.0	9.0	90.0	–
Queen Cakes	680 (18)	40	1 cake	214	2.9	20.0	13.4	9.8	1.7

* Figures in brackets indicate the number.

Nutritive Value of Sweet Snacks (Per Serving)

Preparation	Wt. of cooked preparation g	One Serving Weight g	Measure/ No.	Calories kcal	Protein g	Carbohydrates g	Fat g	Calcium mg	Iron mg
Blanch mange	940	100	2/3 k	195	4.6	34.0	4.5	130.1	0.5
Bread Pudding	2050	125	1 k	260	6.5	23.1	11.2	125.6	1.0
Caramalised Custard	950	100	1 k	165	5.2	23.0	5.7	78.9	0.7
Double Ka Meetha	2500	105	1 k	276	4.1	24.0	17.7	85.3	1.1
Floating Island	1135	95	1 k	131	5.0	15.1	5.6	110.4	0.5
Halwa	533	100	¾ k	322	2.2	42.0	15.9	4.1	1.1
Jelly and Custard	1850	100	1 k	104	4.2	19.0	1.2	33.8	0.2
Payasam	1905	150	1 k	332	8.0	45.0	13.4	81.7	5.6
Pooran Poli	855 (12)*	71	1	270	4.9	39.5	10.3	15.5	3.9
Savian	1240	110	1 k	249	3.2	34.0	11.1	9.8	1.1
Steamed Cake	1500	85	½ k	348	4.5	33.0	22.3	18.5	2.4
Suji Payasam	2330	150	1 k	267	8.2	27.1	14.2	33.2	0.7
Srikhand	1340	100	½ k	382	9.6	41.0	19.7	470.2	0.2
Walnut Pudding	1470	100	¾ k	224	6.9	18.0	13.8	106.8	1.2

* Figures in brackets indicate the number.

Nutritive Value of Chutneys (Per Serving)

Preparation	Wt. of cooked preparation g	One Serving Weight g	Measure/ No.	Calories kcal	Protein g	Carbohydrates g	Fat g	Calcium mg	Iron mg
Coconut Chutney	475	55	12 tbsp.	125	2.0	6.0	10.4	23.0	0.6
Coriander Chutney	200	20	1 tbsp.	47	0.6	1.7	4.2	6.0	0.6
Groundnut Chutney	350	20	1 tbsp.	66	3.0	3.1	4.6	9.6	0.4
Mint Chutney	225	18	1 tbsp.	7	0.3	1.5	0	11.4	0.6
Instant Chutney	185	35	1 tbsp.	62	2.6	6.0	3.0	29.1	0.9
Tamarind Chutney	200	20	1 tbsp.	65	0.2	13.8	0	17.0	1.7
Tomato Chutney	300	50	½ k	32	0.9	5.0	0.9	21.6	0.6

Source: Pasricha Swaran, 1997, count what you eat, National Institute of Nutrition, Hyderabad.

REFERENCES

1. Bamji Mehtab S. et al. (ed), 2002, Textbook of Human Nutrition, Oxford & IBH Publishing Co. Pvt. Ltd., New Delhi.

2. Bell George H et al., 1972. Textbook of Physiology and Biochemistry, ELBS Churchill Livingstone.

3. David A Bender, 2002, Nutritional Biochemistry of the Vitamins, Cambridge University Press, London.

4. Edwards Christopher R. et al. (ed), 1995, Davidson's Principles and practice of Medicine, ELBS Churchill Livingstone.

5. Garrow, J.S., W.P.T. James, A. Ralph, 2000, Human Nutrition and Dietetics, Churchill Living stone, Edinburgh.

6. Groff L. James and Sareen S. Gropper, 1999, Advanced Nutrition and Human Metabolism, Wadsworth/Thomson Learning, Belmont.

7. Guthrie Helen A and Mary Frances Picciano, 1999, Human Nutrition, WCB McGraw Hill, Boston.

8. Guyton Arthur C., 1991, Textbook of Medical Physiology, A Prism Book (Pvt.) Ltd., Bangalore.

9. Mahan Kathleen L and Syliva Escott. Stump (ed), 2000, Krause's Food, Nutrition and diet therapy, W.B. Saunders Company Philadelphia.

10. Oser Bernard, L., 1965, Hawk's physiological chemistry, Tata McGraw Hill Publishing Company Ltd., Bombay.

11. Park, K., 2005, Park's Text book of preventive and social medicine. Banarsidas Bhanot Publishers, Jabalpur, 482 001.

12. Passmore R. and M.A. Eastwood, 1990, Davidson and Passmore, Human Nutrition and Dietetics, ELBS, Churchill Livingstone.

13. Robinson Corinne, H., Marilyn R. Lawler 1982, Normal and Therapeutic Nutrition, Oxford & IBH Publishing Co., New Delhi.

14. Shils, M.E., James A. Olson Moshe Shike, 1999, Modern Nutrition in Health and Disease Lea & Febizer, Philadelphia.

15. Sienkiewicz Frances Sizer and Eleanor Noss Whitney, 2000, Nutrition, concepts and controversies, Wadsworth/Thomson Learning, Belmont.

16. Sinclair, H.M. and G.R. Howat (ed), 1980, World Nutrition and Nutrition education Oxford University Press, New York.

17. Srilakshmi, B., 2005. Dietetics, New Age International (P) Ltd., Publishers, New Delhi.

18. Swaminathan, M., 1998, Essentials of Food and Nutrition, volume I and II. The Bangalore Printing and Publishing Co.Ltd., Bangalore.

19. Williams Sue Rodwell, 1985; Nutrition and Diet therapy, Times Mirror/Mosby College Publishing St. Louis.

APPENDIX-10

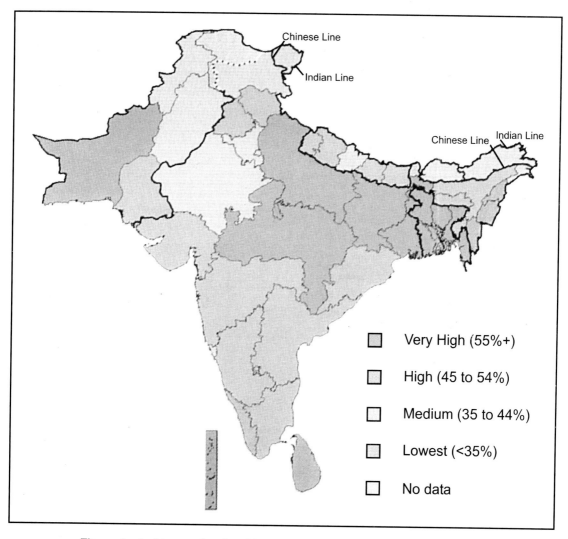

Figure 6a. Incidence of malnutrition in South Asia.

Source: UNICEF, Regional office for South Asia P.O Box 5815, Kathmandu, Nepal, 1996.

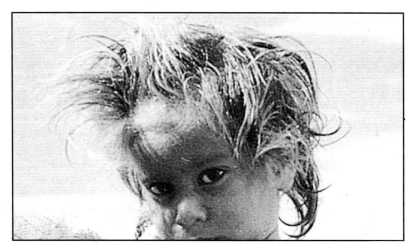

Figure 8d. Changes in colour of hair in PEM—Flag sign

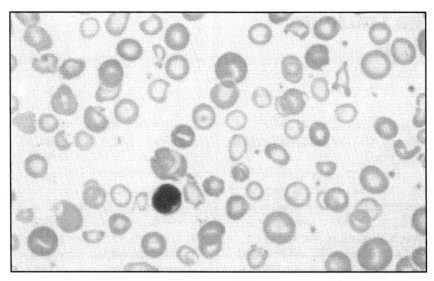

Figure 10d: Microcytic anaemia. This blood smear of a patient with iron deficiency anaemia shows hypochromic, microcytic red blood cells, a few target cells, and red blood cell heterogeneity.

Source: Bergin J. James, Anaemia—microcytic anaemia, Case study, Consultant, **42**, 2002.

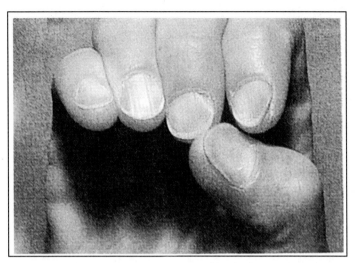

Figure 10e: Koilonychia, thin, concave nails with raised edges, may be seen with iron deficiency anemia. (From Callen WBS, et al. color Atlas of Dermatology. Philadelphia: WB Saunders, 1993). (With permission from WB Saunders, Philadelphia.)

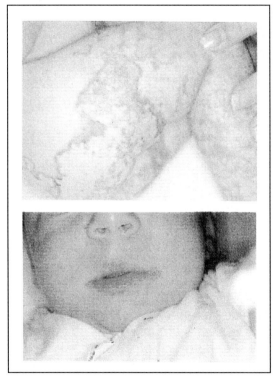

Figure 12f. Cutaneous manifestations of zinc deficiency.

Source: Mahau Kathleen L and Sylvia Escott-stump, (ed), 2000, Krause's food. Nutrition and diet therapy, W.B. Saunders Company, Philadelphia (with permission)

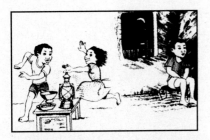

Night blindness

The first symptom of xerophthalmia. A child cannot see after dark or in a dark room.

— Mild deficiency

— Reversible

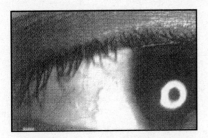

Bitot's spots —

Although Bitot's spots differ somewhat in size, location, and shape, they have a similar appearance. They are accumulations of foamy cheesy material on the conjunctiva, often in association with other signs of xerophthalmia such as night blindness. Bitot's spots showing the white triangular plaques.

— Reversible

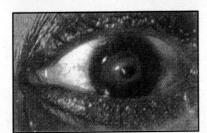

Corneal xerosis/ulceration —

The cornea becomes dry (xerosis). If the disease is not treated, the xerosis can progress within hours to an ulcer of the cornea.

— Not reversible

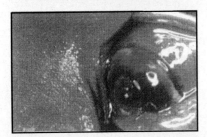

Keratomalacia —

If the disease is not treated, a corneal ulcer can lead to "melting" or "wasting" of the cornea (Keratomalacia).

— Not reversible

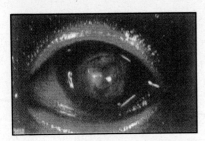

Corneal scar —

Keratomalacia can lead to perforation of the cornea. At this stage, a corneal scar will remain in the eye. The sooner the disease is treated, the smaller the ulcer and the smaller the scar which will remain forever. If treated early, corneal scars and blindness can be prevented.

— Not reversible

Figure 14d. The signs and symptoms of xerophthalmia. Colour plates-Helen Keller Foundation cited from the booklet Prevention and treatment of vitamin A deficiency, Ministry of Health and Family Welfare, Government of India, 1991.

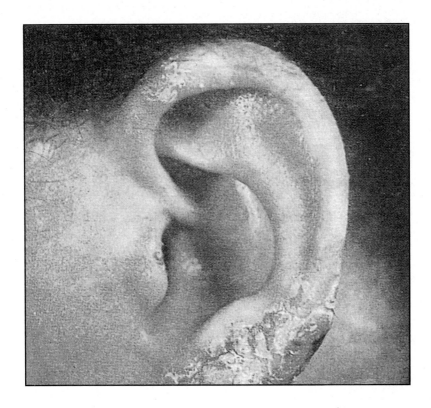

Figure 16g. Riboflavin deficiency

Seborrhoic dermatitis can occur on the forehead, ears and nasolabial groove.

Source: Proudfit T.F., Corinne H. Robinson, 1957, Nutrition and diet therapy. The Macmillan Company, New York.

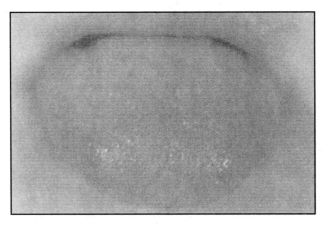

Magenta tongue is a sign of riboflavin deficiency.

Source: Mahan L. Kathleen and Sylvia Escott-Stump, 2000, Kranse's Food, Nutrition and Diet Therapy, W.B. Saunders Company, Philadelphia.

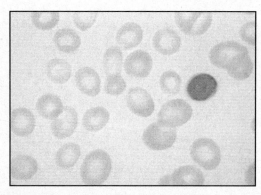

Figure17d: Megaloblastic anaemia–view of red blood cells. This picture shows large, dense, oversized, red blood cells (RBCs) that are seen in megaloblastic anaemia.

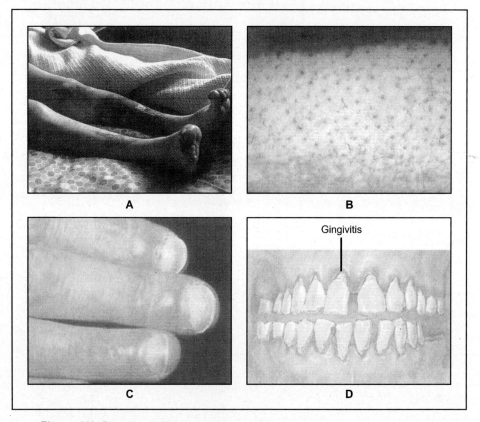

Figure 18i. Scurvy—deficiency of vitamin C.

A: Petechiae—Thighs and shins are common sites.

B, C and **D:** Pinpoint bleeding around the hair follicles, under the nails and along the gums. Note the "cork screw hairs" in Figure **B.**

Source: Shils E. Maurice et al., 1998, Modern nutrition in health and disease, Lippincott Williams & Wilkins, Philadelphia.

http://www.nlm.nih.gov/medlineplus/ency/images